THE MICROCIRCULATION IN CLINICAL MEDICINE

CONTRIBUTORS

Robert L. Dilts
F. A. Elliott
Kenneth H. Falchuk
Roger B. Hickler
Norman K. Hollenberg
Thomas N. James
George K. Massing
John P. Merrill
Francis D. Moore
John R. Murphy
Johannes A. G. Rhodin
Franz Rodríguez-Erdmann
D. D. Stromberg
Roe Wells
Mary P. Wiedeman
C. A. Wiederhielm
James W. Wilson
Sumner Wood

THE MICROCIRCULATION IN CLINICAL MEDICINE

Edited by

ROE WELLS, M.D.
Peter Bent Brigham Hospital and
Harvard Medical School
Boston, Massachusetts

ACADEMIC PRESS New York and London 1973
A Subsidiary of Harcourt Brace Jovanovich, Publishers

ACADEMIC PRESS, INC.
111 Fifth Avenue, New York, New York 10003

United Kingdom Edition published by
ACADEMIC PRESS, INC. (LONDON) LTD.
24/28 Oval Road, London NW1

Library of Congress Cataloging in Publication Data

Wells, Roe.
The microcirculation in clinical medicine.

Includes bibliographies.
1. Microcirculation. 2. Physiology, Pathological.
I. Title. [DNLM: 1. Microcirculation–Pathology.
2. Microcirculation–Physiopathology. QZ170 W455m
1973]
RB113.W43 616.07 72-13609
ISBN 0–12–743750–9

PRINTED IN THE UNITED STATES OF AMERICA

To EUGENE LANDIS, PH.D., M.D.

Professor Emeritus of Physiology
Harvard Medical School

A living pioneer of microvascular research who applied the first systematic quantification of hemodynamics to the microscopic vascular system

CONTENTS

8. Microcirculation in Peripheral Arterial Ischemic Disease

Robert L. Dilts

9. Diseases of Small Coronary Arteries

George K. Massing and Thomas N. James

10. Pulmonary Disease and the Microcirculation

James W. Wilson

11. Systemic Indicators of the Low Flow State: Biochemistry and Metabolism during Tissue Hypoperfusion

Francis D. Moore

LIST OF CONTRIBUTORS

Numbers in parentheses indicate the pages on which the authors' contributions begin.

ROBERT L. DILTS, M.D. (113), Community Hospital, Indianapolis, Indiana

F. A. ELLIOTT, M.D. (289), Department of Neurology, Pennsylvania Hospital, Philadelphia, Pennsylvania

KENNETH H. FALCHUCK, M.D. (95), Department of Medicine, Peter Bent Brigham Hospital, Boston, Massachusetts

ROGER B. HICKLER, M.D. (213), The Memorial Hospital, Worcester, Massachusetts

NORMAN K. HOLLENBERG, M.D., PH.D. (61), Peter Bent Brigham Hospital and Harvard Medical School, Boston, Massachusetts

THOMAS N. JAMES, M.D. (147), Cardiovascular Research and Training Center, University of Alabama School of Medicine, Birmingham, Alabama

GEORGE K. MASSING, M.D. (147), Cardiovascular Research and Training Center, University of Alabama School of Medicine, Birmingham, Alabama

JOHN P. MERRILL, M.D. (81), Cardiovascular Section, Peter Bent Brigham Hospital and Harvard Medical School, Boston, Massachusetts

FRANCIS D. MOORE, M.D. (195), Peter Bent Brigham Hospital, Boston, Massachusetts

JOHN R. MURPHY, M.D. (227), Department of Medicine, University Hospitals of Cleveland, University Circle, Cleveland, Ohio

JOHANNES A. G. RHODIN, M.D., PH.D. (13), Department of Anatomy, New York Medical College, New York, New York

FRANZ RODRÍGUEZ-ERDMANN, M.D.* (253), Peter Bent Brigham Hospital and Harvard Medical School, Boston, Massachusetts

**Present address*: The Abraham Lincoln School of Medicine, University of Illinois at the Medical Center, Chicago, Illinois

Roe Wells, M.D.* (47), Peter Bent Brigham Hospital and Harvard Medical School, Boston, Massachusetts

Mary P. Wiedeman, Ph.D. (1), Department of Physiology, Temple University, School of Medicine, Philadelphia, Pennsylvania

C. A. Wiederhielm, Ph.D. (33), Department of Physiology, University of Washington School of Medicine, Seattle, Washington

James W. Wilson, Ph.D., M.D. (169), Department of Pathology, Duke University, Medical Center, Durham, North Carolina

Sumner Wood, M.D., F.C.A.P. (275), Department of Experimental Pathology, Merck Institute for Therapeutic Research, Rahway, New Jersey

Present address: Massachusetts Rehabilitation Hospital, Boston, Massachusetts.

FOREWORD

The history of medicine illustrates that remote or esoteric studies of the basic science laboratories eventually find their way to the clinical arena, whether by integration into a larger clinical subject or by the development of a clinically feasible test procedure that leads to a whole new series of clinical entities, e.g., the flame photometer and the spectrum of serum electrolyte abnormalities.

Over 50 years ago Augustus Krogh reported his observations of blood flow in the mesenteric membranes of small laboratory animals. Five years later Eugene Landis quantitated the pressures in the microvasculature. Today the clinician is faced with a rapidly increasing flow of laboratory and clinical reports describing microvascular involvement or reactions in a wide variety of important new clinical phenomena. The term microcirculation now appears repeatedly in the literature of shock, transplantation, diabetes, cancer, and many other disorders.

It becomes apparent therefore that some unifying or integrated overview of this vascular system would be of great value to clinicians. This should not only provide a better perspective for those already interested in the subject, but should also provide, as Dr. Wells notes, a broad introduction for clinicians who may not have realized how often they must refer to the microcirculation in their deliberations on the pathophysiology of disease.

I am confident this book will accomplish its purpose of stimulating the clinician to consider the hemodynamics of the microcirculation in his day-to-day thoughts about diagnosis and therapy. It is but another example of how investments in basic science research eventually play a role in better medical care for the consumer and the community.

ROBERT EBERT, M.D.
Harvard Medical School

PREFACE

The clinician who must often consider disease in terms of organ systems has rarely had occasion to think of the microcirculation as either an organ system or as a primary site of pathologic phenomena. This is due to the fact that the microcirculation is not often considered as a functional component of the cardiovascular system. This misconception plus the lack of published information on the clinical aspects of the microcirculation have combined to leave the clinician unprepared to evaluate disease processes in terms of microvascular reactions or pathology. This book is designed to introduce the clinician to the concept that the microcirculation is an important and dynamic vascular system, consideration of which can fruitfully be applied in both differential diagnosis and therapy.

The bulk of the research in this field has generally been reported in the basic science literature, yet it contains many findings that have direct application to contemporary clinical problems such as shock, thrombosis, organ transplantation, and hemoglobinopathies. One of the aims of this work, therefore, is to bring to the clinician's attention contemporary research findings that will be useful to him in the analysis of clinical problems. References are recorded for those wishing to pursue any given subjects in greater detail.

The present rate of accumulation of new knowledge is such that accomplishment of these goals by a single author would occupy such time that a major portion of the material would require revision by the time the last chapter was written. Multiple authorship appears to be the best solution to this problem, acknowledging that it tends to produce variation in style and method of presentation.

The nature of the subject is such that most readers will likely utilize this book with reference to that disease state or organ system which is most pertinent to their primary interest. The possibility of this variable usage notwithstanding, the larger goal remains the illustration that the microcirculation is a dynamic component of the total cardiovascular system and is involved either primarily or secondarily in a wide variety of clinical conditions.

ROE WELLS

1 ANATOMY

MARY P. WIEDEMAN, Ph.D.

I. Historical Introduction

The smallest blood vessels, those that represent the microcirculation, were first mentioned as a concept rather than as a reality. They were conceived in the mind of William Harvey, whose experimental and speculative conclusions were published in 1628 and remained as a product of Harvey's logical reasoning until magnifying lenses in the hands of Marcello Malpighi, a professor of medicine in Bologna in 1661, revealed to him "tubules" through which blood flowed from arterial to venous vessels (Young, 1929).

Information regarding the microcirculation was collected sporadically as interest waxed and waned. Among the notable contributors during the nineteenth century was Leeuwenhoek, who drew the vascular patterns he saw in various aquatic forms and documented the continuity between arteries and veins. Definitive terminology had still not been accepted (as it has not today) in the nineteenth century, which made it difficult for historians to describe the progress that was being made in unraveling the structure and function of microscopic vascular networks (van Leeuwenhoek, 1964).

The first attempt to differentiate between arterioles, capillaries, and venules was made by Marshall Hall in 1831 who defined arterial vessels as those which divided to become smaller and smaller, and venous vessels as those which enlarged as a result of confluences. He saw capillaries as being different from both in that they maintained a uniform diameter. He also reasoned that, functionally, capillaries served as nutritional beds. His observations were made on fishes and frogs. In 1852, T. Wharton Jones presented a paper containing microscopic observations on blood vessels in the wing of the bat and focused his attention on the veins, describing in detail their spontaneous contractile activity and the action of venous valves. Müller, in 1838, published a review of the literature extant at that time and included diameters of capillaries in various tissues. He noted that vascular beds assumed different patterns depending on the tissues, taking on special characteristics to accommodate to specific areas. It must be surprising to current students of microcirculation to discover, in researching the literature, that there is such an extensive and detailed background of descriptive material, and yet, in 300 years of microscopic observations of small blood vessels, there are still many deficiencies in regard to both architecture and function.

After the flurry of activity in the middle 1800's, little of consequence appeared until a new interest was generated by August Krogh whose book "The Anatomy and Physiology of Capillaries," published in 1922, promised to be the source book and the irrefutable reference for all things pertaining to the subject matter, about which, in view of such an encompassing title, all was known, all problems solved. The reaction was not one of total acceptance, however, and a new era of investigation began with more sophisticated equipment and the introduction of new techniques utilizing *in vivo* microscopy. Many of the techniques are in use today.

In general, there are four basic methods. One technique employs the fused quartz rod, fiber optics, or some other means of transmitting light to relatively inaccessible areas, and by this means tissues can be observed *in situ*. Such tissues are lung, spleen, and liver. Another method is the preparation of tissues for transillumination by the implantation of transparent chambers, as has been done in the rabbit ear, the hamster cheek pouch, and the skin of various mammals. A third method consists of the exteriorization of suitable tissues for direct microscopic observation, such as the cecal mesentery of the rat, the omentum and mesentery of the dog and cat, and the cremaster muscle of the rat. A fourth method is the utilization of superficial structures whose vasculature can be easily seen with transmitted or direct light, such as the wing membrane of the bat or conjunctival vessels in man. Detailed descriptions of these and other methods can be found in the current literature (Wiedeman, 1967).

The development of new methods, the refinement of older ones, and their current widespread use in both clinical and basic science laboratories attest to the continued interest in the microcirculation as a site for discovering the solution to problems related to the cardiovascular system.

II. Terminal Vascular Beds

A. Components

The final ramifications of the arterial distribution represents the beginning of the terminal vasculature. Between the large, thick-walled aorta, heavily endowed with elastic and fibrous tissue, and the pure endothelial tube which is the capillary, there is a gradual thinning of elastic and fibrous tissue. Wall thickness decreases and also the diameter of the vessels, from approximately 25 mm in the aorta to 5 μm in the capillary. The relationship between wall thickness and the internal diameter varies with the distribution of smooth muscle and this is determined by the functional role of the different categories of vessels. The details of wall structure will be considered in the chapter dealing with ultrastructure.

The vessels which are recognized as components of the microcirculation are arterioles, terminal arterioles, capillaries, postcapillary venules, and venules.

B. Definition of Components

Although there is no universally accepted nomenclature or list of specific characteristics to use as a guide in defining the vessels of the microcirculation, there are generalizations which can be made to assist in identification.

The term "microcirculation" is used to designate blood flow through small vessels. The microcirculatory bed is that portion of the vascular system which is concerned with the transfer of gases and nutrients and the removal of metabolic waste products and is referred to as the exchange system. The vessels designed to function in the exchange of materials to maintain the life of tissues and cells are considered separately from the vessels of the macrocirculation which are designed for the maintenance of systemic blood pressure to assure the delivery of blood to the microcirculation.

The microcirculatory system begins with arterioles. Branches from arterioles are called terminal arterioles, so named because they terminate in a capillary network and have no vascular communication, such as an anastomosis or arcuate structure, with any other arterial or venous vessel. The increasingly familiar "precapillary sphincter" has almost as many definitions as there are investigators who have needed its functional activity to explain their observations. In general, however, it is the portion of the terminal arteriole that contracts or relaxes to monitor blood flow into the capillary network which lies distal to it. Originally, it was placed at the point of origin of a capillary vessel leaving a "preferential channel." The concept of the preferential channel, proposed in early descriptions of terminal beds (Zweifach and Kossman, 1937), was not given much support by subsequent investigators, but the term appears occasionally in current literature. A vessel called the metarteriole is perhaps its counterpart in current usage. Swedish investigators, headed by Mellander (Mellander and Johnson, 1968) have defined the precapillary sphincter on a functional rather than anatomical basis as the most distal point at which changes in peripheral resistance occur. Since we are dealing with anatomy of the microcirculatory system, perhaps the most acceptable definition for the precapillary sphincter is that it is the final smooth muscle cell that separates arterial and capillary vessels, realizing that its location will vary in different vascular beds and from species to species. It affords the ultimate control of blood flow into the capillary circulation.

Defining a capillary vessel is the easiest. It can be stated without fear of contradiction that a capillary vessel is a pure endothelial tube, lying between distributing arterial vessels and collecting venous vessels. Details regarding the ultrastructure of the different types of capillaries will be discussed in Chapter 2, so it is sufficient to say here that most capillaries originate from terminal arterioles either singly or as a burst of vascular pathways to form interconnecting networks that ultimately end where two vessels converge to form a postcapillary venule. In some instances, the determination of the beginning and ending of a capillary vessel that acts as a conduit between the arterial and venous systems may be difficult when observed with the light microscope because there are vascular connections, sometimes U-shaped and sometimes straight, sometimes long and at other times short, that join a terminal arteriole with a postcapillary venule. Some portion of the vessel is pure endothelium, and by definition, a capillary, but it remains for the electronmicroscopist to identify the proximal and distal limits. It is this configuration, lacking the design of a network, that has been designated as a thoroughfare channel, a preferential channel, or an arteriovenous capillary (Zweifach and Kossman, 1937). The arteriovenous capillaries were described as being muscular throughout and parent vessels for true capillaries. It seems undesirable to introduce additional terminology to the microcirculation, already overladen with descriptions of vessels. In some cases different names have been given to the same vessels and in others the same names have been used for different types of vessels.

The convergence of short capillary vessels marks the formation of the postcapillary venules which may be described as nonmuscular venous vessels whose diameter is noticably larger than that of the capillaries which form them. Each further convergence results in larger diameters, smooth muscle cells reappear, and, finally, with the appearance of venous valves, the venules are reached.

C. Relationships between Arterial and Venular Vessels

There are certain relationships between the components of the microvascular beds that are appropriate to mention here. The information comes from observations made on the vascular bed in the wing membrane of the little brown bat *(Myotis lucifugus)* (Wiedeman, 1962), but, because of general similarities in the vascular beds which have been studied in recent years, may be considered as acceptable for relative relationships in any terminal vascular configuration.

Arterial and venous vessels accompany one another except in the final ramification of the arterial vessels in the capillary network. There are also no arterial counterparts for postcapillary venules. The arterial vessels are smaller in diameter than their venous companions. Arterioles have an average diameter about one-third that of their accompanying venules. Capillary vessels are the smallest in diameter, having an average diameter of 3.7 μm, while the postcapillary venules formed from them average 7.3 μm in diameter. Postcapillary venules convene to form the venules with an average diameter of 21 μm. (See Fig. 1.) It must be made clear that the exact diameter should not be the basis on which a vessel is placed in any

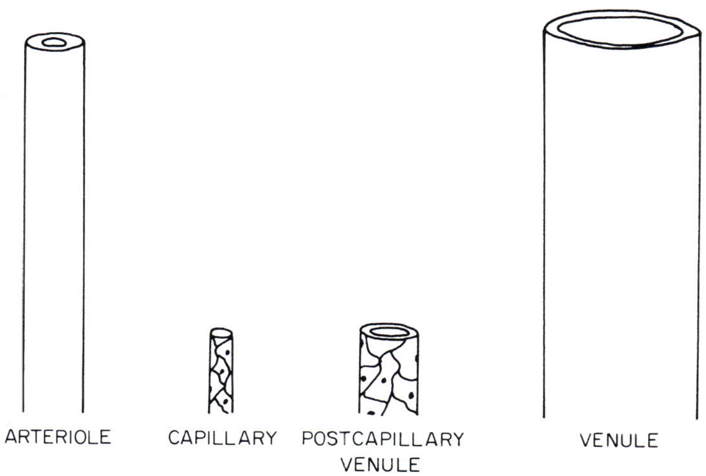

Fig. 1. Comparison of lengths, wall thickness, and diameter of four components of the capillary network.

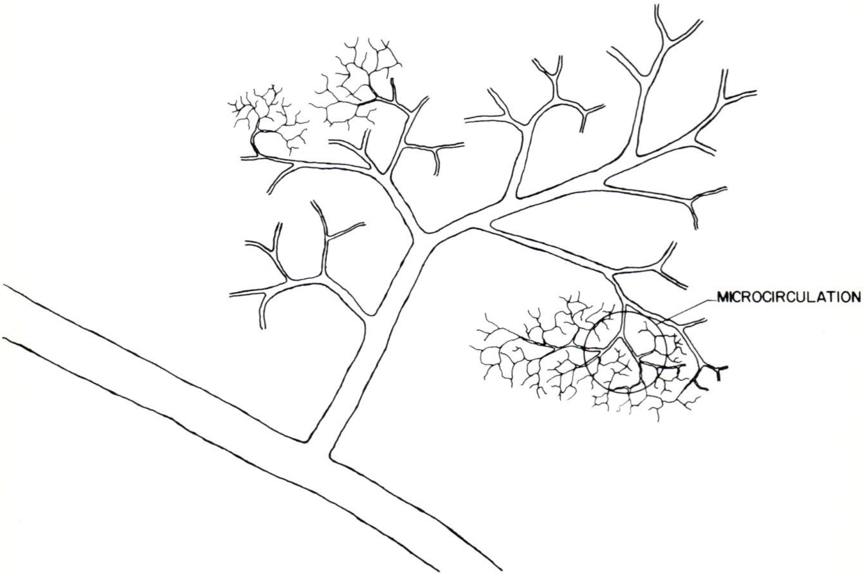

Fig. 2. This diagram represents the final distribution of arteriolar vessels. This architecture is common to many vascular beds except in special glandular tissue.

designated category because the dimensions vary considerably depending on the organ, tissue, or species of mammal being documented. It is more important to consider the location in the vascular distribution, at the same time recognizing that there is great similarity in vascular architecture among all mammals at the level of the final ramifications of the arterial vessels, the capillary network, and the converging venules, and it should be understood that the microcirculatory systems are concerned with the function of exchange as opposed to the maintenance of systemic blood pressure. Figure 2 is a diagrammatic representation showing the termination of arterial distribution. It can be seen by examining the diagram that the arterial vessels of the microcirculation have an arcuate pattern, that the arterial vessels may interconnect before becoming capillaries and, therefore, there are several arterial routes to a capillary network.

Another aspect of the relationships of the different categories of vessels to one another is the total cross-sectional area formed by the vessels. It has recently been established that there is a linear increment in total cross-sectional area from artery to arterial capillary, a marked increase at the postcapillary venules, and that the greatest total cross-sectional area appears at the level of the venules (Wiedeman, 1963). This is a departure from the long-accepted idea that there were only small increases in the total area from artery to arteriole followed by a tremendous increase at the level of the capillaries, an architectural design which gave credence to the thought that the reduced flow velocity in capillary networks which resulted from the marked enlargement of the total cross-sectional area was necessary to permit adequate time for the exchange of nutrients and wastes. While the new information does not negate the concept of a sharply decreased flow rate at the capillary level, it does promote the idea that more vessels should be included in the areas devoted to exchange of materials, notably the postcapillary venules and the venules.

D. Anatomical Shunts

Consideration must be given to the frequent speculation that anatomical shunts exist between arterial and venous vessels, bypassing the capillary network. The apparent need for such an arrangement is to establish a means by which blood can be moved with great rapidity from the arterial side to the venous side, and the idea that such structures exist is substantiated to some extent by investigations utilizing microspheres thought to be too large to pass through capillary beds, microradiographic studies, and analyses of transcapillary exchange of radioactive materials under some conditions. In a recent paper, Hyman (1971), who defines a shunt as a vessel through which blood flows from the arteriolar to the venular side of the circulation without loss of some crystalloid solute, criticizes these methods and explains why they do not conclusively prove the existance of shunts. He does, however, develop the idea that there are two different types of vessels connecting the arterial and venous vessels and refers to nutrition circulation, which includes the microvessels devoted to exchange, and shunt circulation, which includes the microvessels designed to modify total flow.

Anatomical shunts, however, have not been liberally demonstrated by *in vivo* microscopic techniques. Except for numerous arteriovenous anastomoses in the rabbit ear and the dog's paw, both of which are used in temperature regulation of these animals and in organs such as liver and spleen, the evidence that there are such anatomical structures is still controversial. One may easily be swayed by the excellent photographs as shown by Kuprianov and Kozlov (1971), to accept these H-like structures without further ado, but they occur so infrequently in most vascular beds observed *in vivo* that it is hard to believe they can have a truly significant influence on total flow from the arterial to the venous vessels. On the other hand, if a

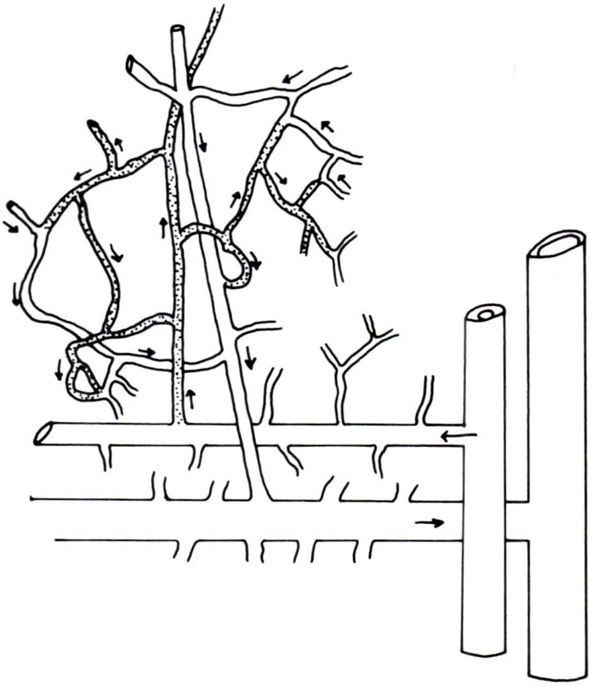

Fig. 3. Detailed architecture of the capillary network indicating alternate routes for blood flow from arterial to venous side.

careful study is made of the structure of terminal vascular beds and the knowledge recently gained regarding control of blood flow through the beds is reviewed, it is apparent that blood can traverse the area between the arterial and venous systems rapidly and effectively and, therefore, satisfy the conditions for which shunts have been postulated. An examination of Fig. 3 depicting a microvascular pattern shows a very short pathway, a pathway of intermediate length, and a long, tortuous route between the arteriolar distribution and the venular convergence. It is a reasonable assumption that both metabolic demands of the tissue and hemodynamic forces subserving the total organism would dictate whether all, some, or only one route would be open at any one time. To move the greatest volume of blood from arterial to venous vessels in the shortest time may require that all of the routes be utilized simultaneously. Because these pathways are outside the macrocirculation and, therefore, not involved in pressure maintenance, the systemic blood pressure need not be compromised.

E. Innervation

There is currently considerable confusion regarding the innervation, or absence of it, in the microvascular beds. However, if one takes cognizance of the voluminous literature describing autoregulation and the theories which have been proposed to explain how resistance vessels can respond to maintain adequate nutritional flow in an organ in the face of changing perfusion pressure, it is evident that nervous control of blood flow at the level of the microcirculation is not mandatory. Neither of the two most acceptable theories of autoregulation are concerned with compensatory diameter changes dependent on central or peripheral nervous control. The myogenic theory of autoregulation (Johnson, 1964) is based on intraluminal pressure changes, while the metabolic theory (Johnson, 1964) calls for variations in metabolic by-products to explain varying vascular diameters which assure constant flow. While not actually denying the presence of autonomic nervous system activity, such investigations support the concept that the microvasculature operates independently of nervous control. Furthermore, other physiological evidence from studies on surgically and chemically denervated vessels in the bat wing (Wiedeman, 1954) strongly suggests that vascular smooth muscle cells which invest the arterioles and terminal arterioles have an inherent, spontaneous, contractile activity that in no way relies on chemical mediators released from postganglionic nerve endings for its initiation, continuation, or variation.

Anatomically, the evidence for innervation of terminal arterioles and precapillary sphincters also is not convincing. In a thorough and excellent study, Rhodin (1967) demonstrated in electron micrographs that nerve fibers closely approximated these vessels and therefore could exert a regulatory influence via synapses *en passage*. Conversely, in a pilot study utilizing electron micrography, Phillips and Wiedeman (1968) reported diminution of nerve fibers in the area of third-order (arterioles) vessels and essentially no nerve fibers near fourth-order (terminal arterioles) vessels.

Therefore, until additional definitive information is supplied to us through further anatomical studies of the ultrastructure and extensive physiological studies of the behavior of denervated and innervated vessels, it is inappropriate to state emphatically whether or not precapillary sphincters and terminal arterioles are innervated. The balance weighs heavily, however, in favor of the proposition that components of the microcirculation involved in maintaining the tissue cells through delivery, exchange, and removal of constituents compatible with life are independent of innervation and, therefore, of the central and peripheral nervous controls and reflexes that regulate total systemic blood pressure.

III. Microcirculatory Patterns in Specific Organs and Tissues

It has been stated in the foregoing pages that, in general, terminal vascular beds throughout the body share numerous common characteristics. The specific characteristics of many organs and tissues have been described in detail within the decade (Wiedeman, 1963), and, therefore, no descriptions will be included here. It was noted at that time that there were more similarities than dissimilarities in the architecture of the vascular distribution, and minor differences in the patterns were most likely associated with the structural organization of the tissues to which the vessels conformed. Additional descriptive papers continue to appear in the current literature, and it is reasonable to assume that in time more concise terminology and specific characteristics of organ systems will be available.

References

Hall, M. (1831). "A Critical and Experimental Essay on the Circulation of the Blood; Especially as Observed in the Minute and Capillary Vessels of the Batrachia and of Fishes." Seeley & Burnside, London.

Harvey, W. (1628). "Movement of the Heart and Blood in Animals" (translated by K. J. Franklin), published in 1957 by Thomas, Springfield, Illinois.

Hyman, C. (1971). Independent control of nutritional and shunt circulation. *M.V.R.* **3,** 89–94.

Johnson, P. C. (1964). Review of previous studies and current theories of autoregulation. *Circ. Res.,* Suppl. **1,** 1–2.

Jones, T. W. (1852). Discovery that the veins of the bat's wing (which are furnished with valves) are endowed with rhythmical contractility, and that onward flow of blood is accelerated by each contraction. *Phil. Trans. Roy. Soc. London* **142,** Part 1, 131–136.

Krogh, A. (1922). "The Anatomy and Physiology of Capillaries." Yale Univ. Press, New Haven, Connecticut.

Kuprianov, V. V., and Kozlov, V. I. (1971). Dynamic structures of the microvascular bed. *M.V.R.* **3,** 22–34.

Mellander, S., and Johnson, B. (1968). Control of resistance exchange and capacitance functions in the peripheral circulation. *Pharmacol. Rev.* **20,** 117–196.

Müller, J. (1838–1842). "Elements of Physiology" (translated by W. Baly), Taylor & Walton, London.

Phillips, S. S., and Wiedeman, M. P. (1968). Nerve distribution patterns along terminal vessels of the bat wing. *Anat. Rec.* **160,** 409.

Rhodin, J. A. (1967). Ultrastructure of mammalian arterioles and precapillary sphincters. *J. Ultrastruct. Res.* **18,** 181–223.

van Leeuwenhoek, A. (1964). The capillary circulation. Fig. 4, *In* "Circulation of the Blood, Men and Ideas" (A. P. Fishman and W. R. Dickinson, eds.), p. 361. Oxford Univ. Press, London and New York.

Wiedeman, M. P. (1954). Reactivity of arterioles following denervation of subcutaneous areas of the bat wing. *Amer. J. Physiol.* **177,** 308–314.

Wiedeman, M. P. (1962). Lengths and diameters of peripheral arterial vessels in the living animal. *Circ. Res.* **10,** 686–690.

Wiedeman, M. P. (1963). Patterns of the A–V pathways. *In* "Handbook of Physiology" (Amer. Physiol. Soc., J. Field, ed.), Sect. 2, Vol. II, p. 891. Williams & Wilkins, Baltimore, Maryland.

Wiedeman, M. P. (1967). A preparation for microscopic observation of circulation in the unanesthetized animal. *In "In Vivo* Techniques in Histology" (G. H. Bourne, ed.), p. 162. Williams & Wilkins, Baltimore, Maryland.

Young, J. (1929). Malpighi's "De Pulmonibus." *Proc. Roy. Soc. Med.* **23,** 1.

Zweifach, B. W., and Kossman, C. E. (1937). Micromanipulation of small blood vessels in the mouse. *Amer. J. Physiol.* **120,** 23–34.

2 ULTRASTRUCTURE OF THE MICROVASCULAR BED

JOHANNES A. G. RHODIN, M.D., Ph.D.

I. Definition of the Term

In this chapter, the structural and ultrastructural components of the microvascular bed will be considered. It is recognized that a short discussion of the term microvascular bed cannot adequately describe, distinctly define, and comprehensively include all variations of this part of the vascular system, or adequately recall the many different opinions voiced by a multitude of authors over the past half century. However, the term "microvascular bed," as I understand it, refers to "arterioles" less than 300 μm in diameter; "precapillary arterioles" (metarterioles or precapillary sphincter area); "capillaries"; "postcapillary venules"; "collecting venules"; and "muscular venules" with a diameter of up to 300 μm.

II. Organ and Tissue Variations in Pattern

It should be recognized that there is a marked difference in the three-dimensional architecture of the microvascular bed depending on the species, the organ, and the tissue (Illig, 1961). In this chapter, no attempt is made to give a detailed description of differences and similarities. Only when I find these at the ultrastructural level and as they relate to components of the walls of the various segments of the bed, will they be discussed. However, in general terms, it must be recognized that the spread of the microvascular bed in essentially a "monolayer" in the mesentery, the subdermal space of the skin, as studied in the "ear chamber" of the rabbit and the cheek pouch of the hamster, is not representative of the "three-dimensional" architectural pattern of microvascular beds in the skeletal muscle, the lung tissue, or the intestinal wall. Yet, there are enough common denominators to justify a generalization of the fine structure of the component parts of the microvascular bed, bearing in mind that structural similarities may not always imply that functional similarities exist. In this chapter, the description is based on ultrastructural analyses of microvascular beds in the hypodermis of the rabbit and in the kidney, intestinal wall, skeletal and cardiac muscles, lung, cerebral cortex, eye, inner ear, ovary, testis, penis, lymph nodes, and spleen of the rat.

III. Microvascular Dimensions

It is generally accepted to use the luminal diameter and the thickness of the vascular wall as a means to help identify a specific vascular segment. *In vivo* observations and recordings of the microvascular bed lend themselves to accurate measurements of these parameters. Histological and electron microscopic techniques have been less useful, but, recently, fixation by vascular perfusion has been adopted, particularly for electron microscopy. I have used this type of vascular fixation extensively, and some of the material presented in this chapter is based on that technique. The state of vessel contraction or dilatation at the moment of fixation is accurately preserved with this technique (Fig. 1). This method introduces a new and more realistic way of looking at the size and shape of the microvascular segments, since many of the earlier histological and electron microscopic investigations reported vascular dimensions of vessels which were contracted or collapsed as a result of termination of blood flow and/or postmortem changes. Unfortunately, biopsied material must also be considered inadequately fixed from the point of view of properly preserving the true vascular dimensions and the true structural topography of cellular organelles.

IV. Technical Approach

As indicated in several chapters of this book, there are many ways of studying the structure and the reactivity of the microvascular bed. The early classic studies by the Clarks (1925, 1934) and by Krogh (1930) utilized essentially the two-dimensional vascular pattern of the frog's toe web, the subdermal vessels of the skin of the ear, or the mesentery. Later investigators used a variety of tissues and technical approaches. For a comprehensive review of these techniques, consult Illig (1961). I have (Rhodin, 1967, 1968) attempted to combine some of the early approaches to observing the microvascular beds *in vivo* with a fixation of the same area for histological and electron microscopic analyses. Method of fixation was the topical application of osmium tetroxide or the intravascular perfusion of glutaraldehyde, followed by a perfusion of osmium tetroxide (Rhodin, 1971b). Both techniques have yielded excellent preservation, both grossly and at the fine structural level.

V. Arterioles

Arbitrarily, microvessels with a luminal diameter of 300 μm or less and a wall thickness of about 5–10 μm are categorized as arterioles. The luminal diameter and the wall thickness gradually decrease to 30 μm and 0.5 μm, respectively, as the vessel approaches the precapillary sphincter area, a segment which varies greatly in length depending on organ and tissue. The wall of the arteriole consists of: (1) endothelium; (2) smooth muscle cells; and (3) connective tissue.

The "endothelium" is generally squamous but attains a cuboidal appearance in highly contracted or collapsed arterioles. The cells are laterally connected by junctions which are local regions of the cellular periphery where the superficial laminae of the opposing cell membranes are brought into close proximity. In certain tissues, i.e., the central nervous system, these junctions display a fusion of the peripheral plasma membrane laminae, which is referred to as a tight junction. In most tissues and organs, microfilaments are numerous in the endothelial cells. Their function is mostly supportive, but contractile properties cannot be excluded. Other organelles are present in limited number with the exception of micropinocytotic vesicles. They occur mostly at the cell surfaces, and to a limited degree within the cell cytoplasm. They represent the structural evidence for metabolic exchange between the cell and its environment and/or may represent one kind of transport vehicle across the endothelium. In the larger arterioles, as a rule, a thin "elastica interna" is present. It has disappeared in most arterioles with a diameter of less than 30 μm, the segment which is referred to here as the precapillary sphincter area. Exception to this is the glomerular afferent arterioles of the kidney (Fig. 2) where an elastica is present even at a luminal diameter of 10–15 μm. The "smooth muscle cells" of the arteriolar wall are thin, spindle-shaped cells with the polar ends divided into many long processes. The cells are arranged circularly or spirally around the long axis of most arterioles. Each cell is invested by a thin basal lamina, except for the "myo-myo junctions," areas of local cellular contact. Connective tissue fibers are present between smooth muscle cells in the larger arterioles. Toward the precapillary sphincter area, smooth muscle cells tend to make lateral contacts over extended areas. It is generally accepted that membranous contacts between smooth muscle cells (myo-myo junctions) are areas which facilitate and participate in propagating contraction impulses within a given smooth muscle. Peripherally to the smooth muscle cells is a thin collar of loose "connective tissue" composed of a few fibroblasts, collagenous and elastic fibrils, occasional macrophages, mast cells, and nonmyelinated nerve fibers. Toward the precapillary sphincter area, this connective tissue is reduced to occasional fibroblasts and a loosely woven network of collagenous fibrils.

VI. Precapillary Sphincter Area

This term is used here to describe both a functional concept and a structure. The classic precapillary sphincter may have been thought of as one or two smooth muscle cells around the entrance to a capillary. However, after analyzing a great number of small arterioles near the end where they

Fig. 1. Microvascular dimensions. Rat skeletal muscle fixed by a vascular perfusion. (1) Arteriole, lumen 60 μm, wall 1.7 μm; (2) precapillary arteriole, lumen 10 μm; (3) precapillary arteriole, lumen 3.5 μm; (4) muscular venules, lumen 50–75 μm, walls 0.8 μm; (5) lymphatic capillary; (6) perineurium of myelinated nerves; (7) capsule of intrafusal muscle fibers (neuromuscular spindle); (8) true capillaries, lumen 3.5 μm, among cross-sectioned striated muscle cells; (9) postcapillary venules, lumen 8–10 μm. Electron micrograph, magnification 600×.

Fig. 2. Cross-sectioned afferent arteriole of rat kidney. (1) Lumen 14 μm; (2) nucleus of smooth muscle cell; (3) nucleus of endothelial cell; (4) thin elastic membrane; (5) cross-sectioned, nonmyelinated nerves; (6) parts of renal tubules. Electron micrograph, magnification 4500×.

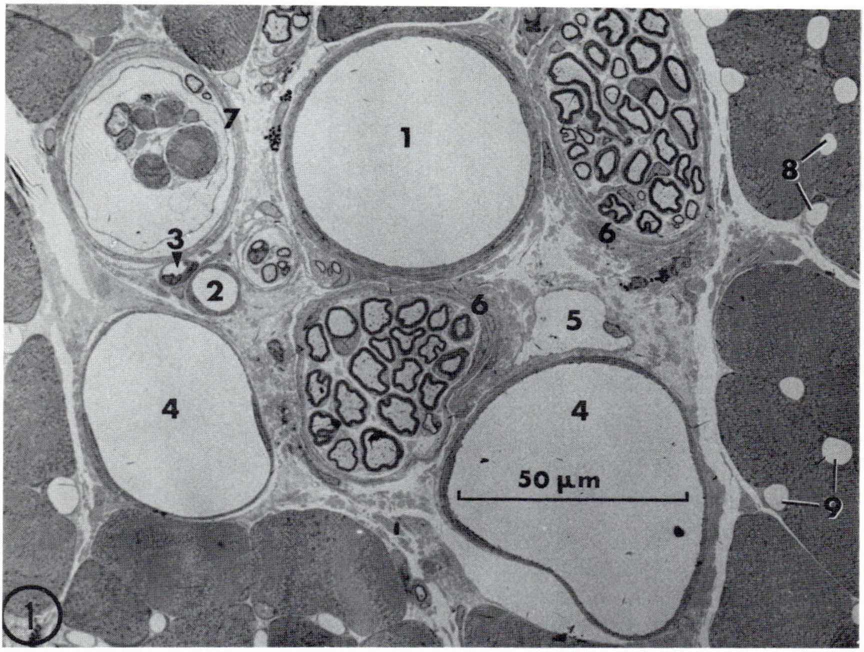
1
2
3
4
4
5
6
6
7
8
9
50 μm
1

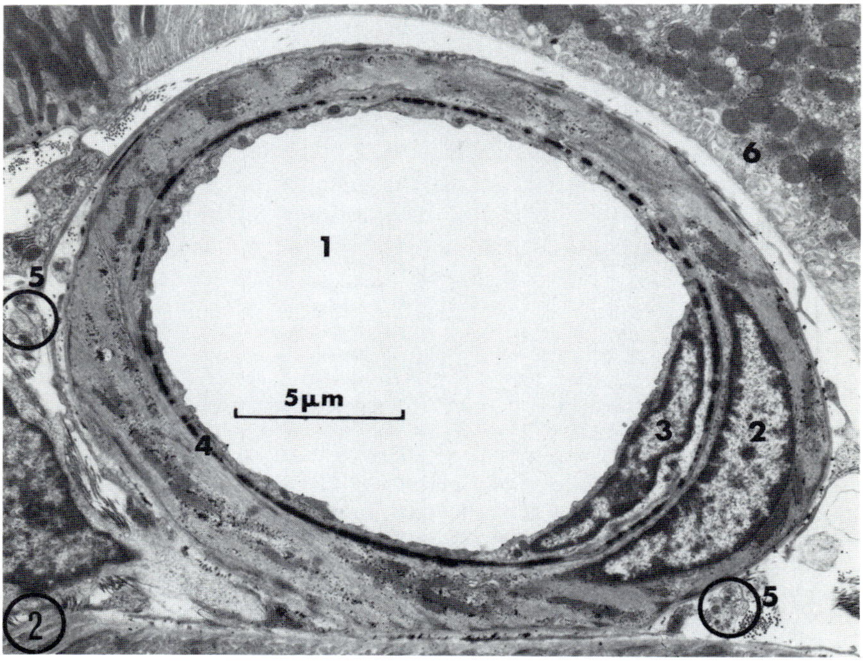
1
2
3
4
5
5
6
5μm
2

connect with, or give off capillaries, one is convinced that the metarteriole concept of Zweifach (1957) and the precapillary sphincter structure are best combined into and expressed as the "precapillary sphincter area." Functionally, it determines what passes through its own channel as well as what passes on to the capillary bed. However, it does this over a segment that may vary from 5 μm to 50–100 μm, rather than at the very end of the arteriole (Fig. 3).

The precapillary sphincter area, then, is variable in length, but generally has a luminal diameter which decreases from about 30 μm to about 5–10 μm. The "endothelium" of this area is similar to that of the larger arterioles. It rests on a thin basal lamina. One exception is the gradually increasing number of "myo-endothelial junctions." These are short, blunt, or narrow processes, emerging either from the endothelium or the neighboring smooth muscle cell and penetrating the basal lamina to make membranous contacts with the opposite cell (Fig. 4). These contacts may, at times, be of the tight variety, in which fusion of the superficial laminae of opposing cell membranes occur. They are particularly numerous just before the capillaries take off from the arteriole. Their function is not known, but it has been suggested that they may facilitate an ionic exchange between endothelium and smooth muscle cell. If so, they may help to initiate contraction of the smooth muscle cells, either by a mechanical stretch of the smooth muscle cell membrane (Bayliss' effect) or by initiating a change in membrane potential. The "smooth muscle cells" are small and few in number. They disappear gradually as the arteriole is transformed into an arterial capillary. In the afferent glomerular arteriole and in the arterioles of the cavernous tissue of the penis, the termination of smooth muscle cells is very abrupt, whereas in organs, such as lung, intestine, and skeletal muscle, there is a gradual decrease in number of smooth muscle cells. The sparse perivascular "connective tissue" merges imperceptively with that present in respective organs. As a rule, there are some nonmyelinated nerve fibers in this connective tissue.

Fig. 3. Longitudinal section of precapillary sphincter area. Dermis of rabbit. Arrows indicate direction of blood flow. (1) Smooth muscle cells surround the arteriole and the area where a 12-μm arteriole branches off from the 30-μm arteriole; (2) this is the point at which the smooth muscle cells form a final sphincterlike arrangement as the capillary emerges with a lumenal diameter of 7.5 μm; (3) endothelial cell nuclei; (4) lymphatic capillary; (5) collagen fibrils; (6) fibroblasts. Electron micrograph, magnification 2200×. [From Rhodin (1967).]

Fig. 4. Enlargement of area similar to the rectangle in Fig. 3, showing detail of wall of arteriole. (1) Lumen; (2) endothelium; (3) smooth muscle cells; (4) myo-endothelial junction; (5) myo-myo junction; (6) basal lamina. Electron micrograph, magnification 44,000×. [From Rhodin (1967).]

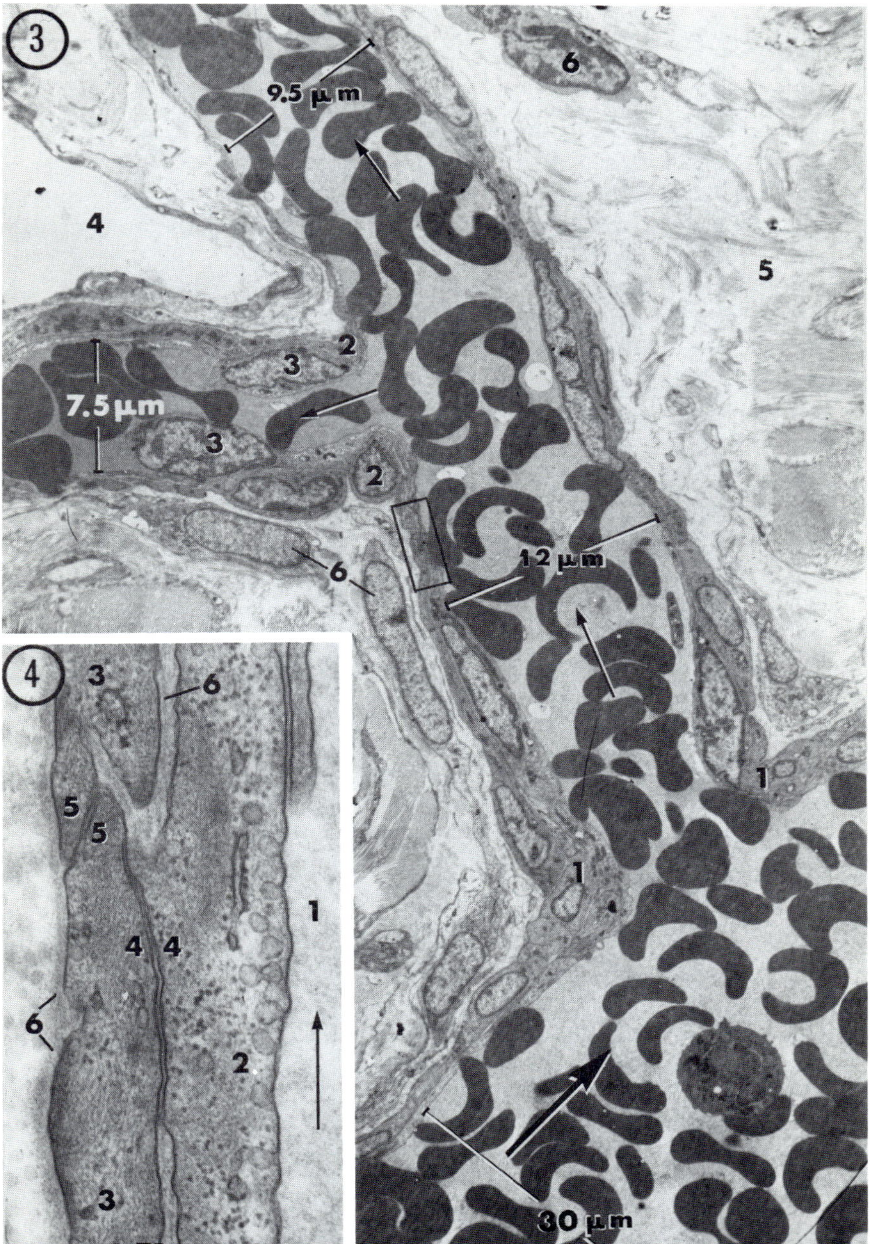
3
9.5 μm
4
5
6
2
3
7.5 μm
3
2
6
12 μm
1
1
30 μm
4
3
6
5
5
4 4
1
6
2
3
0.75 μm

VII. Capillaries

The capillary beds, their structural and ultrastructural components, and the possible relation of these components to some known functions require an extensive discussion in order to present adequately the many varied aspects. For detailed information consult Majno (1965). In this section an attempt is made to summarize some of the recent fine structural analyses. Until recently, it was believed that capillaries had the same general structure, but it is now recognized that there are several types of capillaries and that different organs and different tissues have their own type of capillary. In addition, there are indications that structural differences exist between arterial and venous capillaries in some organs. The average luminal width of a "true capillary" ranges between 3 μm and 7 μm (Fig. 5). I use the term true capillary to mean the narrowest segments of the capillary bed which, in most cases, consist of: (1) endothelium; (2) basal lamina; and (3) occasional pericytes. Each component varies slightly in its ultrastructural architecture, but the subdivision into several types of true capillaries is based largely on the structural design of the endothelium.

A. Endothelium

1. *Continuous Thick Endothelium*

This layer is present in the true capillaries of cardiac, skeletal, and smooth muscle tissue (Fig. 6) and to some extent in testis and ovary. The endothelial cells have an average thickness of 0.2 μm. The endothelial cytoplasm has many micropinocytotic vesicles, both at the surfaces and within the cytoplasm. Some microfilaments and microtubules are present. There is always a thin basal lamina and occasional pericytes.

2. *Continuous Thin Endothelium*

Continuous thin endothelium is present in the true capillaries of the central nervous system (Fig. 7), the lung (Fig. 8), arterial capillaries of the dermis, capillaries of the spleen, thymus, lymph nodes, and bone marrow, and in lymphatic capillaries. The endothelial cells have an average thickness of 0.1 μm. Their cytoplasm contains a small number of micropinocytotic vesicles. Microfilaments are present to a limited degree. A basal

Fig. 5. Longitudinal section of the capillary network in the connective tissue core of a rat intentinal villus. The average luminal diameter of the capillaries is 6 μm. Arrows indicate direction of blood flow. The capillary bed is drained by the post-capillary venule. (1) Endothelial nuclei; (2) pericytes; (3) pericapillary space; (4) fibroblasts; (5) collagen fibrils; (6) plasma cell; (7) macrophage; (8) eosinophil leukocyte; (9) Schwann cell nucleus of nonmyelinated nerve. Electron micrograph, magnification 1800×. [From Rhodin (1971a).]

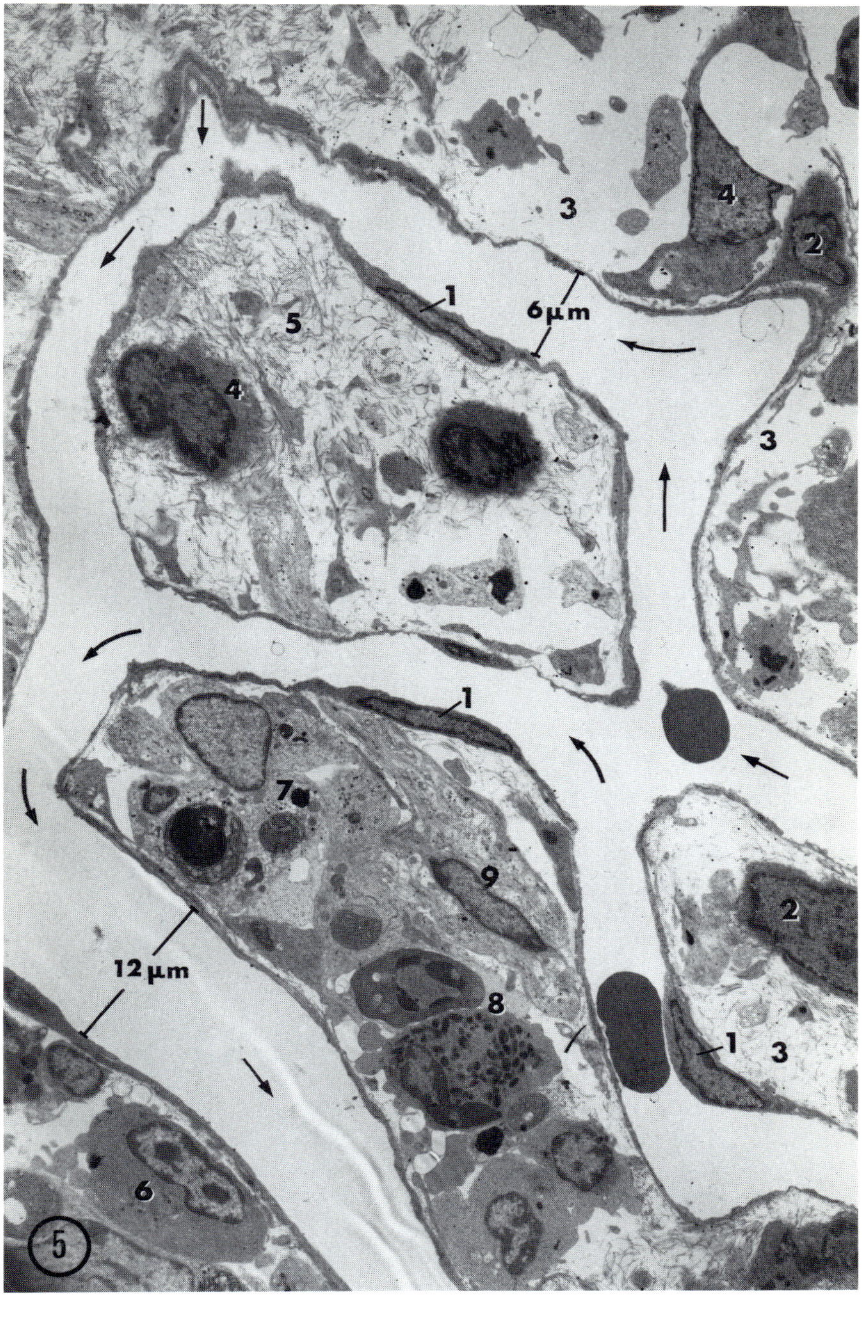
3
4
2
1
6μm
5
4
3
1
7
9
2
12μm
8
1
3
6
5

lamina exists in the lung and the nervous tissues but is missing in the lymphoid and myeloid tissues. Pericytes are largely absent.

3. *Fenestrated Thin Endothelium*

Fenestrated thin endothelium is present in the true capillaries of the urinary system (kidney, bladder) (Figs. 9–10), endocrine organs, choroid plexus of the brain, ciliary body of the eye, the venous capillaries of the dermis, and the intestinal connective tissue (lamina propria of mucous membrane). With the exception of the glomerular capillaries, the fenestrations are closed by a thin single-layered membrane derived from a fusion of the basal and luminal plasma membranes. The endothelium averages 800 Å in thickness. The fenestrations are round with a diameter of about 600 Å. A basal lamina is always present but pericytes are rare.

4. *Discontinuous Endothelium*

Discontinuous endothelium is found only in the sinusoids of the liver parenchyma (Fig. 11). It contains cytoplasmic holes with a diameter ranging between 0.5 μm and 2 μm. Membranes rarely close off these holes. A basal lamina is not present. Occasional pericytes occur.

B. Pericapillary Space

The extent of the pericapillary space and its components varies greatly with the organ. For example, it is generally rather wide around capillaries

Figs. 6–11. A comparison of different types of capillary walls, all shown at a magnification of 50,000×. [From Rhodin (1971a).]

Fig. 6. Rat cardiac muscle. (1) Lumen; (2) endothelium; (3) basal lamina; (4) pericapillary space; (5) pinocytotic vesicle.

Fig. 7. Rat cerebrum. (1) Lumen; (2) endothelium; (3) basal lamina; (6) brain tissue.

Fig. 8. Rat lung. (1) Lumen; (2) endothelium; (3) basal lamina; (5) pinocytotic vesicles; (7) alveolar epithelium; (8) alveolus.

Fig. 9. Rat kidney, peritubular capillary. (1) Lumen; (2) endothelium; (3) basal lamina; (4) pericapillary space; (9) fenestrations closed by a thin membrane.

Fig. 10. Rat kidney, glomerular capillary. (1) Lumen; (2) endothelium; (3) basal lamina; (7) visceral epithelium of Bowman's capsule; (8) urinary space; (9) fenestrations (open).

Fig. 11. Rat liver sinusoid. (1) Lumen; (2) endothelium; (4) pericapillary space (of Disse); (9) large gaps in endothelium; (10) microvilli of hepatic parenchymal cell.

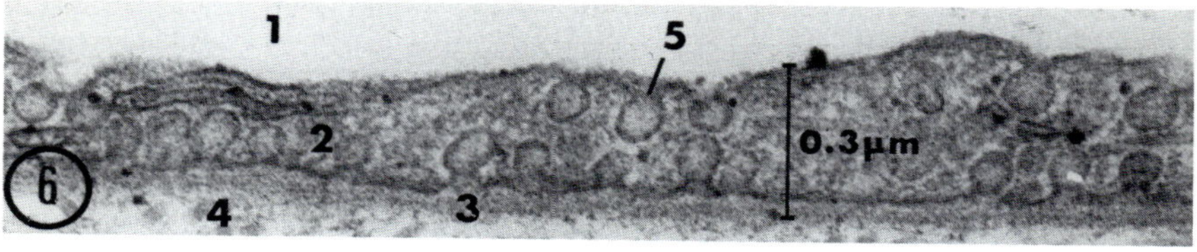
1
5
2
0.3µm
6
4
3

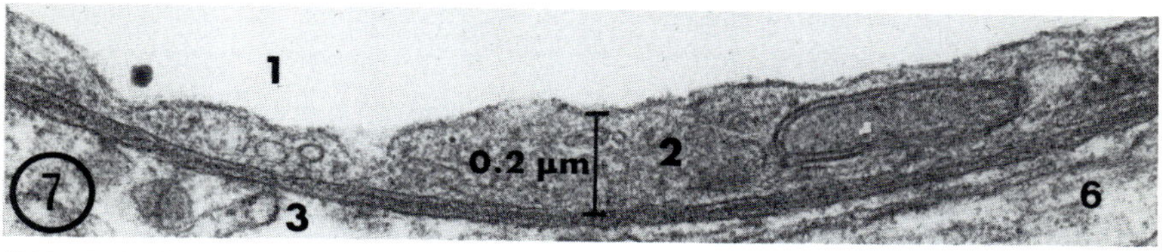
1
0.2 µm
2
7
3
6

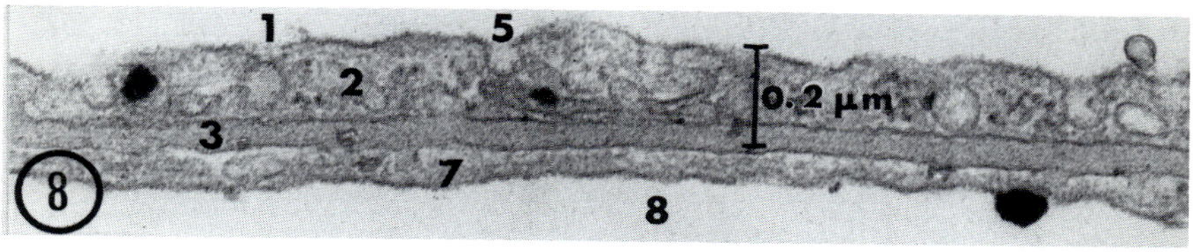
1
5
2
0.2 µm
3
7
8
8

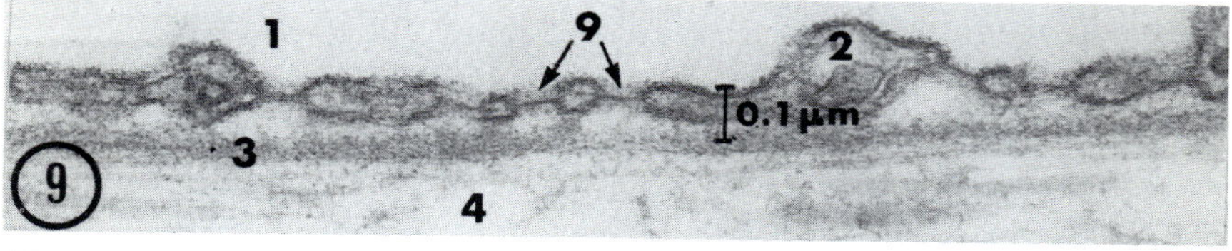
1
9
2
0.1µm
3
9
4

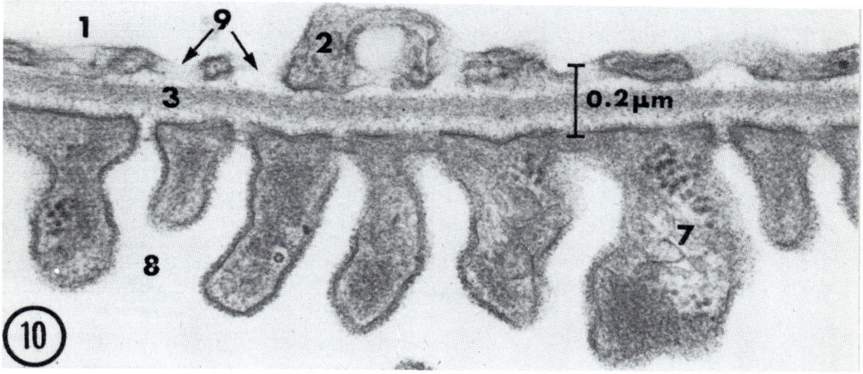
1
9
2
3
0.2µm
7
8
10

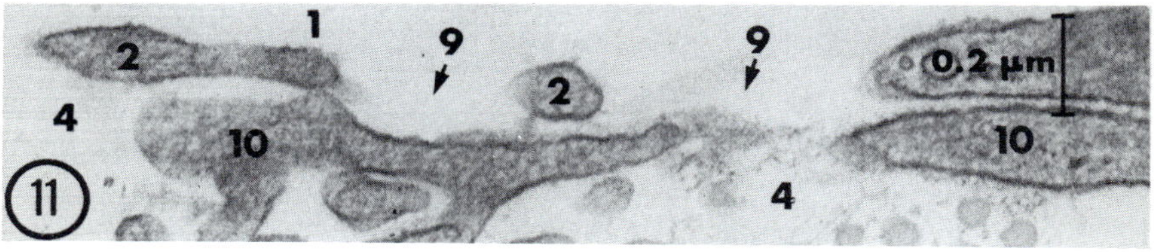
2
1
9
9
0.2 µm
4
2
10
10
11
4

of loose connective tissue [gastrointestinal tract (Fig. 5), endocrine organs, and urinary and reproductive systems] where it contains a loosely woven network of collagen and elastic fibrils. Around liver sinusoids, it is represented by the space of Disse, a narrow space for blood plasma between the endothelial cells and the liver cells. It is practically nonexistent around capillaries of muscle and nervous tissue, and it is very narrow, restricted only to part of the capillary circumference, in the pulmonary capillaries. In the glomerular capillaries of the kidney, it corresponds to the urinary space of Bowman's capsule.

C. Functions

It is generally believed that the "micropinocytotic vesicles" of the continuous endothelium help to carry metabolites, ions, and fluids across the endothelium (Fig. 12). The "fenestrations" probably represent sites of easy diffusion, but experimental data are not available to support this hypothesis. In most capillaries, endothelial cells are held together by "junctions" in which the outer laminae of opposing cell membranes are not fused. This narrow, intercellular gap of about 50 Å may be utilized for endothelial transport. In the brain capillaries, the junctions are closed by a fusion of the cell membranes, possibly creating the so-called blood-brain barrier. The "basal lamina" represents only a very crude barrier to the formed elements of the blood and to large molecular substances. When absent, there is one factor less blocking or interfering with transcapillary passage. The "large holes" of the liver sinusoids clearly offer preferential channels for exchange. Experimental evidence is not available to support the formulation of a hypothesis of whether the capillary "fenestrations" are stationary or transient, and whether they occur more often near the venous segment of a capillary in tissues other than the dermis (Fig. 13) and intestine. The "microfilaments" of the endothelial cytoplasm may indicate a potential contractility of the capillary. If so, this is probably a very slow contraction, more in the nature of ameboid movements than the relatively fast contraction of smooth muscle myofilaments.

VIII. Postcapillary Venules

In most early investigations of the microvascular beds in which the light microscope was used as an investigative tool, microvessels with a diameter of 20 μm and less were collectively referred to as capillaries. However, high speed cinemicrophotography and electron microscopy have clearly shown that there is a segment of the microvascular bed which has a reactivity and an ultrastructure different from the true capillaries. This segment is referred to here as "postcapillary venules."

Ultrastructural analyses show that the postcapillary segment has a luminal diameter which ranges between 8 μm and 30 μm (Fig. 13). The length of this segment varies considerably. It can be as short as 50 μm and as long as 500 μm. The wall of the postcapillary venule consists of: (1) endothelium; (2) basal lamina; (3) pericytes; and (4) fibroblasts (veil cells). The endothelium is thin but continuous at the connection between the venous capillary and the postcapillary venule. It gradually becomes thicker and averages about 0.4 μm. One exception is the lymph node in which the postcapillary venules have an endothelium consisting of cuboidal cells. Micropinocytotic vesicles are present only to a moderate degree.

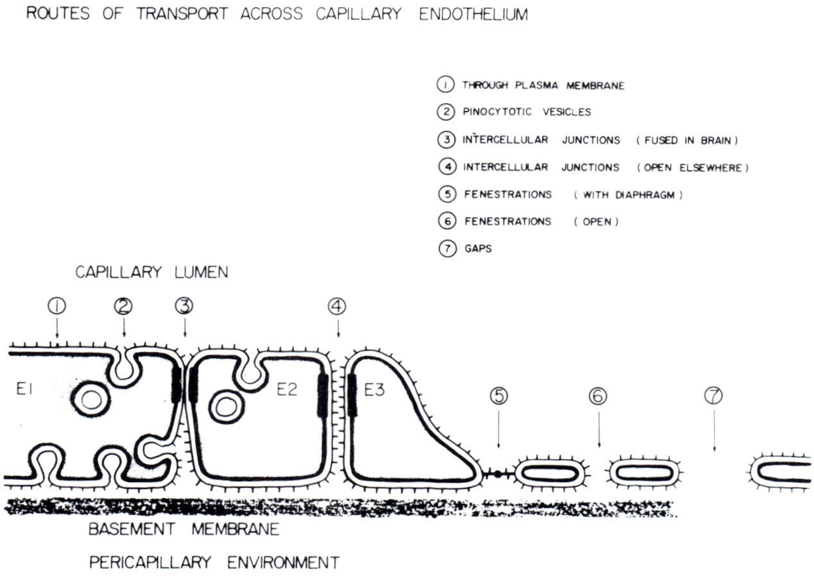

Fig. 12. Different routes of transport across the capillary endothelium are schematized in this composite drawing. The transport may occur from the capillary lumen across the endothelium and the basement membrane (basal lamina) to the pericapillary environment, as well as in the opposite direction. Several endothelial cells, or parts thereof, are represented as E1, E2, and E3. The cell membrane is depicted as composed of a superficial glycoprotein layer (fuzz) and two laminae of electron dense material, surrounding a less electron dense central lamina. The outermost dense laminae of adjacent cells fuse in the cellular junctions of mammalian brain capillaries and in the diaphragm of fenestrated endothelia. The basement membrane is often absent in capillaries with large endothelial gaps. [From Rhodin (1971a).]

Ribosomes are numerous, and profiles of the granular endoplasmic reticulum are more frequent than in the endothelium of true capillaries. Microfilaments are abundant. The endothelial cells overlap each other slightly and are held together by junctions in which fusions of opposing cell membranes are rare. Long and narrow projections of the endothelial cytoplasm penetrate the basal lamina, making membranous contacts with pericytes or extending into the perivenular connective tissue. The pericytes are connective tissue cells with a highly branched cytoplasm embracing the endothelial tube. Near the venous capillary, the pericytes are widely scattered, but increase gradually in number to form an almost complete layer around the distal end of the postcapillary venule. The ultrastructure of the pericyte is very similar to that of a fibroblast, except that the pericyte is invested by its own basal lamina. There are also "fibroblasts" present. They are thin, sheetlike cells, normally referred to as veil cells which together with collagen fibrils form a thin, perivascular collar. It should be kept in mind that pericytes and fibroblasts are mostly associated with postcapillary venules of loose connective tissue, and may be entirely absent in other tissues.

FUNCTIONS

The reactivity of the postcapillary venule is quite different from that of true capillaries. Under normal conditions, this segment of the microvascular bed is probably the site for the diffusion of metabolites, ions, and fluids from the tissue to the blood. However, it is also the most sensitive and vulnerable, since this segment is affected by allergic reactions, inflammation, and extreme temperatures, reacting to these factors by an increase in outward diffusion (edema) and, in extreme cases, by an extravasation of formed elements of the blood. The cells involved in these processes are the endothelial cells and the pericytes, but the exact mechanism is not understood. Normally, the pericyte probably functions as a stabilizer of the endothelial tube, and it may also have some contractile properties. However, there is no indication that it functions as a true postcapillary sphincter. The pericyte may also represent an undifferentiated precursor cell which could develop into smooth muscle cells, fibroblasts, or other types of connective tissue cells.

Fig. 13. Longitudinal section of connection between venous capillary and postcapillary venule in the dermis of the rabbit. Arrows indicate direction of blood flow. (1) Venous capillary; (2) postcapillary venule; (3) endothelial nuclei; (4) nuclei of pericytes; (5) at the junctions of a capillary and a postcapillary venule, smooth muscle cells are not present; processes of pericytic cytoplasm surround the capillary at this point; (6) fibroblast; (7) collagen fibrils; (8) in some parts of the endothelium of a venous capillary in the dermis fenestrations occur. An area similar to the rectangle is enlarged in Fig. 9. Electron micrograph, magnification 2200×.

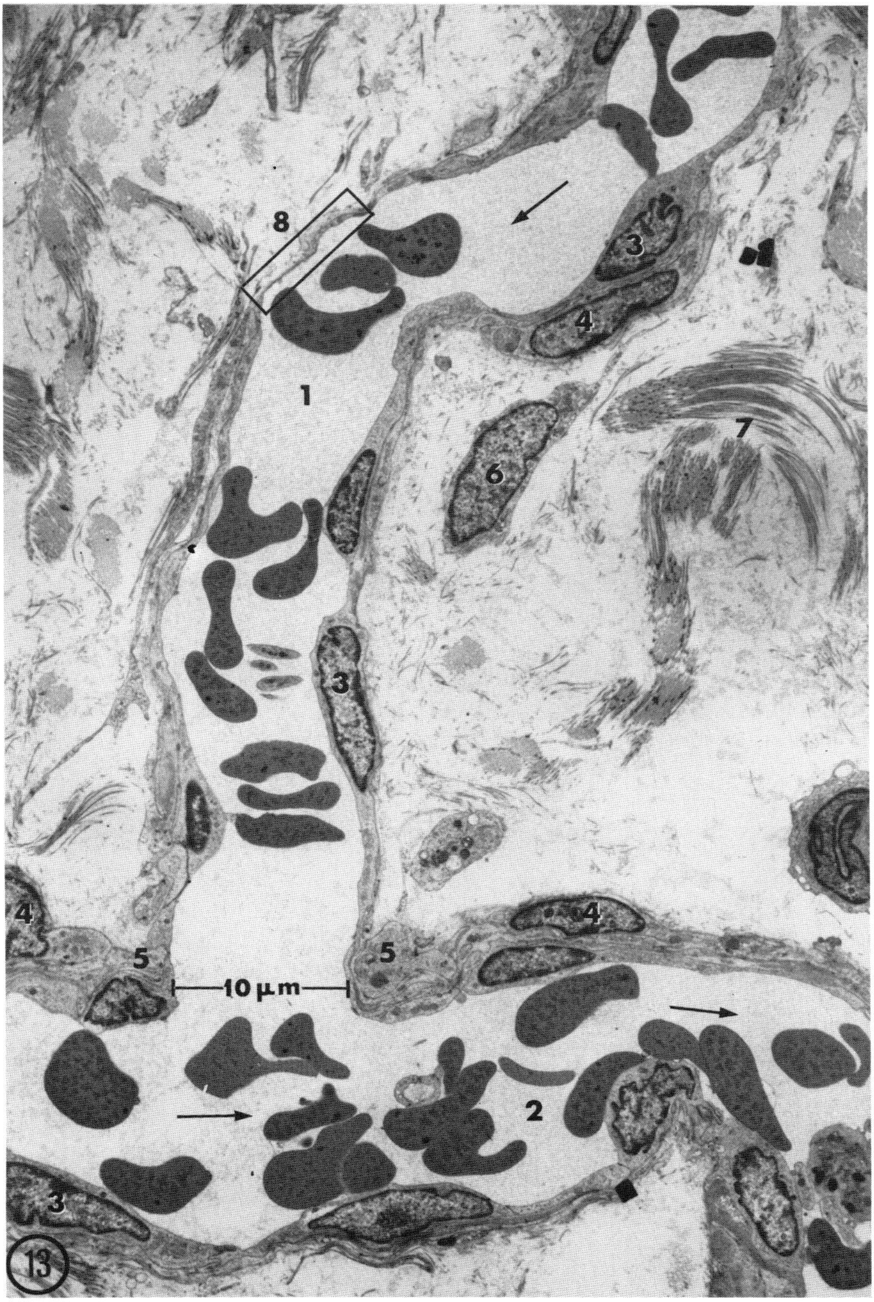
8
3
4
1
6
7
3
4
5
5
4
10 µm
2
3
13

IX. Collecting Venules

The postcapillary venules increase gradually in size from a luminal diameter of 30 μm to about 50 μm. This segment of the microvascular bed varies greatly in length but the structure of the vascular wall is sufficiently different from that of the postcapillary venule to justify the term "collecting venule."

The endothelium and the basal lamina are similar to those of the postcapillary venule. The pericytes form a complete layer around the proximal part of the collecting venule, and there are several layers at the distal end of this segment. Cells occur among the pericytes which ultrastructurally must be classified as "primitive smooth muscle cells" since their cytoplasm contains bundles of filaments with scattered oblong, fusiform densities along the cytoplasmic aspect of the cell membrane and among the bundles of filaments (Fig. 14). There are numerous myo-endothelial junctions, mostly where cytoplasmic processes of the primitive smooth muscle cells contact the endothelium. The fibroblasts (veil cells) also form one or several complete layers around the collecting venule. The function of this segment is not clear, but a potential regulation of the luminal diameter through smooth muscle action is quite possible. In terms of reaction to pathogens or other influencing factors, this segment is far less sensitive than the postcapillary venule.

X. Muscular Venules

Once the luminal diameter of the collecting venules becomes larger than 50 μm, the vascular wall contains only fully differentiated smooth muscle cells (Fig. 15). There is only a very small number of muscle layers, even as the venules reach a luminal diameter of up to 300 μm. Furthermore, there is a great variation in the layering depending upon the tissue and

Fig. 14. Detail of the region where two collecting venules merge (lumenal diameters 30–35 μm). Dermis of rabbit. Arrows indicate direction of blood flow. (1) Lumen; (2) endothelium; (3) erythrocytes; (4) nucleus of primitive smooth muscle cell; (5) long cytoplasmic extensions; (6) fusiform densities along cell membrane; (7) collagen fibrils; (8) basal lamina. Electron micrograph, magnification 14,500×. [From Rhodin (1968).]

Fig. 15. Rat brain muscular venule. Lumenal diameter 100 μm. (1) Lumen; (2) endothelium; (3) gap junction; (4) basal lamina of endothelium; (5) smooth muscle cell with myofilaments, ribosomes, and micropinocytotic vesicles; (6) basal lamina of the smooth muscle cell. Electron micrograph, magnification 58,000×.

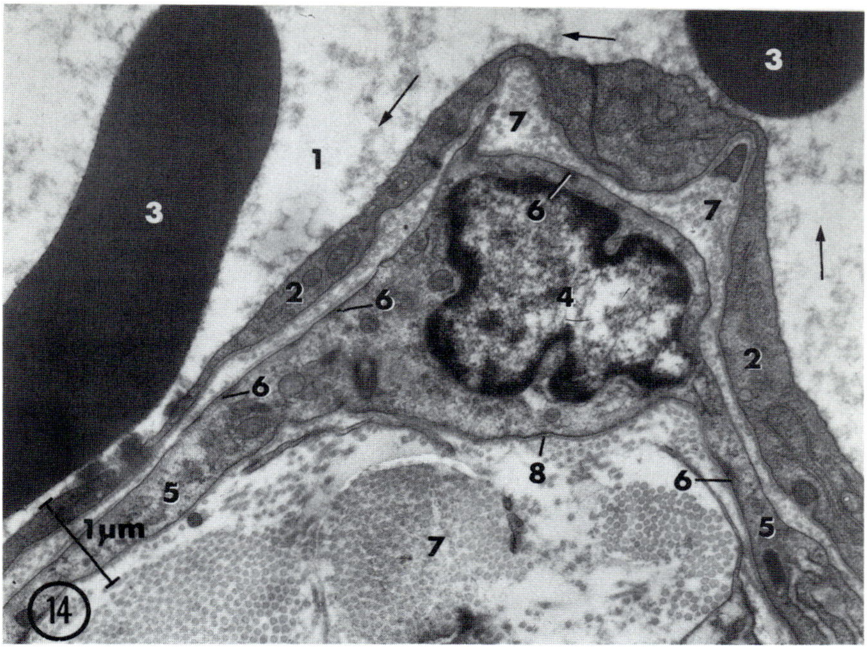
1
2
3
4
5
6
7
8
1µm
14

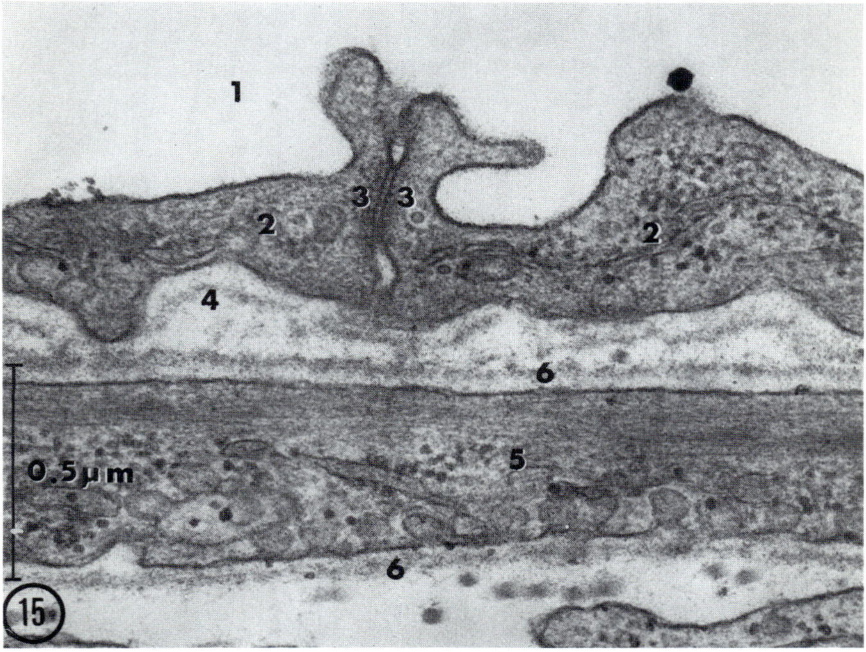
1
2
3
4
5
6
0.5µm
15

the organ. The dermal connective tissue venules and small veins generally have 2–3 layers of smooth muscle cells, whereas corresponding vessels in the kidney may have only one layer, sometimes none. The endothelium is thicker than in the collecting venules, often containing large numbers of specific, membrane-bounded endothelial granules, the function of which is not known. Myo-endothelial junctions are numerous. The fibroblasts form, together with large bundles of collagenous fibers, the beginning of what might be termed an adventitia.

XI. Innervation of the Microvascular Bed

Unmyelinated sympathetic and parasympathetic nerves accompany arterioles, capillaries, and venules throughout the microvascular beds in most organs and tissues. The topographic relationship between these nerves and components of the vascular wall is that of a distant companionship. The nerves do not make membranous contacts with smooth muscle cells, pericytes, or endothelial cells. It is beyond the scope of this chapter to discuss the mechanisms whereby neurotransmitter substances may be released, how they reach the components of the vascular wall, and how they influence the cell membranes of smooth muscle cells, pericytes, and endothelial cells. It should be recalled that neuromuscular junctions exist between autonomic nerves and smooth muscle cells of the ureter and the ductus deferens, but that this kind of membranous junction does not occur in large or small blood vessels. The question of innervation of vascular smooth muscle remains largely unanswered.

Acknowledgments

This chapter is based on works supported by The Westchester Heart Association, Inc., and the U.S. Public Health Service No. HE–10924 and FR–05398.

The very skillful technical assistance by Mrs. Carin Silversmith throughout the many analyses and the invaluable assistance of Mrs. Betsey Stiepock in typing the manuscript are gratefully acknowledged.

References

Bennett, H. S., Luft, J. H., and Hampton, J. C. (1959). Morphological classification of vertebrate blood capillaries. *Amer. J. Physiol.* **196,** 381–390.

Burton, A. C. (1954). Relation of structure to function of the tissues of the wall of blood vessels. *Physiol. Rev.* **34,** 619–642.

Chambers, R., and Zweifach, B. W. (1944). Topography and function of the mesenteric capillary circulation. *Amer. J. Anat.* **75,** 173–205.

Clark, E. R., and Clark, E. L. (1925). The development of adventitial (Rouget) cells on the blood capillaries of amphibian larvae. *Amer. J. Anat.* **35,** 239–264.

Clark, E. R., and Clark, E. L. (1934). Observations on living arteriovenous anastomosis as seen in transplant chambers introduced into the rabbit's ear. *Amer. J. Anat.* **54,** 229–286.

Crone, C., and Lassen, N. A., eds. (1970). "Capillary Permeability." Academic Press, New York.

Fawcett, D. W. (1959). The fine structure of capillaries, arterioles and small arteries. *In* "The Microcirculation" (S. R. M. Reynolds and B. W. Zweifach, eds.), pp. 1–27. Univ. of Illinois Press, Urbana.

Fawcett, D. W. (1963). Comparative observations on the fine structure of blood capillaries. *In* "The Peripheral Blood Vessels" (J. L. Orbison and D. E. Smith, eds.), pp. 17–44. Williams & Wilkins, Baltimore, Maryland.

Illig, L. (1961). "Die terminale Strombahn." Springer-Verlag, Berlin and New York.

Karnovsky, M. J. (1967). The ultrastructural basis of capillary permeability studied with peroxidase as a tracer. *J. Cell Biol.* **35,** 213–236.

Krogh, A. (1930). "The Anatomy and Physiology of Capillaries." Yale Univ. Press, New Haven, Connecticut.

Majno, G. (1965). Ultrastructure of the vascular membrane. *In* "Handbook of Physiology" (Amer. Physiol. Soc., J. Field, ed.), Sect. 2, Vol. III, pp. 2293–2375. Williams & Wilkins, Baltimore, Maryland.

Ratschow, M. (1959). "Angiologie." G. Thieme, Stuttgart.

Reale, E., and Ruska, H. (1965). Die Feinstruktur der Gefässwände. *Angiologica* **2,** 90–142.

Rhodin, J. (1962). Fine structure of vascular walls in mammals with special reference to smooth muscle component. *Physiol. Rev.* **42,** Suppl. 5, 48–87.

Rhodin, J. (1967). The ultrastructure of mammalian arterioles and precapillary sphincters. *J. Ultrastruct. Res.* **18,** 181–223.

Rhodin, J. (1968). Ultrastructure of mammalian venous capillaries, venules and small collecting veins. *J. Ultrastruct. Res.* **25,** 452–500.

Rhodin, J. (1971a). Fine structure of capillaries. *In* "Topics in the Study of Life," BIO Source Book, pp. 215–224. Harper, New York.

Rhodin, J. (1971b). The ultrastructure of the adrenal cortex of the rat under normal and experimental conditions. *J. Ultrastruct. Res.* **34,** 23–71.

Simon, G. (1965). Ultrastructure des capillaires. *Angiologica* **2,** 370–434.

Zweifach, B. W. (1957). General principles governing the behavior of the microcirculation, *Amer. J. Med.* **23,** 684–696.

Zweifach, B. W. (1961). The structural basis of the microcirculation. *In* "Development and Structure of the Cardiovascular System" (A. A. Luisada, ed.), pp. 1–198. McGraw-Hill, New York.

3 FUNCTIONAL ASPECTS OF THE MICROCIRCULATION

D. D. STROMBERG, M.D., Ph.D.
and C. A. WIEDERHIELM, Ph.D.

I. Introductory Aspects

Microcirculation involves blood flow in vessels which by definition can be clearly visualized only through use of a magnifying system. The small size of the components not only increases the challenge of studying them, but by virtue of short distances makes physicochemical processes, such as diffusion, assume considerable significance. This chapter will emphasize the functional and dynamic roles of the microscopic and ultramicroscopic components of the microcirculation. Among the functions with which these components are involved are (1) blood flow control, (2) transcapillary exchange, and (3) interstitial transport.

The caliber of elements of the microvasculature varies in response to a wide variety of stimulations. Such adjustments constitute control of resistance to blood flow and of pressure distribution in the microcirculation.

These adjustments are of paramount importance in overall control of peripheral circulation and in blood flow distribution among different organs and tissues. They also influence capillary hydrostatic pressures and fluid exchange processes within organs and tissues. A number of exquisite control systems are involved in these adjustments.

Most of the fluid exchange functions of the cardiovascular system occur across the thin-walled capillaries. By virtue of their solubility and diffusability in tissue components, including the vascular wall, gases such as CO_2 and O_2 may also exchange directly across larger elements of the microvasculature (Duling and Berne, 1970). Transcapillary exchange results from interactions among opposing forces across the capillary wall. These exchange forces include concentration gradients, hydrostatic pressure gradients, and interactions among osmotically active molecules. Each of these forces is subject to changes in levels of nervous and metabolic activity of a whole organism and particularly to changes in level of activity of various organs and tissues within an organism. Transcapillary exchange is therefore a dynamic, ever-changing process.

Capillaries are separated from cells by volumes of interstitial material which vary in size and composition among different tissues. Transcapillary exchange occurs across the capillary wall between capillary blood and the surrounding interstitium. Properties of the interstitium are significant determinants of transcapillary exchange as well as of subsequent interstitial transport. Characteristics of the interstitium that influence exchange and transport processes in tissues are being increasingly recognized. For example, different kinds of edema formation may involve differential effects on components of the interstitium.

II. Functional Architecture of Microvascular Beds

A. Morphologic Definitions

The microvascular unit shown in Fig. 1 is a generalized one based upon functional morphologic characteristics suggested by Chambers and Zweifach (1946). It is intended to provide a basis for generalization about the functions of the different elements. Some elements, such as the precapillary sphincter, are not demonstrable in all vascular beds.

In Fig. 1, blood enters the microcirculation from an arterial conduit via a muscular "arteriole." A distinguishing feature of the arteriole is the smooth muscle in the wall which consists of one continuous layer wound helically around the arteriole. A "metarteriole," in which the single layer of surrounding smooth muscle is discontinuous, arises from the arteriole.

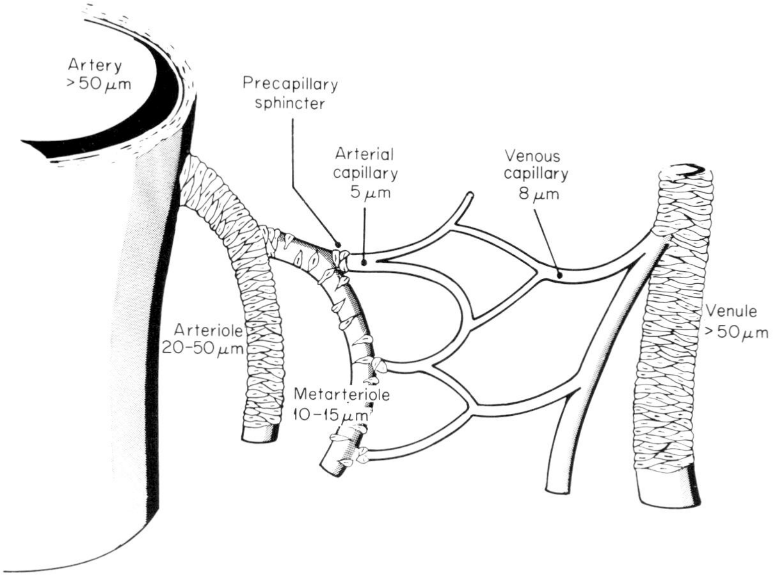

Fig. 1. A simplified anatomic representation based on the morphologic criteria of Chambers and Zweifach (1946). Arteries have several layers of smooth muscle in the wall; arterioles one continuous layer; metarterioles a discontinuous layer. Precapillary sphincters consist of an accumulation of smooth muscle around the origin of the capillary as it arises from the metarteriole. Capillaries consist primarily of an endothelial tube across which occurs most exchange with the surrounding interstitium. This diagram does not correspond in detail to any particular vascular bed.

At the origin of the arterial capillary from the metarteriole there is often a condensation of vascular smooth muscle designated as the "precapillary sphincter." Beyond the precapillary sphincter, the arterial capillaries diverge as thin-walled, nonmuscular channels while similar, larger, thin-walled venous capillaries converge toward the venous channels. The last and largest elements of the microvascular unit are the muscular venules.

B. Roles of the Components

The muscular arterial components comprised of the arterioles, metarterioles, and precapillary sphincters are the primary sites of controlled resistance to blood flow by virtue of their ability to change their caliber actively by changing the tension developed in the smooth muscle in the vessel wall. The capillaries downstream from the precapillary sphincters also undergo caliber changes, but these effects are probably the passive result of changing transmural pressures secondary to caliber changes of the upstream resistance vessels. A major function occurring at the level of the capillaries is exchange of substances between the blood and surrounding tissue. The venules are the return channels which, in addition to playing a possible role in resistance control, also probably serve as volume capacitance vessels of some vascular beds and to control the volume distribution of the blood throughout the body. The role of the microvascular capacitance vessels in the volume shifts occurring during activities such as exercise has not been clearly separated from that of the larger veins.

C. Vasoconstriction

Vasoconstriction is the process of decreasing the caliber of a vessel. It is usually due to a change in the level of active tension developed in the smooth muscle in the vessel wall. During vasoconstriction in an arteriole there is a considerable architectural rearrangement of the elements of the vessel wall. Electron microscopic sections of arterioles during controlled, tapering, localized vasoconstriction show these changes clearly (Phelps and Luft, 1969). The architectural modifications during vasoconstriction result in a "physiologic" thickening of the vessel wall which may be mistaken histologically for pathologic hypertrophy of the wall (Van Citters *et al.*, 1962). Pathologic hypertrophy may be distinguished from physiologic thickening by criteria involving structural rearrangements in the wall during vasoconstriction (Stromberg *et al.*, 1969).

III. Blood Flow Control

Control of peripheral vascular blood flow resistance is largely mediated by those factors influencing the active tension developed by smooth muscle in the walls of the arterioles, metarterioles, and precapillary sphincters. Evidence for this includes the observation that pressure drop, which is a function of resistance to flow, is greatest across these "resistive" elements of the microvasculature (Landis and Pappenheimer, 1963; Wiederhielm, 1967; Wiederhielm and Weston, 1973). A change in caliber of the muscular arterioles, metarterioles, and precapillary sphincters, therefore, has the most profound influence on the amount of pressure dropped as blood flows through the arterial channels between the heart and the capillaries. Postcapillary resistance contributed by the venous vasculature may also contribute to setting the level of capillary hydrostatic pressure (Johnson and Hanson, 1962).

A. Autonomic Control

Autonomic nervous influence on the microvasculature is most evident in the arterioles which have the most completely developed muscular coat of the resistance vessels and are usually richly innervated. Through counter-poised actions producing either vasoconstriction or vasodilation, these influences provide a mechanism for exquisite control of local vascular resistance by the central nervous system. Since arterioles usually supply blood to several capillary networks in the microvasculature, the control exerted on the arterioles by the autonomic nervous system at the microcirculatory level extends to relatively broad blocks of tissue in that increasing or decreasing flow through an arteriole increases or decreases the hydrostatic pressure and the blood available to a number of downstream metarterioles and capillaries. Arterioles are probably capable of complete closure in contrast to larger upstream arteries which probably are not.

B. Other Factors

Metarterioles and precapillary sphincters are probably more directly influenced by local factors, such as differences between intravascular and tissue hydrostatic pressures (transmural pressures) or changes in concentration of local metabolites and metabolic by-products, than are the arterioles (Folkow *et al.,* 1971). Metarterioles occupy an intermediate position both anatomically and functionally. Precapillary sphincters are probably most directly responsive to changes in transmural pressure and in local cellular metabolic activity. Metabolites resulting from local cellular activity have a diffusion distance of a few micrometers to the precapillary sphincter of the local capillary network supplying the cells. This short distance provides rapid, fine control of local capillary blood circulation by way of a localized feedback mechanism. For example, cellular metabolites, possibly operating through a common modality such as osmotic effects (Jonsson, 1970), may act on precapillary sphincter smooth muscle to cause a relaxation of the muscle, an opening of the sphincter, an increase in hydrostatic pressure at the arterial end of the capillary, and, therefore, an increase in very localized capillary blood flow in response to an increase in metabolic activity of nearby cells. Increased local flow "washes out" the accumulated metabolites restoring the local concentrations of metabolites. The variations in capillary hydrostatic pressure shown in Fig. 2 (Wiederhielm and Weston, 1973) may be the result of interactions among the control mechanisms. For example, the local mechanism is subject to modulation by autonomic influences either directly, by transmitter overflow, or by constriction of upstream arterioles reducing or shutting off the blood supplied

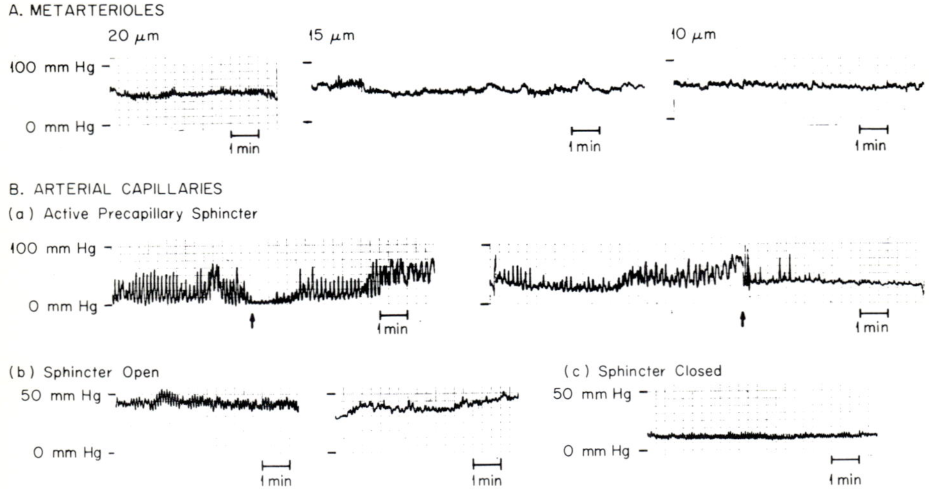

Fig. 2. Variations in intravascular pressures in subcutaneous metarterioles and arterial capillaries of the bat wing subcutaneous tissues. Three different sizes of metarterioles show similar pressures of about 50 mm Hg as indicated in panel A. The arterial capillaries in B include different levels of activity of the precapillary sphincter. Closure of the active sphincter in (a) is represented by the arrows. Note that capillary pressure drops nearly to zero in the first case in section (a), whereas in the second case, parallel connecting capillaries from other open sphincters in the bed probably supplied blood flow through longer, higher resistance, pathways, leading to a decrease in pressure, but not a drop to zero. Rhythmic pressure variations were probably due to cyclic interactions among the controlling variables of the resistance vessels. Such variations should produce cyclic changes in filtration and reabsorption of fluid from the capillaries. (Wiederhielm and Weston, *Am. J. Physiol.* In press.)

to the precapillary sphincter and, therefore, also the pressure applied to the precapillary sphincter. In this way control of vascular resistance probably comprises a hierarchy of controls both anatomically and functionally with the finest local control residing in the precapillary sphincter.

IV. Transcapillary Fluid Exchange

A. Starling-Landis Model

Just before the end of the nineteenth century, E. H. Starling (1896) presented evidence that, contrary to many previous concepts, most of the fluid filtering from the capillaries into the tissues was not returned to the circulation by the lymphatics. A significant portion of filtered tissue fluids was absorbed directly back into the capillary blood. This concept has been confirmed and extended, and is now usually called the Starling-Landis model of transcapillary exchange to acknowledge the additional contributions of E. M. Landis (1926). Landis' work and other evidence for the model and for the concepts involving capillary permeability are well summarized in the review by Landis and Pappenheimer (1963). In the model there are four driving pressures for the movement of fluid between capillary blood and the surrounding interstitium. They consist of (1) hydrostatic pressure in the capillary blood, which tends to push fluid out of the capillary; (2) oncotic pressure developed by the plasma proteins, which attracts fluid from the interstitium into the capillary; (3) hydrostatic pressure in the tissue fluids, which pushes fluid into the capillary; and (4) oncotic pressure developed by plasma proteins and/or other macromolecules or "colloids" in the interstitium, which attracts fluid from the capillaries into the interstitium. It is variation among these pressures which determines the direction and magnitude of fluid exchange across the permeable capillary wall.

1. *Capillary Hydrostatic Pressure*

Capillary hydrostatic pressure is the residual of the energy imparted to the circulating blood by the heart. It is that hydrostatic pressure which remains after the blood has traversed the large feeding arteries and experienced pressure drops, primarily in the muscular arterial portions of the microvasculature. Since the pressures generated by the heart are variable and since with vasomotion the pressure head lost across the arterial microvasculature can vary considerably, capillary hydrostatic pressure is also variable. Changes in venous pressure or postcapillary resistance can also affect capillary pressure (Johnson and Hanson, 1962). Conditions, such as heart failure, in which venous pressure is elevated lead to increased capillary hydrostatic pressure and, therefore, to increased capillary filtration and edema formation.

The factors influencing capillary hydrostatic pressure interact and vary with time. Capillary hydrostatic pressure therefore also varies with time as indicated by the recordings shown in Fig. 2. These variations in pressure are accompanied by variations in fluid flow across the permeable capillary in the dynamic, living microcirculatory system.

2. *Plasma Oncotic Pressure*

In 1896, Starling postulated that the presence of significant protein in the plasma accounted for reabsorption of tissue fluid into capillary blood.

One of his confirmations of this postulate was the direct measurement of the oncotic pressure developed in samples of plasma equilibrated across a peritoneal membrane coated with gelatin against a physiologic salt solution. He found the oncotic pressure developed by the proteins to be about equal to the available estimates of capillary hydrostatic pressure. With refinements of both the oncotic pressure measurements with membrane osmometers and direct measurements of capillary hydrostatic pressure this concept remains established today with only minor modifications and additions.

The capillary wall membrane, which was simulated by the gelatin-coated peritoneal membrane in Starling's experiment, is relatively impermeable to larger molecules, such as plasma proteins, but it does leak. The permeability of the capillary to protein and fluid varies among different organs and tissues and among different sites along the capillary. The venous end of the capillary, in addition to having a larger surface area than the arterial end (Wiederhielm, 1968), contains a few large pores and possibly pinocytotic vesicles (Karnovsky, 1968) which allow protein to leak continuously through to the interstitium. The venous capillary of the mesentery also shows a higher permeability to substances such as water (Intaglietta, 1967; Wiederhielm, 1966).

3. *Tissue Oncotic Pressure*

The effect of this continuous leakage of protein and of the presence of protein in the interstitium was anticipated in Starling's initial hypothesis. He postulated that the protein in the interstitium would offset the oncotic pressure effect of plasma protein on transcapillary fluid exchange and, further, that the concentration of the tissue protein would vary with the rate of transudation of fluid into the tissue. With a greater rate of fluid filtration into the tissues, the tissue protein concentration and, therefore, tissue oncotic pressure should decrease if the rate of protein leakage by the capillaries and removal by the lymphatics remains relatively fixed. This decrease shifts the transcapillary pressures in the direction of reabsorption of fluid into the capillary thus providing an oncotic "buffering" mechanism for controlling fluid exchange at the level of the capillary (Wiederhielm, 1968). Indeed, this buffering is observed clinically in that a substantial decrease in plasma protein concentration is required to induce significant tissue fluid accumulation and edema formation.

4. *Tissue Hydrostatic Pressure*

Hydrostatic pressure in the tissues is another factor in the Starling-Landis model influencing transcapillary fluid exchange. This pressure component is the counterpart of the hydrostatic pressure in the capillary blood but acts in the opposite direction. An increase in tissue hydrostatic pressure enhances reabsorption of fluid by the capillary. The magnitude of tissue hydrostatic pressures has not been definitely established. Measurements in artificially induced fluid spaces in tissues yield subatmospheric pressures (Guyton, 1963; Guyton *et al.,* 1971; Scholander *et al.,* 1968), while those involving puncture techniques generally yield positive pressures (McMaster, 1946; Wiederhielm, 1969). Differences between these results may be due to oncotic effects (Stromberg and Wiederhielm, 1970).

B. Synthesis of the Model

As suggested above, many interacting variables in addition to those in the basic Starling-Landis model are involved in transcapillary exchange. A simulation by Wiederhielm (1968) involved 21 simultaneously interacting equations which were solved using an analog computer and values from the literature for the various parameters and variables. Simulation of phenomena, such as the effects of reducing plasma protein concentration, increasing venous pressure, and accumulating protein in the interstitium, not only predicted many clinical features, such as degree of edema formation, but served a heuristic function. The simulation brought attention to specific areas where our understanding of governing factors is lacking. Among these governing factors is the role of the interstitium in transcapillary fluid exchange.

V. Interstitium

Structure and properties of the interstitium are not the only factors which influence transcapillary exchange, but properties of the components are important determinants of transcapillary pressures. In the two-phase concept shown diagrammatically in Fig. 3, the interstitium consists of islands of gelatinous material surrounded by a sea of free fluid. The gelatinous material is composed of entangled mucopolysaccharides forming a meshwork through which small particles can move relatively freely but which exclude the larger protein molecules (Laurent, 1970). Restricting the volume of interstitium available to proteins influences both the pathways through which proteins move and the effective concentration of protein in the interstitium. Oncotic pressure is a function of macromolecular concentration. The two-phase model implies that there is an interstitial oncotic pressure which is different from the pressure predicted were the interstitium entirely gel or fluid. The concentration of protein and, therefore, the oncotic pressure in a volume of interstitium containing a given quantity of protein

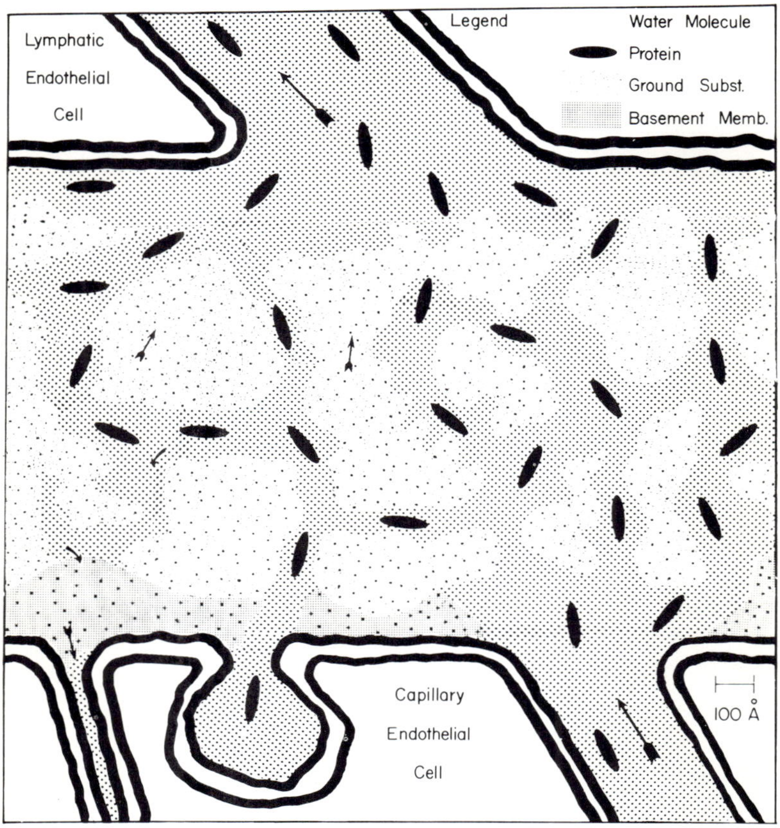

Fig. 3. Schematic representation of the interstitium. A large gap in the endothelium of a lymphatic is shown at the top and a capillary endothelium with a small pore, a pinocytotic vesicle, and a large pore at the bottom. The interstitium is depicted as a two-phase system in which the mucopolysaccharide-rich ground substance, or gel phase, excludes the protein molecules which are therefore restricted to the fluid phase. Water and other small molecules move relatively freely through both phases but with reduced mobility in the gel phase. One result of this model is relative "concentration" of the protein molecules in the interstitium yielding a relatively high interstitial oncotic pressure of about 10 mm Hg (Wiederhielm, 1968).

are effectively increased by the restriction of protein to a fraction of the total volume.

This concept leads to a picture of three basically different methods of edema formation: (1) adding an isotonic salt solution to the interstitium induces an increased volume of both the free fluid and the gel phase; (2)

increasing the amount of protein in the interstitium produces an increase in the free fluid volume due to a shift in fluid from the gel phase to the fluid phase through an oncotic attraction by the protein; (3) similarly, increasing the interstitial concentration of mucopolysaccharides in the interstitium increases the volume of the gel phase at the expense of the free fluid phase. Since the two phases are in equilibrium, their oncotic pressures are equal. This net oncotic pressure of about 10 mm Hg (Wiederhielm, 1968) is the one involved in the Starling-Landis model. The oncotic buffering postulated by Starling, therefore, involves not only the interstitial proteins, but the interaction between those proteins and the gelatinous fraction of the interstitium. These factors were included in the Wiederhielm simulation. The different forms of edema predicted from this model have clinical counterparts in the pitting and nonpitting edemas, e.g., cardiac and nephrotic edema as contrasted with lymphedema and myxedema. In cardiac and nephrotic edema the capillary filtrate is protein poor and the fluid should distribute between the gel phase and the fluid phase with both phases increasing in size. Mobility of fluid moving through the combined phases is relatively low, hence, displacement of fluid under localized pressure yields a residual pit. On the other hand, in lymphedema, protein accumulates in the interstitium increasing the fluid phase volume at the expense of the gel phase due to a shifted oncotic balance. This shift yields the characteristic "rubbery," fluid, nonpitting edema. Fluid is readily displaced by localized pressure in this instance and returns rapidly on release of the pressure due to high fluid mobility in the fluid phase and yields no residual pit. In myxedema the tissue mucopolysaccharide content of the interstitium is supposed to increase. This should increase the volume of the gel phase from which fluid is difficult to displace due to a lower mobility in the dense meshwork, hence, producing the characteristic "brawny," unyielding, nonpitting edema of myxedema.

VI. Summary

Blood flow control is probably distributed among the resistance elements of the microvasculature with neurogenic influence largely exerted on the arterioles and with metabolic and myogenic influences being exerted mostly on the precapillary sphincters. Through their interactions these resistive elements are major determinants of transcapillary fluid exchange variations by means of their influence on capillary hydrostatic pressure. Other factors involved in transcapillary exchange include plasma oncotic pressure and tissue hydrostatic and oncotic pressures. A two-phase structure of the interstitium which restricts protein to a free fluid phase in the interstitium may explain not only the genesis of interstitial oncotic pressure, but may also explain some of the characteristics of different kinds of edema.

References

Chambers R., and Zweifach, B. W. (1946). Functional activity of the blood capillary bed, with special reference to visceral tissue. *Ann. N.Y. Acad. Sci.* **46,** 683–694.

Duling, B. R., and Berne, R. M. (1970). Longitudinal gradients in periarteriolar oxygen tension. A possible mechanism for the participation of oxygen in local regulation of blood flow. *Circ. Res.* **27,** 669–678.

Folkow, B., Sonnenschein, R. R., and Wright, D. L. (1971). Loci of neurogenic and metabolic effects on precapillary vessels of skeletal muscle. *Acta. Physiol. Scand.* **81,** 459–471.

Guyton, A. C. (1963). A concept of negative interstitial pressure based on pressures in implanted perforated capsules. *Circ. Res.* **12,** 399–414.

Guyton, A. C., Granger, H. J., and Taylor, A. E. (1971). Interstitial fluid pressure. *Physiol. Rev.* **51,** 527–563.

Intaglietta, M. (1967). Evidence for a gradient of permeability in frog mesenteric capillaries. *Bibl. Anat.* **9,** 465–468.

Johnson, P. C., and Hanson, K. M. (1962). Effect of arterial pressure on arterial and venous resistance of intestine. *J. Appl. Physiol.* **17,** 503–508.

Jonsson, O. (1970). Extracellular osmolality and vascular smooth muscle activity. *Acta. Physiol. Scand.* (Supp.) **359**: 5–48.

Karnovsky, M. J. (1968). The ultrastructural basis of transcapillary exchanges. *J. Gen. Physiol.* **52,** 64–95.

Landis, E. M. (1926). The capillary pressure in frog mesentery as determined by microinjection methods. *Amer. J. Physiol.* **75,** 548–570.

Landis, E. M., and Pappenheimer, J. R. (1963). Exchange of substances through the capillary walls. *In* "Handbook of Physiology" (Amer. Physiol. Soc., J. Field, ed.), Sect. 2, Vol. II, pp. 961–1034. Williams & Wilkins, Baltimore, Maryland.

Laurent, T. C. (1970). The structure and function of the intercellular polysaccharides in connective tissue. *In* "Capillary Permeability" (C. Crone and N. Lassen, eds.), pp. 261–277. Academic Press, New York.

McMaster, P. D. (1946). The pressure and interstitial resistance prevailing in the normal and edematous skin of animals and man. *J. Exp. Med.* **48,** 473–494.

Phelps, P. C., and Luft, J. H. (1969). Electron microscopical study of relaxation and constriction in frog arterioles. *Amer. J. Anat.* **125,** 399–427.

Scholander, P. F., Hargens, A. R., and Miller, S. L. Negative pressure in the interstitial fluid of animals. *Science* **161,** 321–328.

Starling, E. H. (1896). On the absorption of fluids from the connective tissue spaces. *J. Physiol. (London)* **19,** 312–326.

Stromberg, D. D., and Wiederhielm, C. A. (1970). Effects of oncotic gradients and enzymes on negative pressures in implanted capsules. *Amer. J. Physiol.* **219,** 928–932.

Stromberg, D. D., Phelps, P. C., Rushmer, R. F., and Luft, J. H. (1969). An index for quantitative measurement of vasoconstriction in histologic sections of blood vessels. *Vasc. Surg.* **3,** 68–80.

Van Citters, R. L., Wagner, B. M., and Rushmer, R. F. (1962). Architecture of small arteries during vasoconstriction. *Circ. Res.* **10,** 668–675.

Wiederhielm, C. A. (1966). Transcapillary and interstitial transport phenomena in the mesentery. *Fed. Proc., Fed. Amer. Soc. Exp. Biol.* **25,** 1789–1798.

Wiederhielm, C. A. (1967). Microvascular and lymphatic pressures in the bat wing. *Fed. Proc., Fed. Amer. Soc. Exp. Biol.* **26,** 495 (abstr.).

Wiederhielm, C. A. (1968). Dynamics of transcapillary fluid exchange. *J. Gen. Physiol.* **52,** 29–63.

Wiederhielm, C. A. (1969). The interstitial space and lymphatic pressures in the bat wing. *In* "The Pulmonary Circulation and Interstitial Space" (A. P. Fishman and H. H. Hecht, eds.), pp. 29–41. Univ. of Chicago Press, Chicago, Illinois.

Wiederhielm, C. A., and B. V. Weston (1973). Microvascular, lymphatic and tissue pressures in the unanesthetized mammal. *Am. J. Physiol.* In press.

4 THE MICROCIRCULATION IN DIABETES MELLITUS

ROE WELLS, M.D.

I. Introduction

There is no disease that so uniformly affects the microvasculature as that of diabetes mellitus. One of the more common terminal events of diabetes is renal failure which is the result of a diffuse microvascular lesion of the glomerulus. While an association between vascular disease and diabetes was recorded in the mid-nineteenth century, it was not until after the advent of insulin and the control of coma and ketosis that a clear picture of an accelerated and diffuse vascular and microvascular disease emerged as an integral part of the diabetic process. It is of interest that roughly 10 years after the generalized use of insulin for the management of diabetes and before the reports of a much greater incidence of large vessel disease in diabetes began to appear, the classic paper of Kimmelstiel and Wilson (1936) described the changes in that microvascular entity, the glomerulus. Five years later Dry and Hines (1941) reported on the striking differences in the degree of occlusive vascular disease between diabetics and non-diabetics. Following World War II, the literature blossomed with reports of this accelerated form of arterio- and atherosclerosis in most of the major arteries and especially those of the extremities. The question immediately arose as to whether this was a different phenomenon from the athero-sclerosis of aging. The variables examined most carefully were cholesterol and the lipoproteins. Various investigators did find differences in the lipid composition between diabetic and nondiabetic atheromata (Engelberg *et al.*, 1952) as well as elevated glycoproteins in some patients with diabetes. These chemical differences notwithstanding, it was shown there were no significant differences between the morphologic or cellular details of the atherosclerosis of the diabetic and that found in the nondiabetic—albeit often at a later age (Allen *et al.*, 1959).

II. Basement Membrane Alterations

The idea that the renal lesion might be a distinct microvascular process was introduced in 1941 by Allen. His histologic studies led him to speculate that glomerular nodules were derived from a process involving the basement membrane. He has used what was to become the "magic words," the "basement membrane." The *sine qua non* of the microvascular defect or lesion of diabetes mellitus is a thickened basement membrane. This membrane is actually a homogenous substance located just beneath the endothelium of all vessels (Fig. 1). This material or "membrane" takes up the red dye of the periodic acid-Schiff (PAS) stain, which is an affinity characteristic of glycoproteins. The introduction of the electron microscope revealed that this homogenous layer had a specialized fine structure with reticular fibers or filaments throughout, and that a similar material or membrane lay just beneath the surface of many nonvascular tissues, e.g., the Schwann cell or the sarcolemma of muscle cells. The electron microscope provided more questions than answers, and the primary one remains to the present, namely: What is the cause and/or effect of a thickened basement membrane? All students of the subject can report that diabetes is a disease involving membranes and that in some way insulin plays a role in their function or operates at this location. For the present, or until the biochemist or immunologist can answer this primary question, the basic approach remains the same: diagnose diabetes as early as possible and treat it with optimum control of the blood sugar not only for the welfare of the patient, but also for the containment of the microvascular process as well as the accelerated atherosclerotic phenomenon. It must be noted, however, that while many microvascular lesions have been seen to regress under optimum therapy, there has been no firm evidence that the progressive course of atherosclerosis is altered by therapy. This is as much a reflection on our ability to judge vascular disease *in vivo* as it is on the progression of atherosclerosis. Generally, the well-managed patient develops less severe vascular disease at all levels than the poorly managed

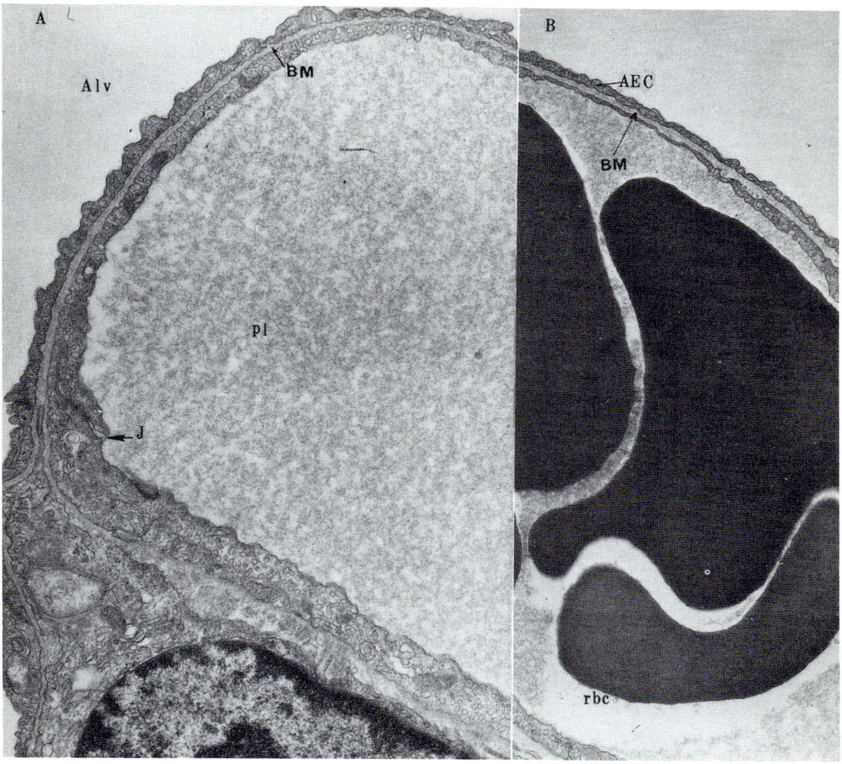

Fig. 1. Two electron micrographs of normal capillary in an alveolus (Alv). Basement membrane (BM) lies between alveolar endothelial cell (AEC) and capillary endothelium. Part A shows plasma (pl) filled vessel, an endothelial junction (J); B a vessel with red cells (rbc). (Photo courtesy of James W. Wilson, M.D.)

or untreated patient. Nevertheless, virtually every capillary in the patient with long-standing diabetes, and especially that originating in the young or juvenile diabetic, will show some degree of basement membrane thickening. The basement membranes of the larger vessels as well as those in nonvascular tissues, e.g., the ciliary process of the eye, Bowman's capsule, or the sarcolemma of the muscle fiber, also show distinct thickening with long-standing disease.

The clinical generality that optimum therapy leads to less vascular disease notwithstanding, there are a number of features of the microvascular aspects of the disease which bear directly upon the clinician's approach to the patient. These relate principally to the kidney and the eye.

III. Diabetic Nephropathy

As noted above, the glomerulus of the kidney appears to be the most heavily involved vascular target in the angiopathy of diabetes. The glomerulus may be involved to different degrees and in different ways in the disease process, but, again, the common denominator is the altered basement membrane. To begin with, the basement membrane of the glomerulus is 10 to 20 times thicker than that of all other systemic capillaries, 2000 to 4000 Å, as compared to 200 Å. The tremendous literature on the subject of basement membrane changes of the glomerulus in diabetes reflects the struggles of many workers who have attempted to answer the question of whether the microvascular changes preceded or followed changes in the metabolic aberrations of the disease. In the more easily analyzed patient material, the juvenile diabetic, the bulk of evidence indicates the basement membrane changes or microangiopathy *follow* the metabolic changes. It is in the long-standing, "mild" diabetic or mature onset diabetic, often with the complication of obesity, that the abnormally thickened basement membrane has been observed at the time of development of abnormal glucose metabolism (Siperstein *et al.,* 1968; Osterby-Hansen and Lundbaek, 1971). Here the pivotal point is what was the thickness of the membrane in the controls. Different groups have presented overlapping ranges of values for the thickness of the basement membranes of their controls, and it is this problem of the degree of thickness of "normals" that underlies the dilemma of how thick is abnormal. In the older age groups, it is very difficult to be certain as to when the diabetic process really started. This question is best dealt with in the reference by Osterby-Hansen and Lundbaek (1971), which is recommended reading for those interested in a comprehensive and contemporary review of the basement membrane changes in diabetes mellitus.

Virtually all of the microvascular changes in the glomerulus of the diabetic are included in the term diabetic glomerulosclerosis. As with all abnormal biologic processes, there are great variations on one theme. There are two relatively well-defined forms of glomerulosclerosis, the nodular form and the diffuse form. The original glomerular microangiopathy described by Kimmelstiel and Wilson concerned a relatively "advanced" stage of a nodular lesion with hyaline masses involving the mesangium and its connective tissue. "Advanced" became advanced because of subsequent electron microscopic studies and the reports of hundreds of subsequent case studies and biopsies. In 1936 such a judgment could not as easily be made with a light microscope. The mesangium or the material that fills the spaces between the convoluted capillaries of a glomerulus is normally made up of almost 50% of a basementlike material, and occupies from 20 to

40% of the total volume or area of the glomerular tuft. It is well documented that in long-established diabetes, the mesangium enlarges or proliferates to occupy more than half of the glomerular unit (Lannigan *et al.*, 1964). Kimmelstiel and his associates through the years have maintained their original position that the nodular lesion begins as a disorder of the mesangium (Kimmelstiel, 1966). The sacredness of Kimmelstiel's position in this field has led to very carefully defended positions that the thickening of the basement membrane of capillaries precedes the changes of the mesangium. In general, however, most agree that it is the change in the basement membrane or basement membranelike material that precedes the appearance of the nodule, its fibrosis, and hyalinization. The problem is not unlike that of the Hamman–Rich syndrome originally described as a diffuse, acute interstitial pneumonitis and fibrosis in 4 patients who rapidly succumbed to their disease. Over the past 25 years, a very wide variety of diffuse forms of fibrosis with alveolocapillary blockage have been referred to as Hamman–Rich syndromes. Many patients with this syndrome survived for many years. The 8 patients of Kimmelstiel and Wilson's original report also followed short courses relative to the modern diabetic in whom renal biopsies indicate that nodular lesions may exist in early disease and may be associated with the diffuse form of glomerulosclerosis (Hatch *et al.,* 1961). Electron microscropy is now the tool most often used in the research of this subject, and it is apparent that maintaining the perspective of the whole nodule is difficult when examining such a small portion of one part of it. The photomontage techniques of Osterby-Hansen (1965) would appear to offer the best method of maintaining a realistic perspective of all the changes.

The diffuse form of glomerulosclerosis is simply a generalized and diffuse thickening of the basement membranes of the capillary vessels often to various degrees in any given segment but with virtually no area free of some degree of basement membrane change. The diffuse changes may resemble the diffuse membranous type of glomerulonephritis seen in the collagen vascular diseases or in its late stages the deposits seen in amyloidosis. From the morphologic standpoint, the question arises as to whether there is a relationship between the nodular form and the diffuse form. Since biology rarely involves only black or white, there are reports recording only the nodular form, only the diffuse form, or mixtures of both. Many have referred to a mixture of the two as a third type of glomerulosclerosis, and appropriately so. The report of Thomsen (1965) is valuable in this respect, where in a study of 581 glomeruli in 32 patients with long-standing diabetes, he found 27% were normal glomeruli, 37% showed diffuse changes, 28% were hyalinized, and 8% showed nodular lesions. Dachs and associates (1964) also observed nodular and diffuse lesions in all the diabetic glomeruli they studied. One may assume the hyalinized lesions were derived from either the diffuse or nodular forms. This late stage process of scarring and hyalinization leads to the terminal event of uremia whether the original lesion was nodular, diffuse, or a mixture of both.

There is one other type of glomerular lesion seen in diabetic nephropathy and, like the membranous form, is not specific for diabetes mellitus. This lesion titled "exudative" is also nodular in form and takes up PAS very strongly, but also gives positive reactions to the Sudan dyes as well as those for fibrin. These precipitated materials are seen within the glomerular capillaries, within the walls of the arterioles, and between Bowman's capsule and the glomerular tuft (Hall, 1952). The identical lesion is also seen in patients with adrenal cortical hyperplasia or in patients receiving large doses of ACTH (Bloodworth and Hamwi, 1956). This exudative lesion is seen principally in the late stage of diabetes. The clinical effects are the same as the other forms of glomerular pathology, namely, leakage of protein and poor renal clearance.

There would appear to be a contradiction of sorts with respect to a membrane that thickens while the functional defect is increased leakage of protein. The explanation may be that the abnormality of this subendothelial substance leads to greater porosity even though it is thicker (Trap-Jensen and Lassen, 1968). Consider also that the capillary with the greatest filtration volume of any in the body has a basement membrane that is 10 to 20 times thicker than that of any other capillary. Does the glomerulus filter 10 to 20 times the fluid of a nonrenal capillary? If the purpose or function of the basement membrane is eventually defined, this information should be one of the important pieces of the puzzle.

There is a limit on available space in the glomerulus so that basement membrane thickening will also lead to loss of the capillary lumen. It has been well established that the human red cell must deform to pass through the capillary as the resting, undeformed erythrocyte is 7 to 8 μm in diameter while the internal diameter of the average capillary is 5 to 6 μm. The normal erythrocyte can pass through pores as small as 3 μm, but the passage time is greatly increased. The other hemodynamic fact relative to glomerular perfusion is that volume flow changes as the fourth power of the radius. This is to say that a one-seventh or 15% reduction in radius will reduce flow in half. Therefore, capillary perfusion and clearance will suffer greatly if basement membrane thickening leads to slight reductions in the size of the capillary lumen. In addition, endothelial hyperplasia has been described for a number of tissues in the diabetic process (Moritz and Oldt, 1937). It is apparent, therefore, that many factors operate to restrict capillary flow in the diabetic.

The changes in the glomerular microcirculation do not end abruptly at the afferent and efferent arterioles. They, too, are involved in the same manner with respect to the basement membrane. Arteriolar nephrosclerosis is a common complication of diabetes, and the progression from basement membrane thickening to scarring and hyalinization is seen in these vessels as well as in the tubules and Bowman's capsules. These changes, as well as the poorly managed diabetic's increased frequency of urinary tract infection and subsequent pyelonephritis, all may lead to total renal failure.

In light of the multitude of these microvascular renal lesions, the question arises for the clinician as to when is a renal biopsy indicated. It can be argued that the modern renal function tests can reasonably well discriminate between glomerular dysfunction and tubular insufficiency, and pragmatists can say once diabetes mellitus is established optimum therapy must be instituted no matter which lesion dominates. This is true, but there will remain a small number of patients whose clinical course and complications, or unprecedented lack of complications, will lead them to the major diabetic speciality centers for tissue studies involving immunologic as well as metabolic testing. Renal biopsy is an important part of this analysis. From this writer's viewpoint, the immunologic aspects of the disease will be the area of study with the greatest rewards. Reactions at membrane surfaces, glycoprotein and mucopolysaccharide biochemistry, other hormone actions, interactions between insulin and basement membranes, and autoimmunity to insulin and insulin products will likely be the "stuff" of the new chapters in this unfolding story (Deckert, 1967). See also the chapter by Falchuk regarding immunologic reactions of the microvasculature.

IV. Diabetic Retinopathy

The other major structure that represents much of the clinical problem is the eye because it, too, depends upon a microcirculation for its primary function. And like the renal glomerulus with its filtration depending upon a specialized microcirculation, the retina is highly vulnerable to very slight changes in the perfusion of its microvasculature. The retinal capillaries, as well as arterioles and venules, all show thickening of the basement membrane in diabetes (Bloodworth, 1964). But the unusual and visible part of the angiopathy of the eye is the capillary microaneurysm of the retina. Electron micrography of these aneurysms has revealed that while there is a saccular or aneurysmal conformation the wall is thicker than the normal capillary; this thickening is due primarily to an increased amount of basement membrane. Another and later form of the microaneurysms, sometimes classified as the hyaline type, appears to be a progression of the sacular type in which red cells, platelets, and fibrin have apparently been incorporated in or about the wall. These elements of a thrombotic process obviously argue for a leakage of blood at the site of the aneurysm. Coïncident with this is the presence of more PAS staining material, often in a laminated form, in addition to the fibrin and old red cells. Besides thrombosis, an inflammatory reaction is also part of the reaction, as exudates can be found adjacent to the aneurysms and localized edema may be seen on slit lamp microscopy. As noted above, basement membrane thickening is associated with increased filterability. Fluorscein infusion during cinephotography of the retinal fundus shows overt leakage of the dye which remains extravascular long after the dye has cleared the veins (Norton and Gutman, 1965). Stereoscopic fundus photography is another method of visualizing the process and is no less difficult to accomplish than the other two procedures (Donaldson, 1965). Obviously this type of retinal injury, when it occurs near the macula, leads to loss of some part of the visual field, albeit in a very patchy way. It is not until the very late stage of retinopathy, which is one of diffuse neovascularization with hemorrhage, retinal separation, and progressive glaucoma, that blindness is clinically overt (Forster, 1956). The new vessel formation often involves the vitreous so that adhesions and scarring between retina and vitreous become apparent. This contraction of the vitreous plus contraction of the retinal surface, combined with the fragility of new capillaries, lead to retinal hemorrhages. It has not been resolved as to why this process is so patchy when the entire capillary network undergoes basement membrane thickening. Some have proposed that the aneurysm formation is an early manifestation of neovascularization or a budding process (Ashton, 1963). The findings of Folkman (1971) on neovascularization in tumor development should be examined with respect to these changes in diabetes.

The cause of the microvascular changes in retinopathy remains unknown. Cogan *et al.* (1961) have suggested that as a result of loss of the mural cell, also called a pericyte, that the capillary wall is weakened and the aneurysm follows. They also speculated that the dilated microvessels seen in association with the aneurysm are shunts between arterioles and venules and that capillary nutrition is thereby compromised. One of the most provocative clinical aspects of this problem concerns the reports of reversal of the microaneurysms and venular dilation after institution of optimal therapy (Keen and Smith, 1959; Dollery and Oakley, 1965).

The conjunctival vessels have also been examined with care, and many have related the degree of abnormality in morphology and flow to the severity or duration of the disease (Ditzel and Sagild, 1954). These microphotographic studies of the conjunctiva have shown, as in the retina, venular dilations, microaneurysms, and arteriolar convolutions (Rees *et al.*, 1964). Heisig (1962) found these changes to better correlate with the degree of arteriosclerosis rather than the state of the diabetes.

With respect to therapy, it must be remembered that diabetic retinopathy is the second most common cause of blindness. Short of the point of visible and progressive neovascularization, optimum control of the disease may still abort the progression of vascular lesions. Once proliferative vascular retinopathy is established, pituitary ablation can be considered. This form of therapy is obviously balanced against the odds of total loss of vision. Proton beam irradiation, which obviates the need for surgery, is often used in preference to the various surgical techniques (Goldberg and Fine, 1968). The most recent successes have been had with the Ruby-Argon Laser for photocoagulation of the retinal lesions (Beetham *et al.*, 1970). If the retinal lesion is beyond repair, i.e., generalized separation and widespread vitreous contraction, the pituitary ablation will likely not reverse the situation (Bradley *et al.*, 1965). Many of the earlier lesions, including neovascularization, may be well managed with photocoagulation, but it cannot be easily applied to those lesions at or very near the macula. As with the reference to optimum therapy and resolution of microaneurysms, pituitary ablation has been seen to reverse the course of neovascularization to the point of its disappearance (Balodimos *et al.*, 1968). Cataract formation and glaucoma, while not directly microvascular phenomena, are important complications of the diabetic process. The microcirculation of the iris and the meshwork at the anterior angle at Schlemm's canal are also often involved in a new vessel formation.

V. Diabetic Neuropathy

The emphasis on the renal and ocular complications of diabetes should not take away from the fact that some patients may be severely disabled by other system failures without significant or clinical involvement of the kidneys or the eyes. It is well established that large vessel disease, especially in the extremities in the form of premature atherosclerosis, is a common and early complication of the disease (Dry and Hines, 1941; LeCompte, 1958). Neurologic disturbances also may be the first clinical manifestation of the disease. Possibly the most common of these is the peripheral neuritis with its paresthesias, numbness, and pain, primarily in the feet and legs. Deep tendon reflexes are depressed or absent and vibratory sense is also reduced or absent. In these patients the physician might first consider a primary neurologic disturbance or a vitamin deficiency syndrome. It is also logical to consider primary vascular insufficiency because large vessel disease and impaired perfusion of the extremity may be the original evidences of the disease. The other and varied manifestations of involvement of the nervous system include neurotrophic ulcers of the skin, usually on the foot, Charcot-type joint changes in ankles and wrists, cordlike bladder, impotence, gastrointestinal dysfunction, diarrhea, incontinence, absorption deficiency syndromes, paralysis of extraocular muscles, autonomic nerve dysfunction with vasomotor instability, anhidrosis, postural syncope, and edma (Ellenberg, 1964; Pirart, 1965). The primary question to all this is whether these neuropathic phenomena arise as a result of a direct metabolic influence upon nerve function. The original reports of Fagerberg (1959) showed a good correlation between small vessel changes within the nerve and the degree of diabetic neuropathy. Subsequent studies have supported this relationship. Other studies of nervous tissues in diabetics have been interpreted as histological changes not associated with vascular insufficiency (Gregerson, 1968), but these have not been documented with electron microscopy of the intraneural vessels. Metabolic abnormalities have been shown to exist in the Schwann cell in the nerves of diabetic animals (Gabbay and O'Sullivan, 1968). Some have argued that a metabolic etiology is supported by the observation that the neurologic changes are patchy and sometimes reversible with ideal therapy. These are imperfect arguments since microvascular lesions have been reversed and microangiopathic lesions also may be patchy. It is not the desire of this writer to argue for a unitarian basis for all the changes in diabetes, but in the case of the neurologic processes many more sophisticated histologic studies must be done before a strong case can be made that the neuropathy is not causally related to the microangiopathy.

VI. Microangiopathy of Other Organ Systems

Microvascular changes of diabetes have also been well reported for muscle, skin (including gingiva), fat, GI tract, liver, pancreas, endometrium, placenta, and, as noted, all vascular tissues from heart to aorta to capillary including the vasa vasorum. The best literature review of this entire subject is that of Starry (1966). Relative to the changes in skin and muscle, it is unfortunate that the greatest variation in microvascular changes resides in these tissues for they are the most convenient and accessible for routine and continuing study. There would appear to be as many reports showing uniform changes of basement membrane thickening as those where significant differences from the normal could not be demonstrated. The majority of reports, however, do show that a single needle-punch biopsy may reveal relatively few abnormal vessels while immediately adjacent there may be a large number of abnormal vessels. The focal or localized nature of the changes in the skin cannot be overemphasized. The pros and cons of this aspect of the problem and the limitation of analysis by electron microscopy are nicely reviewed by Osterby-Hansen and Lundbaek (1971).

It is apparent from this brief survey of the microvascular aspects of diabetes mellitus that we are but near the end of the second of four phases in the conquest of this disease. The first concerned the definition and development of therapeutic insulin, the second the elucidation of the fundamental microvascular lesion, the third the relationship of insulin and carbohydrate metabolism to the vascular changes, and the fourth the application of the information of phase three to the prevention and control of the disease. The purpose of this chapter is simply to bring to the clinician's attention the history and recent developments with respect to phase two since he is the one who must apply this information to the clinical management of his patients.

References

Allen, A. C. (1941). So-called intercapillary glomerulosclerosis—A lesion associated with diabetes mellitus. *Arch. Pathol.* **32,** 33.

Allen, E. V., Barker, N. W., and Hines, E. A., Jr. (1959). "Peripheral Vascular Disease." Saunders, Philadelphia, Pennsylvania.

Ashton, N. (1963). Studies of the retinal capillaries in relation to diabetic and other retinopathies. *Brit. J. Ophthalmol.* **47,** 521.

Balodimos, M. C., Rees, S. B., Aiello, L. M., Bradley, R. F., and Marble, A. (1968). Fluorscein photography in proliferative diabetic retinopathy treated by pituitary ablation. *In* "Treatment of Diabetic Retinopathy," pp. 153–169. U.S. Public Health Service, Arlington, Virginia.

Beetham, W. P., Aiello, L. M., Balodimos, M. C., and Koncz, L. (1970). Ruby laser photocoagulation of early diabetic neovascular retinopathy. *Arch. Ophthalmol.* **83,** 261–272.

Bloodworth, J. M. B., Jr., and Hamwi, G. J. (1956). Experimental diabetic glomerulosclerosis. *Diabetes,* **5,** 37.

Bloodworth, J. M. B., Jr. (1964). Histochemistry and electron microscopy of diabetic retinopathy. *In* "Diabetes Mellitus" (M. D. Siperstein, A. R. Colwell, Sr., and K. Meyer, eds.), pp. 81–88. Amer. Inst. Biol. Sci., Washington, D.C.

Bradley, R. F., Rees, S. B., and Fager, C. A. (1965). Pituitary ablation in the treatment of diabetic retinopathy. *Med. Clin. N. Amer.* **49,** 1105.

Cogan, D. G., Toussaint, D., and Kuwabara, T. (1961). Retinal vascular patterns. IV. Diabetic retinopathy. *Arch. Ophthalmol.* **66,** 366.

Dachs, S., Churg, J., Mautner, W., and Grisham, E. (1964). Diabetic nephropathy. *Amer. J. Pathol.* **44,** 155.

Deckert, T. (1967). Autoimmunologic aspects of diabetes mellitus. *Acta Med. Scand.* **176,** 29 (Suppl. 476).

Ditzel, J., and Sagild, U. (1954). Morphologic and hemodynamic changes in the smaller blood vessels in diabetes mellitus. *N. Engl. J. Med.* **250,** 587.

Dollery, C. T., and Oakley, N. W. (1965). Reversal of retinal vascular changes in diabetes. *Diabetes* **14,** 121.

Donaldson, D. (1965). A new camera for stereoscopic fundus photography. *Arch. Ophthalmol.* **73,** 253.

Dry, T. J., and Hines, E. A., Jr. (1941). The role of diabetes in the development of degenerative vascular disease: With special reference to the incidence of retinitis and peripheral neuritis. *Ann. Intern. Med.* **14,** 1893.

Ellenberg, M. (1964). Diabetic neuropathy. *In* "Diabetes Mellitus: Diagnosis and Treatment" (T. S. Danowski, ed.), pp. 171–193. Amer. Diabetes Ass., New York.

Engelberg, H., Gofman, J. W., and Jones, H. (1952). Serum lipids and lipoproteins in diabetic glomerulosclerosis. *Metabolism* **1,** 300.

Fagerberg, S. E. (1959). Diabetic neuropathy. A clinical and histological study on the significance of vascular affections. *Acta. Med. Scand.* **164** (Suppl. 345).

Folkman, J. (1971). Tumor angiogenesis: Therapeutic implications. *N. Engl. J. Med.* **285,** 1182.

Forster, H. W., Jr. (1956). Ocular diabetes. *Med. Clin. N. Amer.* **40,** 1641.

Gabbay, K., and O'Sullivan, J. B. (1968). The sorbitol pathway. *Diabetes* **17,** 239.

Goldberg, M. F., and Fine, S. L. (1968). "Treatment of Diabetic Retinopathy." U.S. Public Health Service, Arlington, Virginia.

Gregerson, G. (1968). A study of the peripheral nerves in diabetic subjects during ischemia. *J. Neurol., Neurosurg. Psychiat.* [N.S.] **31,** 175.

Hall, G. F. M. (1952). The significance of atheroma of the renal arteries in Kimmelstiel-Wilson's Syndrome. *J. Pathol. Bacteriol.* **64,** 103.

Hatch, F. E., Watt, M. F., Kramer, N. C., Parrish, A. E., and Howe, J. S. (1961). Diabetic glomerulosclerosis: A long term follow up study based on renal biopsies. *Amer. J. Med.* **31,** 216.

Heisig, N. (1962). Contribution to the morphology of the terminal vascular system in man. Studies in normal persons, arteriosclerotics and diabetics. *Deut. Arch. Klin. Med.* **208,** 421.

Keen, H., and Smith, R. (1959). Vitamin B_{12} and the cause of diabetic retinopathy. *Lancet* **1,** 849.

Kimmelstiel, P. (1966). Basement membrane in diabetic glomerulosclerosis. *Diabetes* **15,** 61.

Kimmelstiel, P., and Wilson, C. (1936). Intercapillary lesions in the glomeruli of the kidney. *Amer. J. Pathol.* **12,** 83.

Lannigan, R., Blainey, J. D., and Brewer, D. B. (1964). Electron microscopy of the diffuse glomerular lesions in diabetes mellitus with special reference to early changes. *J. Pathol. Bacteriol.* **88,** 255.

LeCompte, P. M. (1958). The "Kimmelstiel-Wilson" lesion. *Diabetes* **7,** 495.

Moritz, A. R., and Oldt, M. R. (1937). Arteriolar sclerosis in hypertensive and non-hypertensive individuals. *Amer. J. Pathol.* **13,** 679.

Norton, E. W. D., and Gutman, F. (1965). Diabetic retinopathy studied by fluorscein angiography. *Ophthalmologica* **150,** 5.

Osterby-Hansen, R. (1965). A quantitative estimate of the peripheral glomerular basement membrane in recent juvenile diabetes. *Diabetologia* **1,** 97.

Osterby-Hansen, R., and Lundbaek, K. (1971). The basement membrane morphology in diabetes mellitus. *In* "Diabetes Mellitus: Theory and Practice" (M. Ellenberg and H. Rifkin, eds.), pp. 178–209. McGraw-Hill, New York.

Pirart, J. (1965). Diabetic neuropathy: A metabolic or a vascular disease? *Diabetes* **14,** 1.

Rees, S. B., Camerini-Davalos, R. A., Caulfield, J. B., Lozano–Castenada, O., Cervantes-Amezcus, A., Taton, J., Pometta, D., Kranthammer, J. P., and Marble, A. (1964). Pathophysiology of microangiopathy in diabetes mellitus. *In* "Aetiology of Diabetes Mellitus and Its Complications" (M. P. Cameron and M. O'Connor, eds.), pp. 315–329. Little, Brown, Boston, Massachusetts.

Siperstein, M. D., Unger, R. H., and Madison, L. L. (1968). Studies of muscle capillary basement membranes in normal subjects, diabetic and prediabetic patients. *J. Clin. Invest.* **47,** 1973–1999.

Stary, H. C. (1966). Disease of small blood vessels in diabetes mellitus. *Amer. J. Med. Sci.* **252,** 357.

Thomsen, A. C. (1965). "The kidney in Diabetes Mellitus: A Clinical and Histological Investigation Based on Renal Biopsy Material." Munksgaard, Copenhagen.

Trap-Jensen, J., and Lassen, N. A. (1968). Increased capillary diffusion capacity for small ions in skeletal muscle in long term diabetics. *Scand. J. Clin. Lab. Invest.* **21,** 116.

5 RENAL DISEASE

NORMAN K. HOLLENBERG, M.D., Ph.D.

I. Introduction

The renal microvasculature provides a striking example of the relationship between anatomic organization and functional economy. The kidney is an extremely well-perfused organ; 300 gm of tissue receive over 20% of the cardiac output, resulting in an average flow per gram of approximately 4 ml/min. This level of perfusion, as shown in Fig. 1, is about four times that in such metabolically active organs as the heart, brain, liver, and skeletal muscle during exercise. Thus it clearly exceeds the "grocery function" of a vascular supply in providing oxygen and substrate for oxidative processes. In fact, the kidney is unique in that blood flow is ultimately one of the determinants of oxygen utilization. An increase in renal blood flow frequently results in an increase in oxygen consumption. The major metabolic cost of renal function is the support of active tubular transport processes. These processes are responsible for the reabsorption of sodium and other critical components of the internal milieu from the tubular lumen. An increase in renal blood flow which increases the rate of glomerular filtration results in an increase in total solute reabsorption, and thus, in oxygen consumption (Thurau, 1964).

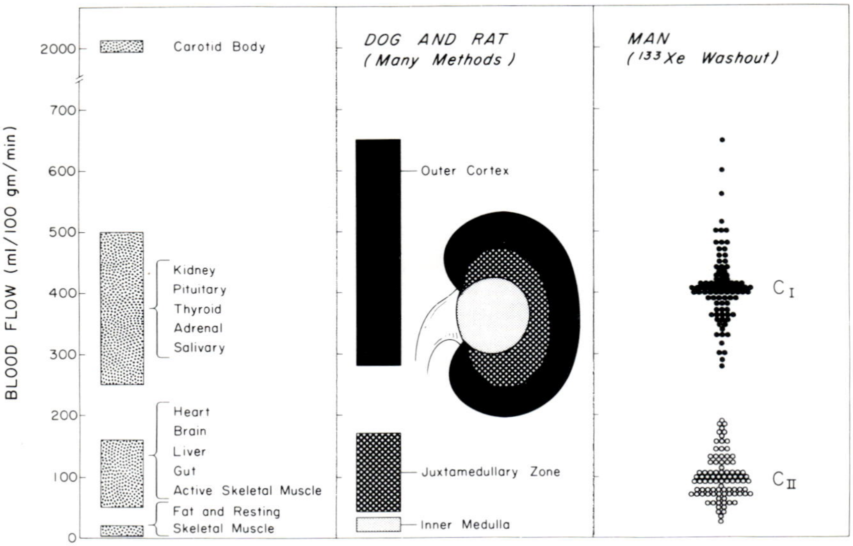

Fig. 1. Blood flow is normalized on the ordinate to 100 gm of tissue so that small and large organs can be compared. On the left, it is apparent that a number of metabolically active organs function well with a blood flow in the neighborhood of 100 ml/100 gm/min. A number of other organs, including the kidney, have flows which exceed this value considerably. In each case the very high flow is related to a specific function of the organ or to the delivery of a specific substrate which is present in blood in only a low concentration. In the center figure, the distribution of flow within the kidney is shown. Note that inner medullary flow is somewhat lower than values for active metabolic organs. On the right, the flow values derived from compartmental analysis of xenon washout in normal potential kidney donors are shown. Note the similarity between the flow rates in C_I, the "cortical component" and values for cortical flow found in animals with many direct methods. The second component corresponds well with juxtamedullary blood flow.

Trueta and collaborators during the 1940's were the first to delineate an apparently independent control of the circulation through the renal cortex and medulla (Trueta *et al.*, 1947). A number of techniques were used to assess the renal circulation in the rabbit, but blood flow was never measured directly. Several types of manipulation induced a clear reduction in cortical perfusion, which they attributed to the diversion of an unchanged total renal blood flow from the cortical to the medullary circulation. Their use of the terms "bypass" and "diversion" leaves little doubt that a shunt mechanism was postulated. A prodigious literature on the subject appeared during the next several years, leaving a consensus of opinion that a true shunt was not present in the kidney (Smith, 1951). Trueta's colleagues continued to work in the area and later clearly dissociated themselves from the shunt concept, while continuing to point out that the maneuvers they utilized resulted in a preferential reduction in cortical perfusion (Daniel *et al.*, 1952). The repeated failure of most investigators to demonstrate a shunt mechanism, however, resulted in a hiatus of interest in the subject for some time.

In the late 1950's as the functional implications of the countercurrent anatomic arrangement of the tubular and vascular elements in the medulla became apparent, it also became apparent that medullary perfusion must differ from that in the renal cortex. The kidney's ability to generate hypertonic urine, a critical function in water conservation, was dependent on the creation of a hypertonic inner medullary milieu. The characteristics of the countercurrent system made it clear that medullary perfusion had to operate at rather lower levels than that of the whole kidney to prevent washout of the osmolal gradiant (Thurau, 1964). Abundant evidence that medullary blood flow is considerably less than that in the renal cortex soon became available (Thorburn *et al.*, 1963; Thurau, 1964). The range is shown in Fig. 1. Blood flow in the renal papilla, in the neighborhood of 30 ml/100 gm/min, was found to be less than that in most metabolically active organs. In addition, oxygen is lipid soluble and tends to "shunt" directly from vessels entering the renal medulla to vessels leaving it. This combination of factors results in a precarious, relatively hypoxic state of even the normal renal papilla. The development of papillary necrosis in a number of clinical settings including the nephropathies of analgesic abuse and of diabetes has been attributed to impairment of an already marginal papillary blood supply (Kincaid-Smith *et al.*, 1968). In sickle cell disease, as described in Chapter 10, the most effective stimulants for the sickling phenomenon include hypoxia and hypertonicity. It is not surprising, therefore, that abnormalities of renal medullary function occur in this setting. These range from inability to elaborate a concentrated urine to local tissue destruction presenting as pernicious hematuria or papillary necrosis (Welt and Lyle, 1963).

The extremely high perfusion level usually associated with the kidney is, in fact, confined to the renal cortex, as shown in Fig. 1 (Barger, 1960; Blaufox *et al.*, 1970; Carriere *et al.*, 1966; Thorburn *et al.*, 1963; Thurau, 1964). This provides not only the large volumes of plasma for glomerular filtration but also the force promoting filtration; glomerular capillary pressure is estimated to be at least 60 mm Hg, clearly the highest capillary pressure in the body. A reduction in renal perfusion, therefore, frequently expresses itself as a reduction in the rate of glomerular filtration. Several lines of evidence, reviewed in detail below, suggest that the life threatening failure of renal function which occurs in a number of clinical settings can be accounted for on the basis of a failure of glomerular filtration due to a critical reduction in cortical perfusion (Carriere *et al.*, 1966; Daniel *et al.*, 1952; Epstein *et al.*, 1970; Hollenberg, 1965; Hollenberg *et al.*, 1968a, b, 1969a, b, 1970a).

During the past decade many methods have been devised for the assessment of regional intrarenal perfusion and the intrarenal distribution of blood flow. Only one of these methods, the inert gas washout technique first applied to the canine kidney by Barger and co-workers (Barger, 1960; Blaufox *et al.*, 1970; Hollenberg *et al.*, 1968a; Thorburn *et al.*, 1963), is sufficiently atraumatic to allow application in man. Because the method demands the intraarterial injection of the isotope, it is necessary in man to carry out the study at the time of selective renal arteriography. Radioactive xenon in saline solution, the most widely used indicator in man, is injected into the renal artery through the selective catheter and its disappearance from the kidney is monitored by external counting techniques. The resultant complex curves can be analyzed in a number of ways. Examples are shown in Fig. 2, and the range defined in normal man in Fig. 1. From the initial disappearance slope it is possible to calculate mean renal blood flow. Also, graphical peeling methods make it possible to analyze the curve as the sum of a series of damped exponential functions. From the zero-time intercepts of each exponential component one can calculate the distribution of isotope and, by inference, the distribution of blood flow within the compartments of the kidney. The slopes of the components allow the calculation of the flow rate per unit tissue mass in each compartment. The results of serial radioautographic studies suggest that in the normal dog kidney the compartments described by this approach represent different anatomical zones, each defined by its characteristic blood flow. The most rapid flow component represents the blood flow to the renal cortex, and the next most rapid, outer medullary blood flow.

It has been possible to define intrarenal hemodynamics in normal man despite the requirement for selective renal arterial catheterization because potential kidney donors in the Peter Bent Brigham Hospital transplant program require selective renal arteriography as part of their assessment. The xenon washout curve in normal man bears a striking resemblance to that in the dog. The most rapid flow component, cortical blood flow in the dog, represents 60 to 90% of the total renal blood flow in man with a flow rate ranging from 300 to 550 ml/100 gm/min. Several lines of evidence support the hypothesis that the rapid flow component also represents cortical perfusion in man. It is absent in the presence of cortical necrosis (Hollenberg *et al.*, 1968a), and shows a close correlation with

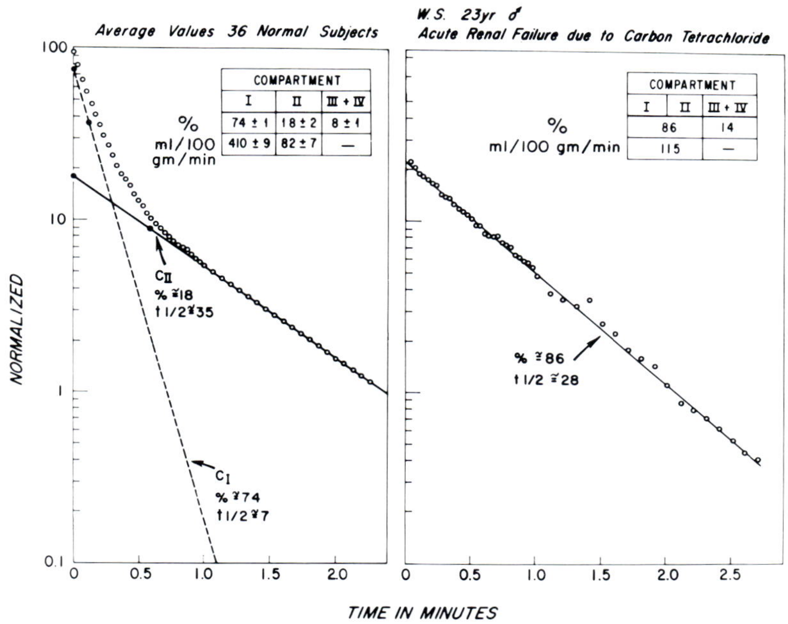

Fig. 2. Average values for the early rapid flow components of xenon disappearance from the kidney in normal subjects (left) compared with xenon disappearance from the kidney in a patient with acute renal failure which followed exposure to carbon-tetrachloride (right). Note that the two early components which characterize the normal kidney have been replaced by a monoexponential with a half time which resembles the second compartment (C_{II}) more than the first (C_{I}). Reprinted with the kind permission of the *New England Journal of Medicine*. Hollenberg *et al.* (1970a).

glomerular filtration rate in the transplanted human kidney (Hollenberg *et al.*, 1968b). When there is angiographic evidence to suggest a major decrease in cortical flow in patients with various diseases (Hollenberg *et al.*, 1969b), or after the induction of transient cortical ischemia with epinephrine (Hollenberg *et al.*, 1968a), the rapid flow component is reduced or absent. Strong supportive evidence for the conclusion that the rapid flow component reflects cortical perfusion has come, recently, from studies carried out with the scintillation camera on xenon transit through the human kidney. This instrument, which makes it possible to visualize the isotope as it moves through the kidney, has made it clear that transit through the human renal cortex is much more rapid than through the rest of the kidney and that isotope has disappeared from the cortex when the rapid flow component becomes small (Blaufox *et al.*, 1970). Much of the following review will be based on results obtained from the application of the xenon washout technique in man because, while imperfect, it has provided new insights which can be obtained in no other way at present.

The microvasculature, as defined in the introduction, is made up of blood vessels which are less than 300 μm in diameter. These vessels, in the absence of a significant stenosis of a major artery, are the critical determinants of flow in a vascular bed. At present, renal angiography cannot visualize vessels this small directly. Despite the physical limitations of available roentgen systems, they have provided useful insights into the renal microvasculatures' contribution to human disease in a number of settings. This contribution of angiography, reviewed below, has been possible because of a number of factors. The interlobar and arcuate arteries, which can be visualized well, tend to mirror more distal events. The cortical nephrogram, which does not depend on visualizing individual vessels, is a function of cortical vascular dynamics. The interlobular arteries in the cortex are theoretically too small to be visualized directly. A penumbra of these vessels is sufficiently well visualized in many normal subjects, however, that failure to demonstrate them routinely in some pathological states, reviewed below, has had pathogenetic implications.

When considering the relationship of renal hemodynamics to renal function in a number of clinical settings it is useful to classify the disease states into two broad categories, functional and organic. In organic vascular disease, gross and histological examination reveals structural vascular alterations adequate to account for the abnormalities of renal perfusion and function. There are a number of other conditions in which the renal vessels are histologically normal but in which more subtle, necessarily indirect evidence suggests that an element of active vasoconstriction and the resultant pattern of intrarenal hemodynamics play a major role in the abnormalities of renal function. The latter syndromes, which are classified as functional for this review, include "prerenal azotemia," "acute tubular necrosis," "the hepatorenal syndrome," and a number of states characterized by sodium retention.

Necessary editorial restrictions on length have made it impossible to provide a detailed review of all the clinically relevant areas in which renal perfusion possibly, probably, or clearly plays a central role. Attention has, therefore, been focused on areas in which recent advances have provided new insights, especially when related to common clinical phenomena. The documentation has been restricted for the same reason, so that in many cases primary references have not been given. In every case, however, the relevant references can be found in the papers that have been cited.

II. Abnormalities of Rental Perfusion with a Functional Pathogenesis

A. Prerenal Azotemia

Depletion of extracellular or plasma volume results in a reversible loss of renal function which is related to the size of the volume deficit. The reduction in glomerular filtration rate in this setting is characteristically corrected rapidly by appropriate replacement of the volume deficit. The volume losses may be due to hemorrhage, burns, diarrhea, vomiting, diaphoresis or to leakage into third space regions of the body, such as gangrenous bowel or traumatized muscle. The central pathogenetic feature appears to be a critical reduction in blood volume, and thus in venous return to the heart and cardiac output. The oliguria is in part due to tubular responses to antidiuretic hormone and aldosterone, the effects of which are potentiated by a major hemodynamic response which results in a decrease in glomerular filtration rate. If severe hypotension occurs, it will clearly contribute to the renal hemodynamic response. Hypotension is not necessary, however, to induce quantitatively important renal vascular responses.

Hemorrhage-induced volume depletion has been the most widely studied model of the prerenal syndrome. While scattered observations suggest that volume depletion induced in this way may not mimic in all details the effects of more gradual volume depletion associated with dehydration, attention will be focused on the effects of hemorrhage because they are best understood and reasonably representative. The dominant feature in the renal vascular response to hemorrhage is a major reduction in renal cortical perfusion, probably mediated in a large part through intense activation of the sympathetic nerve supply to the renal vessels (Barger, 1960; Carriere *et al.*, 1966; Hollenberg *et al.*, 1968a; Thurau, 1964). The effects of moderate hemorrhage are strikingly similar to those induced by direct stimulation of the sympathetic nerves (Pomeranz *et al.*, 1968). At lower levels of stimulation the vasoconstriction appears to be confined largely to the outer cortex, with a reduction in local perfusion rate (Pomeranz *et al.*, 1968). More severe hemorrhage and increasing frequencies of stimulation also result in a reduction in medullary perfusion. The vasa recta lack both an identifiable smooth muscle coat and an autonomic innervation (Gosling and Dixon, 1969; Thurau, 1964) so that the reduction in medullary perfusion is presumably mediated through a reduction in flow through inner cortical glomeruli, the afferent vessels of which are clearly innervated (Gosling and Dixon, 1969). There is continuing debate concerning the possibility of sympathetic innervation of the efferent arterioles. The evidence for a major role of the sympathetic nerves in the pathogenesis of the renal response to a volume deficit comes primarily from assessment of the effects of denervation or alpha-adrenergic blocking agents in experimental animals (Hollenberg, 1965) and the effect of the latter agents in man. Phenoxybenzamine, the most active of the alpha adrenergic blocking agents available for administration in man, frequently results in a dramatic diuresis in patients with prerenal azotemia (Nickerson, 1962).

There has been debate concerning the overall renal vascular response to moderate hemorrhage, some investigators having reported an initial decrease in resistance, while others found an increase. The differences in the reported results are probably related to specific details in the experimental protocols. A decrease in resistance has been reported in association with a relatively rapid hemorrhage at a time when other vascular beds show active and intense vasoconstriction. More gradual hemorrhage routinely results in an increase in resistance, which is mediated by the sympathetic nerves (Hollenberg, 1965). A well-maintained blood flow during the rapid development of hypotension presumably reflects the net effects of an interaction between forces promoting autoregulation and factors which would ordinarily result in an active vasoconstriction. The fact that the rate of hemorrhage is a determinant of the net renal vascular response suggests that especially intense renal vascular responses might be expected when the volume deficit occurs very slowly, as in many forms of dehydration.

The response of the renal vasculature differs from that of other major vascular beds in a number of other ways. At a fixed arterial pressure during hemorrhagic hypotension, the kidney suffers a progressive reduction in blood flow, whereas the response of other vascular beds tends to plateau (Hollenberg, 1965). This trend is extended through the period of cardiovascular recovery associated with reinfusion of the shed blood (Hollenberg, 1965; Kramer, 1962). Most vascular beds respond to the recovery of cardiac output and blood pressure with prompt and dramatic vasodilatation. The renal vasculature, on the other hand, shows a persistent increase in resistance which appears to be related to the degree and duration of the stress (Hollenberg, 1965; Kramer, 1962). If renal blood flow fails to exceed approximately 50% of normal on reinfusion, the animal remains oliguric. Larger increases in renal perfusion, whether spontaneous or induced by denervation or adrenergic blockade, result in a diuresis.

The unique response of the kidney to severe and prolonged stress, an increase in vascular resistance sufficient to sustain oliguria, persisting when other vascular beds have recovered from the effects of hemorrhagic typotension, raises interesting possibilities with regard to the pathogenesis of "acute tubular necrosis." The kidney is especially vulnerable to the effects of a prolonged volume deficit, perhaps related to the special characteristics of its vascular response.

We have had a number of opportunities to assess the renal vascular response to volume depletion in man. The description is necessarily anecdotal because formal protocols designed to induce depletion of extracellular and plasma volume in normal man have not been utilized. On several occasions, however, a constellation of events has resulted in a moderate to large deficit of sodium and water in patients with otherwise healthy kidneys who came to study. In one patient, an especially dedicated potential kidney donor who was resolved to hide her active regional enteritis, the retrospective estimated daily sodium losses in her stools exceeded 200 mEq. She was placed on a sodium restricted diet as part of a research protocol and came to study with a 10% loss of body weight and a deficit of several hundred milliequivalents of sodium. A second potential donor achieved a similar salt and water deficit because of an unusual selective inability of the kidney to retain sodium. Renal function was otherwise normal when he was on his usual, unrestricted diet. A third potential donor developed severe dehydration and sodium depletion because of repeated cathartics and enemas administered inadvertently in preparation for an intravenous pyelogram (IVP) which was deferred on three successive days. She was on a restricted salt diet and was not allowed fluids by mouth for a large part of each day because of the IVP. In each patient the volume deficit was associated with a very large reduction in renal blood flow to levels between one third and one half of normal despite a well-maintained arterial pressure. The flow pattern was similar to that described above for the effects of hemorrhage and sympathetic nerve activity in animal models. The cortical component of flow became very small or unrecognizable. In the third patient, acetylcholine was infused into the renal artery, resulting in a large increase in renal blood flow and normalization of both the intrarenal flow pattern and the selective renal arteriogram. Thus, the information available in man suggests strongly that the renal vascular response to a volume deficit is strikingly similar to that in experimental models.

B. Acute Tubular Necrosis

Fixed acute oliguric renal failure which is unresponsive to volume loading is a frequent and unfortunate complication of prerenal azotemia and occurs as well in response to a number of nephrotoxins and as a consequence of any cause of prolonged renal ischemia. It is one of the most dramatic and puzzling events in medicine—puzzling because of the frequent disproportion between the total loss of function and the associated minimal abnormality of renal structure. In experimental acute renal failure models, generally induced with nephrotoxins, there is frequently evidence of severe tubular necrosis. In patients with acute renal failure, however, such gross distortions of structure are much less common, and even electron microscopic studies may reveal only minimal damage. In one careful study, experienced renal pathologists were unable to identify renal tissue from patients with "acute tubular necrosis" when the sections were coded and presented in random order among sections from patients with normal renal function (Finckh *et al.*, 1962).

The hypotheses which have been elaborated to account for the failure of function can be classified into three broad categories, which appear to cover all of the logical possibilities. The most frequently cited hypothesis suggests that the loss of function is due to the cessation of glomerular filtration, secondary to a renal hemodynamic abnormality (Flanigan and Oken, 1965). The other hypotheses propose either that the failure of filtration is due to the intrarenal obstruction of tubules with debris or by edema or that filtration continues, but the failure of urine output is due to loss of integrity of tubular structures resulting in the back diffusion of filtered fluid into the blood stream. In view of the frequent paucity of histologic abnormalities in the kidneys of patients with acute renal failure, as cited above, the latter two hypotheses seem unlikely. More direct evidence from several animal models has been provided by micropuncture, which revealed a low proximal tubular pressure and a decrease in single nephron glomerular filtration rate (Flanigan and Oken, 1965). These findings are consistent only with the vascular hypotheses.

The first assessment of renal hemodynamics carried out in patients with acute renal failure by Bull and co-workers (1950) suggested the vascular hypothesis: the clearance of PAH—used as a measure of effective renal plasma flow—was reduced to 10% of normal or less. However, it has since become apparent that clearance methods are not reliable in oliguric patients, and independent studies with methods which do not require urine output to measure renal blood flow have shown that renal perfusion is only reduced to between 25 and 50% of normal in such patients (Hollenberg *et al.*, 1968a, 1970a). Many patients with chronic renal failure or congestive heart failure have a similar reduction in total renal blood flow and yet have a normal urine output and a rate of glomerular filtration adequate to maintain life. The direct assessment of renal hemodynamics in patients with acute renal failure was, therefore, not consistent with the vascular hypothesis favored by other lines of evidence.

The application of renal arteriography and the xenon washout method for assessing the intrarenal distribution of blood flow to the study of the renal vasculature in patients with acute renal failure has resolved this apparent dilemma. Patients with acute renal failure, independent of the primary etiology, showed the absence of the rapid flow component of xenon washout from the kidney, an observation indicative of a diffuse and even reduction in cortical perfusion (Hollenberg *et al.*, 1968a, 1970a). An example is shown in Fig. 2. Patients with chronic renal failure, in whom a similar reduction in mean flow was found, had a small rapid component indicative of the presence of regional areas of more normal cortical perfusion. Thus, acute and chronic renal failure differ in the intrarenal distribution of blood flow, and, therefore, in overall renal function. The diffuse and even reduction in cortical perfusion in the patient with acute renal failure is sufficient to account for the failure of function on the basis of a glomerular capillary pressure which is too low to maintain filtration (Hollenberg *et al.*, 1968a). In the patient with chronic renal failure, small areas within the cortex retain a blood supply apparently adequate to maintain capillary pressure and filtration.

A characteristic triad of abnormalities in the selective renal arteriogram of patients with acute renal failure included the absence of a distinct cortical nephrogram and of identifiable arterial vessels beyond the arcuate artery level (i.e., in the cortex), attenuation of the interlobar and arcuate arteries, and a prolongation of transit time of contrast medium through the kidney. These observations, too, suggest a preferential and diffuse reduction of cortical perfusion. The prolongation of the transit time is not consistent with the "shunt" hypothesis elaborated by Trueta and co-workers which was based on the early appearance of contrast in the renal vein. Patients with chronic renal failure had patchy areas of maintained cortical vascular filling in the selective renal arteriogram. This finding supports the hypothesis that small areas in the renal cortex were perfused at a rate sufficient to promote and maintain glomerular filtration, despite the similar large reduction in renal blood flow.

The remarkable similarity of the hemodynamic and angiographic characteristics of acute renal failure which follows a number of classic causes, including shock, hemolysis, the prolonged mechanical reduction in blood flow associated with allograft transplantation, and a host of pharmacologically and chemically unrelated nephrotoxins in man, has suggested that the renal vascular response represents a pathogenetic common pathway (Hollenberg *et al.*, 1970a). The possibility that all of these etiologic factors activate an intrinsic renal vasoconstrictor system and that reversal of the vasoconstriction with appropriate agents will result in the recovery of renal function requires assessment.

C. Acute Renal Allograft Rejection

Allograft rejection provides another acute renal failure state which is described in detail in another chapter. The angiographic and hemodynamic features of the renal vascular response in man are strikingly similar in many respects to those in acute tubular necrosis. The rapid flow component of xenon washout from the kidney is absent in severe acute allograft rejection, and the angiographic features include a delay in transit of contrast medium, marked attenuation of the distal interlobar and arcuate arteries, and a diminution in the cortical nephrogram. An additional feature, tortuosity and irregularity of the interlobar and arcuate arteries, is also frequently seen. The most severe form, hyperacute rejection due to prior sensitization, results in cortical necrosis. Here renal blood flow is even more sharply reduced, to levels frequently less than 15% of normal. The arteriogram reveals filling defects in the larger intrarenal arteries, indicative of thrombus formation, and there is a total disappearance of the nephrogram effect (Hollenberg *et al.*, 1968a). Chronic, delayed allograft rejection results in an approximately parallel reduction in filtration rate, mean renal flow, and the flow rate in the cortical component (Hollenberg *et al.*, 1968b), the significance of which is discussed in Section III, B.

D. The Hepatorenal Syndrome

The "hepatorenal" syndrome is an important, frequently preterminal complication of advanced cirrhosis and hepatic failure (Epstein *et al.*, 1970). Such patients often develop a form of progressive, oliguric renal failure which differs functionally from acute tubular necrosis in several respects. Despite progressive azotemia and oliguria, they frequently retain an astonishing ability to lower their urine sodium concentration and to concentrate the urine. Responses to a volume load tend to be incomplete and evanescent despite the functional similarity to the prerenal syndromes. The abnormalities of the renal vasculature identified in selective renal arteriograms and the characteristics of xenon washout in these patients also differ in several respects from those noted in acute tubular necrosis. In the patient with the hepatorenal syndrome, the interlobar arterial attenuation is more severe, and frequently these vessels show an irregular "beaded" appearance. These abnormalities are not demonstrable on postmortem injection of the renal vasculature with contrast agent, and the vessels are normal on histologic examination. The hemodynamic abnormality in hepatorenal syndrome is striking and unique: blood flow is both very reduced and extremely labile, suggesting the presence of a mediator which is capable of inducing intense, phasic vasoconstriction. Tubular function appears to be much better maintained in this syndrome than in acute tubular necrosis, despite the remarkable reduction in renal perfusion. Mean renal blood flow in hepatorenal syndrome is significantly lower than that in acute tubular necrosis.

E. Sodium Retaining States

The remarkably precise control of sodium excretion exerted by the normal kidney appears to involve a number of extremely well-integrated vascular and tubular processes. Current concepts suggest that the renal microvasculature makes its contribution to this homeostatic process, potentially, through at least three mechanisms. Renal perfusion is a major determinant of overall glomerular filtration rate, which provides the tubular load of sodium for reabsorption. A decrease in the filtered load results in a decrease in sodium excretion, other things being equal. In addition, recent evidence has suggested that perfusion can contribute to renal salt handling in other ways. Nephron heterogeneity, the inner cortical nephrons showing a greater potential for sodium reabsorption than the smaller nephrons in the outer cortex, raises the possibility that the distribution of glomerular filtrate within the kidney is a major determinant of sodium handling (Barger, 1960; Carriere *et al.*, 1966; Pomeranz *et al.*, 1968; Hollenberg *et al.*, 1970b). A redistribution of blood flow and filtration from outer to inner cortical nephrons—such as occurs in the prerenal syndromes described above—would result in an increase in sodium reabsorption. Certainly all of the situations characterized by sodium retention share this renal hemodynamic picture. It also seems likely that physical forces in the peritubular capillaries, through their influence on the rate of removal of solute and water reabsorbed from the proximal tubule, may be the rate-limiting factors in the active transport process in some settings. Thus, if the filtration rate is 120 ml/min, and only 1 ml/min is being excreted, 119 ml/min must be removed from the peritubular space to allow the process to continue. Two factors enhance the reabsorption of this fluid into the peritubular capillaries. Hydrostatic pressure in this network is among the lowest in the body, the blood having passed two arteriolar levels. The intravascular oncotic pressure is increased approximately 20% by the removal of an ultrafiltrate in the glomerulus.

Abnormalities of renal perfusion are well documented in congestive heart failure (Barger, 1960). It seems likely that these abnormalities in perfusion, acting through the mechanisms described above, play an important role in the abnormalities of sodium homeostasis in a number of states characterized by salt retention including heart failure, cirrhosis of the liver, and the nephrotic syndrome. Ethacrynic acid and furosemide, two of the most active natriuretic agents known, also appear to act, at least in part, through their effects on intrarenal hemodynamics (Epstein *et al.*, 1971).

III. Organic Abnormalities of the Renal Microvasculature

A. Benign Nephrosclerosis

Nephrosclerosis is the most common form of nephropathy, identified in 70% of necropsy examinations after the age of 60 years. The resultant loss of renal function in most patients is important clinically only as there is a reduction in renal reserve and in the metabolism of a number of drugs which depend upon glomerular filtration for excretion. The potentiation of this process in the occasional patient with hypertension or diabetes can result in clinically important renal failure.

Nephrosclerosis is responsible for the normal effects of increasing age on the kidney. A progressive reduction in renal mass, renal blood flow, and glomerular filtration rate becomes apparent after the age of 40 years (Shock, 1967). If the reduction in renal mass and blood flow were parallel, the result would be independent of age with this method. We have found in healthy, potential kidney donors that renal blood flow, as assessed by xenon washout, does show a significant reduction with increasing age. A normal renal blood flow of 382 ± 20 ml/100 gm/min in the 20's falls to a level of 310 ± 19 in the 40's and 243 ± 21 in subjects over the age of 60 years. The reduction in blood flow must exceed the reduction in tissue mass. It is thus reasonable to conclude that the reduction in mass reflects tissue atrophy consequent to a critical reduction in renal perfusion. The pathogenesis of the vascular abnormality is not clear. The possibility that a functional component plays a role in the reduction in blood flow is unlikely because the response of the renal vasculature to vasodilators, such as acetylcholine, appears to be blunted by increasing age.

There is little doubt that hypertension potentiates the progress of this vascular process. Examination of the renal vasculature by necropsy and angiography shows an increased prevalence and severity of nephrosclerosis at all ages, the effects being related to both the severity and duration of the hypertension (Hollenberg *et al.*, 1969a). The intrarenal distribution of the process has been of considerable interest. The presence of patchy areas of atrophy suggests a nonuniform distribution of the vascular lesion, an interpretation which derived strong support from the observations of Smith and co-workers (Smith *et al.*, 1943). They carried out an elegant series of studies of renal function assessed by tubular saturation techniques, especially the tubular maximal capacity for glucose reabsorption. The reduction in glomerular filtration was not uniformly distributed in patients with nephrosclerosis. A bimodal distribution of glomerular abnormalities was suggested. Some glomeruli appeared to be essentially normal, while others showed the effects of a considerable reduction in perfusion. More recently, it has been suggested on the basis of local indicator dilution curves of a nondiffusable indicator through the kidney that the reduction in perfusion is uniform (Lowenstein *et al.*, 1967). This interpretation is inconsistent with earlier observations and is of considerable importance because such a reduction would best be attributed to diffuse arteriolar vasoconstriction, an abnormality which could be a primary pathogenetic step in the development of essential hypertension, rather than a consequence. The observations derived from radioxenon washout from the kidney are most consistent with more direct observations cited above. The characteristic abnormality is a reduction in the percentage of flow entering the rapid flow component, with a normal flow rate in that compartment. Such an abnormality would not be expected on the basis of a diffuse reduction in cortical perfusion induced by arteriolar vasoconstriction. Rather, the observation suggests that areas within the renal cortex retain a normal flow rate, while other areas have a sufficiently large perfusion defect that the exponential disappearance of xenon in these regions is indistinguishable from that area of normal lower flow in the medulla of the kidney. The interpretation of such patterns is explored in greater detail in the next section.

Is renal blood flow always abnormal in essential hypertension? The classic experiments of Goldblatt and co-workers raised the possibility that essential hypertension represented the effects of segmental renal ischemia, the equivalent of a large number of small Goldblatt clamps on the intrarenal vessels. However, many patients with essential hypertension have a normal renal blood flow. The coefficient of variation for this measurement is 20% so that the normal range of renal blood flow is from 700 to 1700 ml/min. Thus, a very large reduction could be present without flow falling to below the lower level of normal. Assessment of renal perfusion with PAH clearance, indocyanine transit, and xenon washout have all revealed a significant subpopulation of young essential hypertensives in whom renal blood flow exceeds considerably the upper limit of normal (Hollenberg *et al.*, 1969a). This observation makes the hypothesis of renal ischemia as a central pathogenetic feature of essential hypertension untenable. Our parallel observations that the renal hemodynamic response in this subpopulation is resistant to the effect of sodium restriction, raises the tantilizing possibility of a primary disorder of volume homeostasis. It seems unlikely, however, that essential hypertension represents a single disease process.

Two lines of evidence suggest strongly that there is an abnormality of vasomotor tone involving the renal vasculature in many patients with essential hypertension. It has been reported that the two kidneys in essential hypertensives show a larger difference of renal perfusion than do normal subjects (Baldwin *et al.*, 1960). We have corroborated that observation and extended it to sequential studies on the same kidney. The same degree of variability of renal blood flow exists in sequential studies, a phenomenon incompatible with an organic vascular abnormality, but rather suggestive of an unstable increase in vascular tone. This interpretation has been corroborated by studies in progress which reveal, in essential hypertensives, a much larger flow increase in response to a vasodilator, acetylcholine, infused into the renal artery. Such a potentiation of vasodilatation would be expected on the basis of an increase in resting vascular tone. The angiogram of such patients shows moderate small vessel disease which disappears with acetylcholine. In patients with advanced nephrosclerosis the acetylcholine vasodilator responses are blunted and the angiogram does not show reversal of the arterial abnormality, demonstrating that with advanced hypertension and its complications the vascular abnormality is largely organic and fixed.

B. Advanced Renal Parenchymal Disease

It has long been known from studies with clearance techniques that patients with chronic renal parenchymal disease have a large decrease in renal blood flow, slightly greater than the reduction in glomerular filtration rate, so that the calculated filtration fraction is increased (Bradley *et al.*, 1950). This observation has been made in patients with chronic glomerulonephritis, pyelonephritis, diabetic glomerulosclerosis, polycystic kidney disease, advanced nephrosclerosis (whether due to uncomplicated long-standing hypertension or hypertension in the accelerated phase), and chronic renal allograft rejection. The destruction of renal parenchyma and reduction of blood flow and function in the patient with chronic glomerulonephritis are due to progressive obliteration of the glomerular capillary bed. In the patient with chronic pyelonephritis, these phenomena are due to the development of scar formation and patchy areas of major parenchymal destruction. The patient with diabetic glomerulosclerosis also shows obliteration of the glomerular capillary bed, but, in addition, shows major areas of scar formation related to the virtually universal presence of interstitial nephritis. In polycystic kidney disease, the loss of renal function is presumably on the basis of the gross distortion of renal architecture with elongation, stretching, and tortuosity of the intrarenal vessels. Nephrosclerosis results in renal parenchymal destruction and reduction in the blood flow due to a variable degree of stenosis of smaller intrarenal arteries; the latter phenomenon is frequently also present in the other syndromes presumably due to the long-standing hypertension in most of the patients described above. Chronic allograft rejection reflects elements of all of these processes. The obvious heterogeneity of the pathological processes makes the observation of a similar relationship among the reduction in blood flow, filtration rate, and the characteristics of xenon washout especially astonishing. The pattern of xenon washout, alluded to both in the section on acute renal failure and on nephrosclerosis, is characterized by a reduction in the percentage of flow in the rapid flow component which is in approximate proportion to the decrease in renal function (Hollenberg *et al.*, 1968a, b, 1969a, b). There is a reciprocal increase in the percentage of flow in the second component. The reduction in the volume of the rapid flow component, interpreted in the light of the parallel selective arteriogram and histologic examination of the renal cortex in many of the patients, has suggested strongly that this reflects a patchy reduction in cortical perfusion. The interpretation of the relative increase in the second component is not as straightforward. It seems likely that in the chronically diseased kidney, with a severe distortion of structure, that many areas within the renal cortex are perfused at a reduced rate. The flow in these regions results in an exponential component of xenon washout whose rate constant is indistinguishable from that of the usual second or medullary flow component. It cannot be assumed, therefore, that the increased volume in the second component represents an increase in medullary blood flow. It is much more likely to be a passive effect of reduced blood flow in the most severely involved areas in the renal cortex.

There has been considerable discussion of the pathophysiology of chronic, advanced renal failure (Bricker *et al.*, 1971). A popular, but not universally accepted hypothesis is based on the "intact nephron." This hypothesis suggests that residual renal function in the chronically diseased kidney is not uniformly distributed through all of the nephrons. Rather, the kidney can be divided conceptually into two parts: diseased and spared nephrons. The diseased nephron contributes little or nothing to renal function, and the relatively spared nephron provides the bulk of the residual renal function. According to this hypothesis, the abnormalities of specific renal function which are found in the chronically diseased kidney, such as the inability to concentrate the urine or retain sodium, are not related so much to a specific abnormality of tubular function in the remaining nephrons, but rather to the effects of a continuing osmotic diuresis in a few residual nephrons. The well-known ability of the kidney to hypertrophy in response to the loss of renal mass suggests that part of the compensatory mechanism in this setting involves hypertrophy of residual nephrons so that individual nephron filtration rate rises. An increase in the flow rate in the residual areas of rather well-maintained cortical function might, therefore, be expected to account for an increase in local glomerular filtration rate. Unfortunately, such an interpretation of xenon washout data cannot be relied upon at present. When a large decrease in the percentage of flow in the rapid component occurs, the analysis of first component flow rate becomes unreliable (Hollenberg, 1972). We are therefore dependent on advances in methodology to further our understanding of the process.

In summary, the renal microvasculature provides a striking example of the precise relationship between perfusion and function. Many physiological and pathological processes with a major clinical relevance can only be understood on the basis of microvascular responses. While many advances have been made in the last decade, we are probably only at the threshold of a complete understanding of the system.

References

Baldwin, D. S., Hulet, W. H., Biggs, A. W., Gombos, E. A., and Chasis, H. (1960). Renal function in the separate kidneys of man. II. Hemodynamics and excretion of solute and water in essential hypertension. *J. Clin. Invest.* **39,** 395–404.

Barger, A. C. (1960). Renal hemodynamic factors in congestive heart failure. *Ann. N. Y. Acad. Sci.* **139,** 276–284.

Blaufox, M. D., Fromowitz, A., Gruskin, A., Meng, C-H., and Elkin, M. (1970). Validation of the use of xenon 133 to measure intrarenal distubution of blood flow. *Amer. J. Physiol.* **219,** 440–444.

Bradley, G. P., Bradley, C. J., Tyson, C. J., Curry, J. J., and Blake, W. D. (1950). Renal function in renal disease. *Amer. J. Med.* **9,** 766–798.

Bricker, N. S., Klahr, S., Lubowitz, H., and Slatopolsky, E. (1971). The pathophysiology of renal insufficiency. On the functional transformation in the residual nephrons with advancing disease *Ped. Clin.N.A.* **18,** 595.

Bull, G. M., Joekes, A. M., and Lowe, K. G. (1950). Renal function studies in acute tubular necrosis. *Clin. Sci.* **9,** 379–404.

Carriere, S., Thorburn, G. D., O'Morchoe, C. C., and Barger, A. C. (1966). Intrarenal distribution of blood flow in dogs during hemorrhagic hypotension. *Circ. Res.* **19,** 167–179.

Daniel, P. M., Peabody, C. N., and Pritchard, M. M. L. (1952). Cortical ischaemia of the kidney with maintained blood flow through the medulla. *Quart. J. Exp. Cog. Med. Sci. Physiol.* **37,** 11.

Epstein, M., Berk, D. P., Hollenberg, N. K., Adams, D. F., Chalmers, T. C., Abrams, H. L., and Merrill, J. P. (1970). Renal failure in the patient with cirrhosis. The role of active vasoconstriction. *Amer. J. Med.* **49,** 175–185.

Epstein, M., Hollenberg, N. K., Guttmann, R. D., Conroy, M., Basch, R. I., and Merrill, J. P. (1971). Effect of ethacrynic acid and chlorothiazide on intrarenal hemodynamics in normal man. *Amer. J. Physiol.* **220,** 482–487.

Finckh, E. S., Jeremy, K., and Whyte, H. M. (1962). Structural renal damage and its relation to clinical features in acute oliguric renal failure. *Quart J. Med.* **31,** 429–446.

Flanigan, W. J., and Oken, D. E. (1965). Renal micropuncture study of the development of anuria in the rat with mercury-induced acute renal failure. *J. Clin. Invest.* **44,** 482.

Gosling, J. A., and Dixon, J. S. (1969). The fine structure of the vasa recta and associated nerves in the rabbit kidney. *Anat. Rec.* **165,** 503–513.

Hollenberg, N. K. (1965). The role of the sympathetic nervous system in the development of decompensation during hemorrhagic shock. Doctoral Thesis, University of Manitoba Press.

Hollenberg, N. K., Epstein, M., Rosen, S. M., Basch, R. I., Oken, D. E., and Merrill, J. P. (1968a). Acute oliguric renal failure in man: Evidence for preferential renal cortical ischemia. *Medicine* (*Baltimore*) **47,** 455–474.

Hollenberg, N. K., Epstein, M., Rosen, S. M., and Dammin, G. J. (1968b). Vascular lesions of the transplanted human kidney-morphologic and hemodynamic studies in chronic rejection. *Trans Ass. Amer. Physicians* **81,** 274–287.

Hollenberg, N. K. (1972). *In* "Progress in Nuclear Medicine" (M. D. Blaufox, ed.), Vol. 2, Chapter 10, pp. 200–234.

Hollenberg, N. K., Epstein, M., Basch, R. I., and Merrill, J. P. (1969a). "No Man's Land" of the renal vasculature. An arteriographic and hemodynamic assessment of the interlobar and arcuate arteries in essential and accelerated hypertension. *Amer. J. Med.* **47,** 845–854.

Hollenberg, N. K., Epstein, M., Basch, R. I., Merrill, J. P., and Hickler, R. B. (1969b). Renin secretion in the patient with hypertension. Relationship to intrarenal blood flow distribution. *Circ. Res.* **24** (Suppl. 1), 113–122.

Hollenberg, N. K., Adams, D. F., Oken, D. E., Abrams, H. L., and Merrill, J. P. (1970a). Acute renal failure due to nephrotoxins. *N. Eng. J. Med.* **282,** 1329–1334.

Hollenberg, N. K., Epstein, M., Guttmann, R. D., Conroy, M., Basch, R. I., and Merrill, J. P. (1970b). Effect of sodium balance on intrarenal distribution of blood flow in normal man. *J. Appl. Physiol.* **28,** 312–317.

Kincaid-Smith, P., Saker, B. M., and McKenzie, I. F. L. (1968). Lesions in the vasa recta in experimental analgesic nephropathy. *Lancet* **1,** 24.

Kramer, K. (1962). *In* "Shock: Pathogenesis and Therapy" (K. D. Bock, ed)., pp. 134–144. Springer-Verlag, Berlin and New York.

Lowenstein, J., Steinmetz, P. R., Effros, R. M., Demeester, M., Chasis, H., Baldwin, D. S., and Gomez, D. M. (1967). The distribution of intrarenal blood flow in normal and hypertensive man. *Circulation* **35,** 250–259.

Nickerson, M. (1962). *In* "Shock: Pathogenesis and Therapy" (K. D. Bock, ed.), pp. 356–370. Springer-Verlag, Berlin and New York.

Pomeranz, B. H., Birtch, A. G., and Barger, A. C. (1968). Neural control of intrarenal blood flow. *Amer. J. Physiol.* **215,** 1067–1081.

Shock, N. W. (1967). Current trends in reserach on the physiological aspects of aging. *J. Amer. Geriat. Soc.* **15,** 995–1000.

Smith, H. W., ed. (1951). "Structure and Function in Health and Disease" Oxford Univ. Press, London and New York.

Smith, H. W., Goldring, W., Chasis, H., Ranges, H. A., and Bradley, S. E. (1943). The application of saturation methods to the study of glomerular and tubular function in the human kidney. *J. Mt. Sinai Hosp., New York* **10,** 59–108.

Thorburn, G. D., Kopald, H. H., Herd, J. A., Hollenberg, M., O'Morchoe, C. C., and Barger, A. C. (1963). Intrarenal distribution of nutrient blood flow determined with krypton 85 in the unanesthetized dog. *Circ. Res.* **13,** 290–307.

Thurau, K. (1964). Renal hemodynamics. *Amer. J. Med.* **36,** 698–719.

Trueta, J., Barclay, A. E. Daniel, P. M., Franklin, K. J., and Pritchard, M. M. L. (1947). "Studies of the Renal Circulation." Thomas, Springfield, Illinois.

Welt, L. G., and Lyle, C. B. (1963). *In* "Diseases of the Kidney" (M. B. Strauss and L. G. Welt, eds.), pp. 894–900. Little, Brown, Boston, Massachusetts.

6 ROLE OF THE MICROVASCULATURE IN THE REJECTION OF TISSUE TRANSPLANTS

JOHN P. MERRILL, M.D.

I. Introduction

The role of the microvasculature in the rejection of transplanted tissues and organs was not generally appreciated in the early years of study of this problem. Descriptions of skin, kidneys, and other organs which had been transplanted stressed the role of round cell infiltration. Loeb (1945) believed that tissues had individual differences and that with strong degrees of differences, body fluids exerted a "strongly injurious effect" on the grafted tissue. He felt that the lymphocyte senses or recognizes the finest degrees of these differences, and on this basis he accounted for the round cell infiltration accompanying the rejection of a graft. Later, Medawar and his colleagues pointed out that the rejection of a skin transplant was the result of the foreign antigen of the donor skin stimulating an immune response by the recipient (Medawar, 1944). In this sense then, the lymphocytes which infiltrated the tissue were thought to be antibody-containing cells which caused destruction of the graft. This emphasis upon the role of the round cells seen in the rejected allograft formed the basis for considerable discussion and dispute about the role of "cell-bound" versus the classic "humoral" antibodies in graft destruction. It is now quite evident that both are involved and that the effect of both in damaging the microvasculature of the graft plays the predominant role in graft rejection.

II. Pathology of Rejection

In the early days of transplantation research, the destruction of the graft was measured by observation of the gross appearance. If a first piece of skin was placed upon a recipient who had never been exposed to the antigens of the donor before, the graft was vascularized and became pink. The microcirculation and, indeed, the gross appearance of the graft appeared quite normal at about day six. Shortly thereafter the graft became edematous, cyanotic, blotchy, and eventually underwent necrosis. In a series of studies done by our group, the earliest histologic appearance of rejection of a human skin graft was the appearance of round cells about the small venules of the graft (Henry *et al.*, 1962). However, previous evidence of a more dynamic nature had been presented by Rapaport and his group (1960). These workers, using stereomicroscopy to observe the small vessels of the graft, noted slowing of flow through the vessels, sludging of the blood, and eventual thrombosis which undoubtedly resulted in the gross changes observed. It is of some interest in the light of more recent evidence that thrombosis and increased permeability of the vessel with resultant edema are all part of a classic immune reaction.

More precise evidence regarding the role of the vasculature in the destruction of the graft during rejection was made by observations of the so-called "second set skin graft." When a recipient has been sensitized to donor tissues by previous exposure to and rejection of the antigens of these tissues, he is immunized at the time a second graft is placed. Under these circumstances the graft is destroyed in a more rapid and dramatic fashion. Here, vascular thrombosis and necrosis of the graft appears within 3 days and, indeed, if the circumstances are timed accurately, the graft may be destroyed as a "white graft" (Marshall *et al.*, 1962). The term "white graft" here indicates that vascular thrombosis has occurred with such rapidity that the graft never becomes vascularized. Here again is evidence of the important role of damage to the microvasculature in the rejection of transplanted skin.

The rejection of the transplanted kidney is also accompanied by marked infiltration with round cells (Hume *et al.*, 1955). Vascular lesions have also been seen, but in the early descriptions of renal allograft rejections, the glomeruli are almost universally stated to be "normal." This is at present of great interest in view of the fact that glomerular lesions occurring in long surviving allografts in the human constitute a major problem in this area. Since the glomerular capillary bed constitutes a major part of the microvasculature, its involvement in the immune reaction is critically important.

A. Evidence of Rejection from Human Kidney Transplantation

One of the earliest and most striking observations made which attests to the importance of the microvasculature was that reported by Oeconomos and his colleagues (1953) in which a young man previously healthy had a single normal kidney removed following trauma. Shortly thereafter he received a kidney transplant from his mother. The kidney functioned quite normally for a period of 21 days and then suddenly became anuric. The glomeruli were bloodless and the vessels engorged with some interstitial hemorrhage. The authors attributed this process to sudden "vascular failure."

With the advent of immunosuppressive therapy renal allografting in the human was undertaken on an increasingly large scale. Frequently the transplanted kidney would function well for the first 2 or 3 weeks and then a "rejection" episode occurred. When the kidney had been functioning normally prior to this rejection episode, the early evidences of rejection were oliguria, decreased sodium concentration, and increased osmolality of the urine—the same phenomenon which represents partial obstruction of a major renal vessel in renovascular hypertension. In this case, however, the problem was multiple obstructive lesions of minor renal vessels caused by the immunologic damage.

B. Evidence of Rejection in Inbred Animal Strains

Great strides have been made in our knowledge of the role of the microvasculature in the rejection process in animal transplantation. It is possible to transplant kidneys between inbred strains of rats. In these inbred strains, members of each strain are antigenically similar enough one to the other to constitute virtual identical twins. Therefore, the results of the transplantation from inbred strain A to inbred strain B is unaffected by variations in antigenic differences between donor and recipient, which so often confuse work with the dog and the human. In our own laboratory, the transplantation of a kidney from an (Lewis by BN) F_1 hybrid into a Lewis rat results in rejection of the kidney by day 7 in all of the cases. This rejection is determined by cessation of effective renal plasma flow as measured by the plasma disappearance rate of [^{125}I] hippuran; a fact which attests again to the importance of the rejection response upon the vasculature of the kidney (Guttmann *et al.*, 1967). The sequence of events which follows transplantation in these inbred strains is so predictable that serial biopsies can detect the earliest effect. Thus, sacrificing the animal at sequential times clearly delineates the nature of the lesion. Two days after transplantation, collections of mononuclear cells have already surrounded cortical vessels. By 3 days, the cellular infiltrates, still confined to the perivascular areas, are most apparent. In some instances, cells are adherent to the endothelial lining of these vessels and cells are occasionally seen protruding through the capillary walls. At 5 days, vascular endothelium of arteries contains large vesicular nuclei and swollen cytoplasm. The lumina of small cortical arteries are occasionally occluded by mononuclear cells. At 2 to 3 weeks, fibrinoid necrosis involves the walls of many vessels, and the endothelial cells are large and several layers thick (Guttmann *et al.*, 1967). Utilizing the technique of immunofluorescence the antibody to the animal's own immunoglobin is tagged with fluorescein and injected; one can then find the distribution and location of the immune process occurring with the rejection. Again the earliest lesion is seen around the small venules and in the peritubular capillaries (Guttmann *et al.,* 1967). Characteristically, in the untreated control allograft, mononuclear cells accumulate around interlobular blood vessels; glomerular capillaries are hypocellular and occluded by fibrin and platelets.

Although immunosuppressive therapy with azathioprine may slightly prolong function in these animals, one again notes glomerular capillaries occluded by fibrin and platelets and glomerular cells which are necrotic and decreased in number. However, the striking morphologic feature in this group is the extreme paucity of pyroninophilic mononuclear cells which are the characteristic and prominent feature of allograft rejection in modified recipients. Here then, immunosuppressive therapy has obliterated the striking effects of mononuclear infiltration first observed in untreated recipients and allowed the effect on the microvasculature to become more apparent (Shehadeh *et al.*, 1970).

III. Changes in Partition of Blood Flow during Rejection

It is now possible to measure not only total renal blood flow through the kidney, but the distribution of blood between various vascular compartments by the technique of xenon washout. In such studies, a bolus of radioactive xenon or krypton is injected into the kidney and by external counting a disappearance curve can be constructed whose slope represents the rate of blood flow and, thus, of disappearance of the radioactive material from the kidney. The curve can be analyzed so as to measure several compartments of which the cortical and corticomedullary compartments are the two most important (Thorburn *et al.*, 1963). It can be shown that the earliest effect of the rejection process on a transplanted kidney in the dog is a relative decrease in cortical flow and an increase in that of the corticomedullary area (Rosen *et al.*, 1967; Retik *et al.*, 1967). Radioautographs made of dog kidneys have shown that there is a patchy decrease in cortical flow with the rejection which is identical to that seen in hemorrhagic hypotension. The studies of Rosen and his colleagues (1967) on the transplanted dog kidney show clearly that this redistribution of renal blood flow occurs before marked elevation of blood urea nitrogen, and they conclude that "the reduction of cortical blood flow produced by immunological mechanisms may play a predominant role in the ensuing renal failure." Here again the effect on the vasculature of the rejection process must be evident. The magnificent injection studies of Gardner *et al.* (1968) on the rejecting rat kidney show very clearly the patchy nature of the vascular lesion and the failure of cortical perfusion (Figs. 1 and 2).

IV. The Microvasculature in Hyperacute Rejection

Most patients who are candidates for renal transplants are maintained by dialysis on the artificial kidney for some period prior to transplantation. During the course of this treatment it is customary to transfuse them. Such transfusions contain platelets and white cells which constitute human antigen. It is thus possible by transfusion to sensitize a prospective recipient by previous exposure to human tissue antigens which might cross-react with the donor. Thus, the recipient is immunized to the donor at the time of transplantation. Under these circumstances a "hyperacute" rejection of the kidney occurs (Kissmeyer–Nielsen *et al.*, 1966; Starzl *et al.*, 1968; Williams *et al.*, 1967; Myburgh *et al.*, 1969; Colman *et al.*, 1969). This is characterized by platelet and fibrin deposition, occlusion of the small vessels, acute thrombosis particularly of the afferent arterioles of the glomeruli, and sudden and dramatic failure of renal function. This hyperacute rejection process is primarily an effect in the microvasculature of the kidney and is one of the most dramatic and catastrophic events in human organ transplantation.

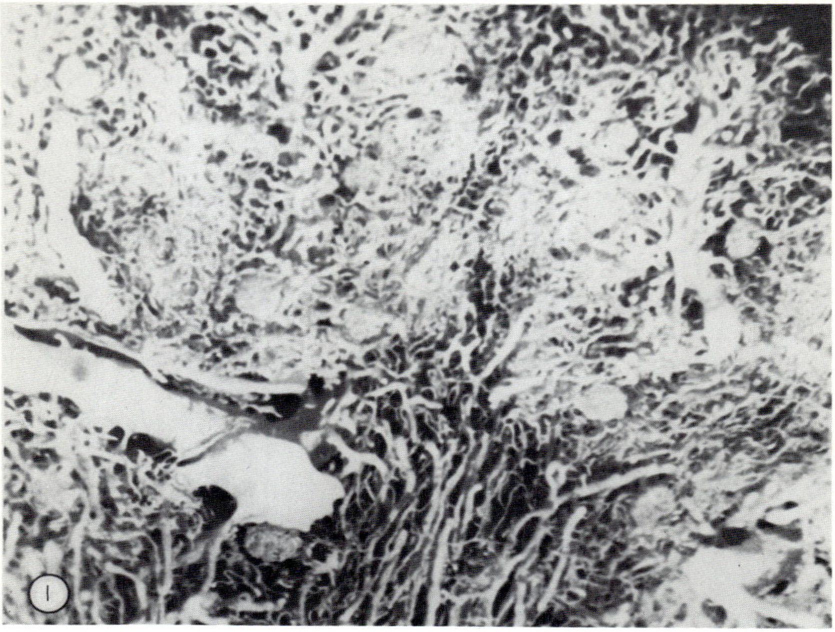

Fig. 1. Silastic injection of kidney from a normal rat. Glomeruli, afferent and efferent arterioles, pertubular capillaries, and vasa rectae are well demonstrated in an evenly perfused pattern. (From Gardner *et al.*, 1968).

V. Role of the Clotting Mechanism

The role of the clotting mechanism in acute and hyperacute rejection has been discussed. Characteristically, in rat renal allografts, fibrin deposition also appears to be the pathogenetic mechanism producing glomerulopathy in long-surviving renal allografts (Figs. 3–5) (Lindquist *et al.*, 1970). In the human, too, platelet aggregation and fibrin deposition appear to play an important role, although the acuteness of this reaction varies with the degree of presensitivity and with the antigenic difference between donor and recipient. However, characteristically, fibrin split products are found in the urine of a rejecting transplant, suggesting that fibrin deposition has occurred and the fibrinolytic mechanism activated (Braun and Merrill, 1968). The role of the involvement of the microvasculature in occlusion by fibrin and platelet deposition has been strikingly described by Lichtman (Lichtman *et al.*, 1968), who has demonstrated typical deformed erythrocytes of microangiopathy in two rejecting transplants which

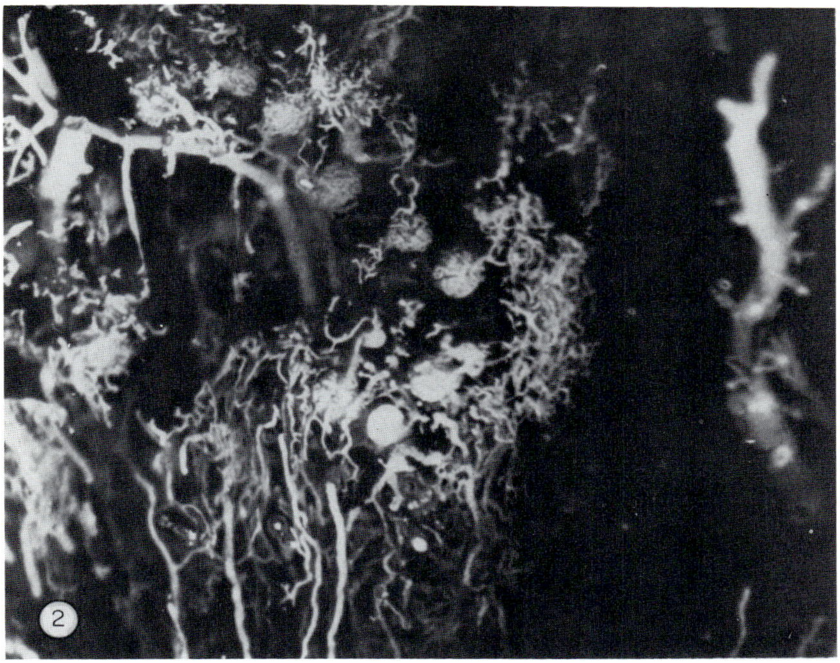

Fig. 2. Wedge-shaped areas of no perfusion and numerous smaller areas of unperfused subcapsular cortex. Deeper, partially perfused areas of cortex show reduced numbers of glomeruli and a correspondingly decreased pertitubular network. (Reprinted with permission from Gardner *et al.*, 1968.)

showed prominent proliferative vasculature lesions by biopsy. The hemolytic anemia and erythrocyte deformation seen in these instances is characteristic of trauma to an erythrocyte which, moving with sufficient velocity, encounters an obstruction small in size in relation to the erythrocyte. The erythrocyte will become arrested and folded about the obstruction. The passage of other erythrocytes around the arrested cell may cause its release or fragmentation. Here again is striking evidence for the involvement of the microvasculature in the rejecting human renal allograft.

VI. Vascular Changes in Human Renal Allografts

Rosen *et al.* (1968) and Hollenberg *et al.* (1968a) have applied the technique utilized in the animal to this study of the rejecting human renal allograft. Hollenberg's studies have correlated the morphologic lesions and

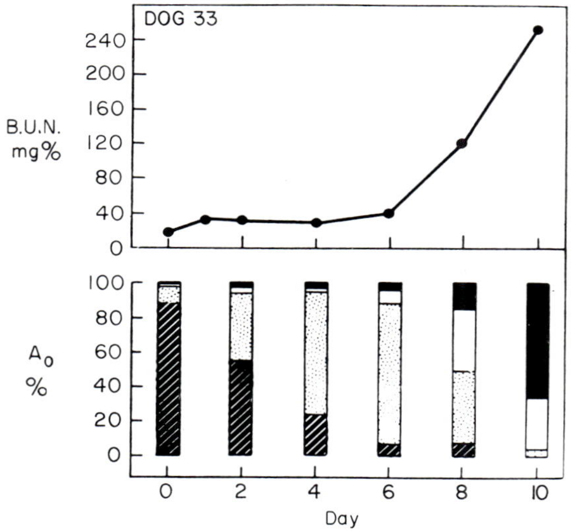

Fig. 3. Serial measurements of intrarenal distribution of blood flow in the homotransplanted kidney of a bilaterally nephrectomized dog. Percentages of total blood received by components 1, 2, 3, and 4 are represented by cross-hatched, dotted, white, and black blocks, respectively. Note that marked decrease in component 1 or cortical flow occurred before elevation of blood urea nitrogen. (Reprinted with permission from Rosen *et al.*, 1967.)

the abnormalities of hemodynamics in chronic rejection in the human kidney. Hemodynamically significant lesions at the arteriolar level were considerably less severe than lesions of small arteries, suggesting that a minimal to moderate arteriolar lesion may well contribute more to abnormal hemodynamics than a more severe lesion at the intralobular artery level. Cortical arteriolar involvement was associated with the decrease in the flow rate within the cortex without a redistribution of blood flow, suggesting an even distribution of disease involving all vessels at the arteriolar level. In addition, these authors found, as did Rosen, a variability of flow suggesting a functional component in the development of abnormal hemodynamics in allograft rejection. Previous work had shown an increase in sensitivity to vasodilator agents during allograft rejection of the renal blood vessels (Hollenberg *et al.*, 1968b). This suggests an element of active vasoconstriction prior to the development of morphologic lesions. Again, the critically important role of the microvasculature both dynamically and morphologically is illustrated by these findings. Renal angio-

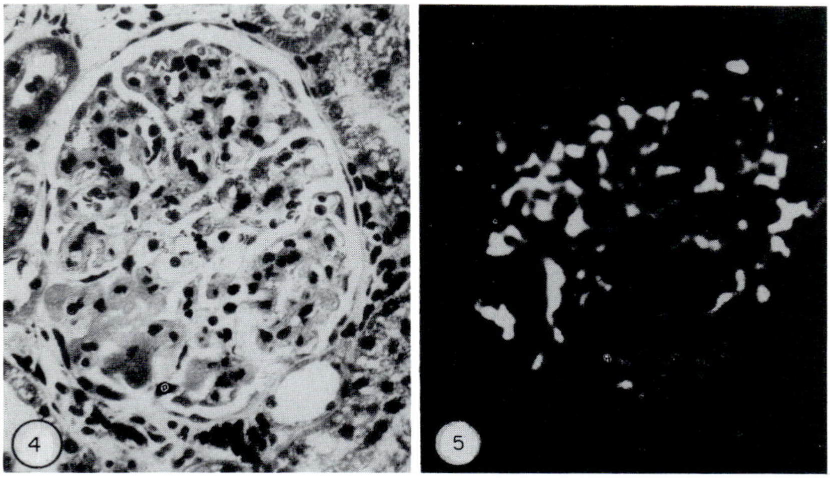

Fig. 4. Glomerulopathy in a long-surviving renal allograft. The capillary walls are irregularly thickened. Some glomerular capillaries are completely occluded and the mesangium is expanded (H & E; magnification 163×). Reprinted with permission from Lindquist *et al.,* 1970.)

Fig. 5. Fibrin localization in a long-surviving LF344 F_1 arrow L renal allograft. Fibrin is deposited in and around glomerular capillaries and in the mesangium (FITC, rabbit-anti-rat-fibrin. Magnification 163×). (Reprinted with permission from Lindquist *et al.,* 1970.)

grams in the acutely rejecting kidney show a characteristic pruning of the small cortical vessels and in the chronically rejecting kidney, the interlobular and arcuate vessels are involved in an irregular occlusive process. The radio-labeled hippuran renogram which measures among other things the delivery of blood to secreting renal tissue and the secretion of hippuran by the renal tubules may show striking aberrations during the rejection process and dramatic improvement with reversal of the rejection process by appropriate immunosuppressive therapy.

VII. Rejection of Xenografts

A number of xenografts, that is, transplanted kidneys from other than human species, have been made in human recipients. Almost universally, baboon kidneys transplanted to humans are rejected with evidence of acute and fulminating vasculitis (Starzl *et al.*, 1964). In one instance, transplantation of the chimpanzee kidney has succeeded for a number of months, but invariably this has been rejected with evidence of vascular involvement (Reemtsma *et al.*, 1964). Ballantyne and his colleagues (1969) studying the effect of modification of the immune process by the use of massive rather than small xenografts from rabbit to rats have again stressed the fact that "on the third day following transplantation most of the small standard xenografts appeared completely vascularized by an extensive network of dilated vessels with active blood circulation. No detectable blood flow was observed in one graft before the sixth day. The earliest indication of the rejection of small xenografts was increased distention of graft vessels followed rapidly by complete cessation of blood circulation and vasculature disruption usually between the sixth and eighth day. Three days after surgery the massive grafts developed a moderate extensive vascular system of slightly dilated vessels which were filled but not engorged with erythrocytes. During the next two days the caliber of vessels and massive grafts were slightly larger but there was no stereomicroscopic evidence of progressive increase in number and ramification of these vessels similar to that previously described for autografts and allografts." The importance placed by these authors on observations of microvasculature as an index of rejection needs no further emphasis.

VIII. Rejection of Organs Other than Kidney

Rejection of the transplanted heart is accompanied by infiltration of the myocardium with large mononuclear cells and deposits of IgG as well as complement components and fibrin in the myocardium (Stastny, 1970). Nora *et al.* (1969) reported that in 3 patients with cardiac transplants who died between the 7th and 13th postoperative days, microscopic examination revealed not only the myocardial interstitial infiltrate but an increased concentration of this infiltrate in the perivascular areas and a similar infiltrate in the thickened intima of the coronary arteries. In patients dying later of more chronic rejection, the classic finding is intimal thickening and fibrosis of the coronary arteries with infiltrating lymphocytes. Varying degrees of obstruction of the coronary arteries occur with acidophilic degenerative changes present in the tunica media of the medium and small coronary arteries. Indeed, in the long-surviving cases, the classic lesion is coronary artery sclerosis which may almost exactly resemble that of the naturally occurring vascular disease.

In human liver transplantation, involvement of the vasculature is a a common cause of failure. Starzl (Starzl *et al.,* 1966) reported that

7 of his 14 recipients of orthotopic liver homografts developed occlusive clots in part of the homograft blood supply. In early rejection, this tended to involve large vessels rather than the microvasculature. However, diffuse vascular lesions were noted in some of the longer survivors in which thickening of the intima of the small branches of the hepatic arteries occurred. The thickened intima had many large cells with abundant cytoplasma containing fine droplets of fat. Frequently the internal elastic lamina was ruptured.

IX. Summary

The process responsible for the rejection of both allografts and xenografts in the mammalian species studied depends in large part on damage to the vasculature with ischemic changes in other structures secondary. The histologic picture depends in large part on the acuteness and vigor of the rejection process which, in turn, depends in part on the difference in tissue antigens between donor and recipient. A special case in which violent rejection of the graft characterized by fibrinoid necrosis and thrombosis of the small vessels occurs is one in which the recipient is already sensitized to tissues of the donor. The role of the microvasculature in all these processes, whether acute or chronic, appears to be critically important.

References

Ballantyne, D. L., Jr., Uhlschmid, G. K., and Converse, J. M. (1969). Massive rabbit skin xenografts in rats. *Transplantation* **7,** 274–280.

Braun, W. E., and Merrill, J. P. (1968). Urine fibrinogen fragments in human renal allografts. A possible mechanism of renal unjury. *N. Engl. J. Med.* **278,** 366–1391.

Colman, R. W., Braun, W. E., Busch, G. J., Dammin, G. J., and Merrill, J. P. (1969). Coagulation studies in the hyperacute and other forms of renal allograft rejection. *N. Engl. J. Med.* **281,** 685–691.

Gardner, L. B., Guttman, R. D., and Merrill, J. P. (1968). Renal transplantation in the inbred rat. IV. Alterations in the microvasculature in acute unmodified rejection. *Transplantation* **6,** 411–418.

Guttmann, R. D., Lindquist, R. R., Parker, R. M., Carpenter, C. B., and Merrill, J. P. (1967). Renal transplantation in the inbred rat. I. Morphologic, immunologic and functional alterations during acute rejection. *Transplantation* **5,** 668–681.

Henry, L., Marshall, D. C., Friedman, E., Dammin, G. J., and Merrill, J. P. (1962). The rejection of skin homografts in the normal human subject. Part II. Histological findings. *J. Clin. Invest.* **41,** 420–446.

Hollenberg, N. K., Epstein, M., Rosen, S. M., Dammin, G. J., and Merrill, J. P. (1968a). Vascular lesions of the transplanted human kidney—morphologic and hemodynamic studies in chronic rejection. *Trans. Ass. Amer. Physicians* **81,** 274–287.

Hollenberg, N. K., Retik, A. B., Rosen, S. M., Murray, J. E., and Merrill, J. P. (1968b). The role of vasoconstriction in the ischemia of renal allograft rejection. *Transplantation* **6,** 59–69.

Hume, D. M., Merrill, J. P., Miller, B. F., and Thorn, G. W. (1955). Experiences with renal homotransplantation in the human: Report on nine cases. *J. Clin. Invest.* **34,** 327–382.

Kissmeyer–Nielsen, F., Olsen, S., Petersen, V. P., and Fjeldborg, O. (1966). Hyperacute rejection of kidney allografts associated with pre-existing humoral antibodies against donor cells. *Lancet* **2,** 662–665.

Lichtman, M. A., Hoyer, L. W., and Sears, D. A. (1968). Erythrocyte deformation and hemolytic anemia coincident with the microvascular disease of rejecting renal homotransplants *Amer. J. Med. Sci.* **256,** 239–246.

Lindquist, R. R., Guttmann, R. D., and Mahabir, R. N. (1970). Fibrin deposition as a pathogenetic mechanism producing glomerulopathy in long surviving renal allografts. *Transplantation* **9,** 65–68.

Loeb, L. (1945)." The Biological Basis of Individuality." Thomas, Springfield, Illinois.

Marshall, D. C., Friedman, E. A., Goldstein, D. P., Henry, L., and Merrill, J. P. (1962). The rejection of skin homografts in the normal human subject. Part I. Clinical observations. *J. Clin. Invest.* **41,** 411–419.

Medawar, P. B. (1944). The behaviour and fate of skin autografts and skin homografts in rabbits. *J. Anat.* **78,** 176–199.

Myburgh, J. A., Cohen, I., Meyers, A. M., Gecelter, L., Abrahams, C., Furman, K. I., Goldberg, B., and Van Blerk, P. J. P. (1969). Hyperacute rejection in human-kidney allografts—Shwartzman or Arthus reaction? *N. Engl. J. Med.* **281,** 131–135.

Nora, J. J., Cooley, D. A., Fernbach, D. J., Rochelle, D. G., Milam, J. D., Montgomery, J. R., Leachman, R. D., Butler, W. T., Rossen, R. D., Bloodwell, R. D., Hallman, G. L., and Trentin, J. J. (1969). Rejection of the transplanted human heart. Indexes of recognition and problems in prevention. *N. Engl. J. Med.* **280,** 1079–1086.

Oeconomos, N., Hamburger, J., Delinotte, P., Vaysse, J., Richet, G., Antoine, B., Elmelik, E., and Perrin, C. (1953). Tentative d'homogreffe renale (rein maternel) après nephrectomie pour traumatisme d'un rein unique *Mem. Acad. Chir.* **79,** 642–652.

Rapaport, F. T., Thomas, L., Converse, J. M., and Lawrence, H. S. (1960). The specificity of skin homograft rejection in man. *Ann. N. Y. Acad. Sci.* **87,** 217–222.

Reemtsma, K., McCracken, B. H., and Schlegel, J. U. (1964). Renal heterotransplantation in man. *Ann. Surg.* **160,** 384–410.

Retik, A. B., Hollenberg, N. K., Rosen, S. M., Merrill, J. P., and Murry, J. E. (1967). Cortical ischemia in renal allograft rejection. *Surg., Gynecol. Obstet.* **124,** 989–998.

Rosen, S. M., Truniger, B. P., Kriek, H. R., Murray, J. E., and Merrill, J. P. (1967). Intrarenal distribution of blood flow in the transplanted dog kidney. Effect of denervation and rejection. *J. Clin. Invest.* **46,** 1239–1263.

Rosen, S. M., Hollenberg, N. K., Dealy, J. B., Jr., and Merrill, J. P. (1968). Measurement of the distribution of blood flow in the human kidney using intra-arterial injection of ^{133}Xe relationship to function in the normal and transplanted kidney. *Clin. Sci.* **34,** 287–302.

Shehadeh, I. H., Guttmann, R. D., and Lindquist, R. R. (1970). Renal transplantation in the inbred rat. XV. An assay study of three immunosuppressive drugs. *Transplantation* **10,** 66–79.

Starzl, T. E., Marchioro, T. L., and Peters, G. N. (1964). Renal heterotransplantation from baboon–to–man: Experience with 6 cases. *Transplantation* **2,** 752–776.

Starzl, T. E., Marchioro, T. L., and Faris, T. D. (1966). *In* "Transplantation of the Liver. Homotransplantation Kidney and Other Tissues *Proc. Natl. Kidney Found.* (Jack Metcoff, ed.), p 122.

Starzl, T. E., Lerner, R. A., and Dixon, J. F. (1968). Shwartzman reaction after human renal homotransplantation. *N. Engl. J. Med.* **278,** 642-648.

Stastny, P. (1970). Bound immunoglobulin and complement in heart allografts under-going rejection. *Transplantation* **10,** 248–257.

Thorburn, G. D., Kopald, H. H., Herd, J. A., Hollenberg, M., O'Morchoe, C. C., and Barger, A. C. (1963). Intrarenal distribution of nutrient blood flow determined with krypton 85 in the unanesthetized dog. *Circ. Res.* **13,** 290–307.

Williams, G. M. *et al.* (1967). Studies in hyperacute and chronic renal homograft rejection in man. *Surgery* **62,** 204–212.

7 COLLAGEN VASCULAR DISORDERS

KENNETH H. FALCHUK, M.D.

I. Introduction

The microcirculatory system maintains effective perfusion at the tissue level. The degree of perfusion varies for each tissue and is regulated at the precapillary level by sphincter muscles. This regulation is responsible for the adequate flow and distribution of blood to tissues with varying requirements. For example, a constant glomerular filtration rate is a function, in part, of adequate perfusion pressure in the glomerular capillaries. This pressure is controlled by the pre- and postglomerular sphincters. An increase in acid secretion by the stomach requires an increase in mucosal blood flow, which is achieved by a reduction in microvascular resistance. The required increase in the rate of removal of lactic acid and delivery of oxygen to exercising muscles necessitates an increase in regional blood flow; this selectivity is accomplished by simultaneously increasing the resistance in the vessels of the abdominal organs and decreasing the resistance of the vessels in the exercising muscles. The critical functions of precapillary sphincter mechanisms, in turn, are responsive both to central nervous and, particularly, local factors, such as hydrogen ion concentration, partial pressures of oxygen, and carbon dioxide, histamine, serotonin, and other vasoactive substances.

The wide alterations in metabolic demand and the differences in functions of the various tissues require that local flow and distribution of blood be optimized in relation to activity in order to remain functionally intact. However, adequate blood flow does not ensure adequate cellular activity since there are barriers (such as the vascular membrane, the connective tissues of the interstitial space, the distance over which diffusion of substances must occur, and the chemical gradients that exist between plasma and interstitial and cellular water) that separate blood and its components from cells. If affected by disease, these barriers can have marked effects on the normal activity of tissues. Changes in the thickness of the vessel wall such as basement membrane thickening, endothelial proliferation, or fibrosis may cause alterations in membrane permeability or increase diffusion pathways and thereby result in impaired exchange of metabolites between cells and blood. The abnormal exchange may be present despite quantitative increases in blood flow to the diseased tissue. Cellular activity, therefore, is dependent on an intact vascular anatomy as well as on adequate regulation of blood flow.

Pathologic changes of vascular anatomy and of the interstitial space are caused primarily by trauma, hemorrhage, infections, etc. As a result of the intimate contact between tissues and the microcirculatory system, the latter can transport to affected areas chemical and cellular components to protect both tissues and the vasculature from damage. These components include the clotting, antibody forming and complement systems, and such cells as polymorphonuclear leukocytes, eosinophils, macrophages, lymphocytes, and plasma cells. These protective systems localize their function to the site which has been altered. Failure to localize, or extensive activation of these mechanisms, is associated with a series of events (described in Section II), which may cause harm to normal tissues. These two broad areas, then, encompass the primary roles of the microcirculation—to maintain adequate perfusion and to protect the tissues from injurious disturbances. Any dysfunction in these roles will have grave consequences to the organism.

The connective tissue disorders are syndromes where abnormalities of the microvasculature are quite prominent. Damaged vessels are found in many organ systems. Histologically, this damage (see Section II) not only involves the vessel walls but also can affect the surrounding tissues. The vessel pathology can be shown to exist in association with plasma factors known to cause the activation of the complement system. Since abnormal activation of the complement system within blood vessels is known to cause vascular and tissue dysfunction, it has been postulated that a similar mechanism may be responsible for the pathology observed in some of the collagen vascular disorders to be discussed in Section III. In the following sections, the vascular lesions observed in these syndromes will be reviewed. Evidence for the possible etiological link between excessive activation of the complement system by antigen-antibody complexes and vascular damage will be presented. What will remain obscure, for lack of experimental evidence, are the effects of these lesions on the primary function of the microcirculation, the balanced relationship between regional blood flow and cellular activity.

II. Vascular Lesions Due to Hypersensitivity Reactions

The role which the microcirculation plays in transporting to affected areas cellular and chemical components to cope with foreign organisms, trauma, hemorrhage, etc., has been alluded to in the introduction. The consequences of the localization and activation of these cellular and chemical components are the destruction of offending organisms, or substances, or the healing of trauma. No damage to the surrounding, uninvolved tissues results. During special circumstances, such as occurs after the repeated presence of the same foreign substance or organisms, the consequences may become quantitatively greater, with important effects on the surrounding tissues. This abnormal, excessive response has been termed hypersensitivity (Rich, 1946–1947). The phenomenon of hypersensitivity can manifest itself through different mechanisms depending on the initiating event. We shall discuss those reactions associated with immune complexes in the serum and with delayed type hypersensitivity. Both these phenomena are associated with vascular and tissue lesions.

A lesion of the hypersensitivity type induced by immune complexes requires the precipitation on a vessel wall of a humoral antibody complexed with the appropriate antigenic substance (Rich, 1946–1947; Stetson, 1951; Ward and Cochrane, 1965). This condition results in the activation of the complement system, which consists of nine serum proteins having enzymatic activity. The initiation of complement activation by antigen-antibody complexes implies both binding of complement by the antigen-antibody and the release of biologically active fragments. Excessive activation of the system leads to the formation of a classic vascular lesion known as the Arthus phenomenon (Arthus, 1903). The vascular lesion will result if (a) the antigen and antibody form a complex in the serum, and then, localize in the vessel wall; or (b) the antigen first fixes to portions of the vessel wall, followed by antibody attachment. The former requires the presence of chemical mediators, such as histamine and serotonin, in order to localize in the vessel wall (Henson and Cochrane, 1971; Jensen, 1967). Histologically, the lesion consists of necrosis of the vessel wall, marked interstitial edema, infiltration with polymorphonuclear leukocytes, and, often, thrombosis of the vessel lumen. Frequently, a type of necrosis termed fibrinoid is present (Movat and More, 1957).

The sequence of complement activation has been reviewed recently (Austen, 1971), but we shall concentrate on those factors which are most relevant to the production of vascular damage. A small molecular weight fragment, anaphylotoxin, is released following activation of the third component (Cochrane and Müller–Eberhard, 1968; Dias de Silva and Lepow, 1967; Jensen, 1967). This fragment increases capillary permeability and probably enhances entry of plasma into the interstitium. The fragment complexed to the antigen antibody causes an increase in the phagocytosis of the antigen-antibody complex, as well as endowing the system with a property called immune adherence. Activation of the fifth component then produces a fragment of larger molecular weight than the third component fraction (Jensen, 1967), which also increases permeability and has the properties of a chemotactic factor (Ward and Newman, 1969). The trimolecular complex of the fifth, sixth, and seventh components also is chemotactic for polymorphonuclear leukocytes (Ward *et al.*, 1966). Activation of these chemotactic factors within the vessel wall is associated with infiltration and accumulation of white cells in the interstitium surrounding the vessel. At this point, proteolytic enzymes from the cytoplasm of white cells are released into the extracellular spaces. The mechanisms for release of lysozymes are variable and not well understood, some requiring complement as in the formation of this type of lesion, while others do not (Waksman, 1961). Lysozymes derived from white cells appear to be important in creating the damage, since no lesion is produced in the absence of white cells, despite the presence of both antibody and activation of complement (Sokoloff and Bunin, 1957; Ward and Cochrane, 1965). The increase in vascular permeability, with the associated edema around the vessel wall, the disruption of the vessel wall due to lysozymal activity, and the profuse infiltration with polymorphonuclear leukocytes destroy the functional capability of the vessel segment involved. This loss of function can cause secondary ischemic damage to the surrounding tissue.

The vascular lesions which result from complement activation are quite similar histologically. However, since activation of the system can be produced by different immunoglobulins of the IgG or IgM type (Stelos and Talmage, 1957; Talmage *et al.*, 1956) complexed with numerous distinct antigens, it should be emphasized that identical histological findings in two damaged vessels cannot be interpreted as having identical etiologic origins.

The mechanism for the production of vascular lesions associated with delayed type of hypersensitivity is less well understood. This system differs from the immune complex-induced type of hypersensitivity in that there is no requirement for the circulating type of antibody. Instead, the mechanism for complexing antigen is accomplished directly by interaction of mononuclear cells with antigen. When interaction with antigen occurs, substances are released causing monocytes and macrophages to adhere to the vessel wall (Uhr, 1966; Waksman, 1960, 1961). The combination of antigen with cell results in discrete lesions of blood vessels. In these lesions, the majority of cells that infiltrate and surround the blood vessel (particularly venules) are of the lymphocytic and mononuclear type, though eosinophils and polymorphonuclear leukocytes also are present (Uhr, 1966; Waksman, 1960). This lesion differs from the lesion of the immune complex type of hypersensitivity in which polymorphonuclear leukocytes predominate. The damage to the blood vessels is quite variable. The lesions may demonstrate mild or moderate inflammatory changes or even necrosis of both the vessel wall and the surrounding tissue. The mechanism for destruction does not require complement and probably is dependent on substances, such as lysozymes, released from cellular elements by undefined mechanisms. The effect on the physiologic function of the vessel is similar to that described for the immediate type lesion. The perivascular cellular infiltration and the vessel and parenchymal destruction all lead to ischemic necrosis of the surrounding tissues (Waksman, 1961) and, hence, increase the effect of the pathologic process to a greater area.

It is conceivable that a vascular reaction, which may begin as a result of immune complex type of hypersensitivity, may subsequently form at the site of tissue damage the antigenic stimulus for the development of delayed hypersensitivity. A tissue where such reactions have occurred may demonstrate vascular lesions with histochemical traits characteristic of either or both types of hypersensitivity damage.

III. Collagen Vascular Disorders

The syndromes that are classified under the term "collagen diseases" are characterized by vascular damage. The histologic and immunologic nature of much of the vascular damage is analogous to the lesions observed in hypersensitivity type reactions in that immune complexes are often found in the serum of patients with these syndromes; antibody and complement as well as cellular infiltration are present in many of the lesions. Despite these similarities in vessel pathology, however, there are major clinical differences among each of these disorders. These may result from

TABLE I

Comparison of Pathology and Serum Factors in Three Types of Collagen Vascular Diseases

Disease	Size and distribution	Serum factors	Complement	Vascular damage	Tissue pathology
Hypersensitivity angiitis	Capillaries	Increase in serum globulins	Present in vascular lesions	Acute vasculitis	Secondary to vascular pathology
	Venules			Lesions in same stage of development	
Systemic lupus erythematosus	Small arteries	Nuclear material	Normal or decreased in serum. Present in vascular lesions	Acute vasculitis	Secondary to vascular pathology
	Capillaries	Antinuclear antibody		Lesions in different stages of development	
	Venules	Rheumatoid factor			Direct damage
Rheumatoid arthritis	Small arteries	Rheumatoid factor	Decreased in joint fluids. Present in some vascular lesions	Mixed lesions in different stages of development.	Secondary to vascular pathology
	Arterioles			Acute vasculitis	
	Capillaries	Antinuclear antibodies		? Delayed hypersensitivity	Synovial pathology unrelated to vessel damage?
	Venules				

differences in the distribution and size of vessels damaged, the antigens which initiate the disease, the type of antibody involved, the plasma concentration of the antigen-antibody complex, or the ratio of antigen to antibody in the plasma. The following section will describe three general syndromes (Table I) where these differences are exemplified. In the first, immune complex type of hypersensitivity reactions may occur, involving blood vessels of different sizes. In the second, similar vessel pathology occurs, but direct damage to the parenchyma is also present. In the third, direct tissue damage, immune complexes, and delayed type of hypersensitivity reactions may occur in the same patient.

A. Hypersensitivity Angiitis

Acute vasculitis is the hallmark of a number of syndromes which are categorized under the term hypersensitivity angiitis (Opie, 1924; Clark and Kaplan, 1937; Hawn and Janeway, 1947; McCombs *et al.*, 1956; Rich and Follis, 1940; Rich, 1946–1947). Some of these disorders are caused by the administration of drugs, such as penicillin, sulfonamides, and horse serum, whereas, in others the initiating agent is unknown. Clinically, many organ systems are involved, including skin, kidney, and muscle. Biopsy of the involved tissues may show acute necrotizing vascular lesions involving both capillaries and venules. Precipitating antibody may be found within the wall of involved vessels (McCombs *et al.*, 1956). A large number of polymorphonuclear leukocytes concentrate in the interstitium. There is involvement of the endothelium, the elastica, and the media, with marked disruption and necrosis of all these elements. The interstitium is edematous and, not infrequently, there is thrombosis within the vascular lumen. Hemorrhage into the interstitium is often associated with these findings (McCombs *et al.*, 1956). Release of lysozymes from white cells is presumed to cause injury to the vessel wall (Fell and Dingle, 1963). Fibrinoid necrosis is often present and consists, in part, of the breakdown of collagen fibers (Movat and More, 1957). As described in the previous section, the experimentally produced lesions of immune complex type of hypersensitivity reactions are identical to these lesions. The vasculitis of both the experimentally produced and the drug-induced human disease involves the same size vessels, capillaries, and venules. The lesions are frequently in the same stage of development. No new lesions are found simultaneously with healed, recanalized lesions. It has been assumed, on the basis of these similarities, that the syndromes of drug or serum-induced angiitis probably represent classic manifestations of diffuse immune complex type of hypersensitivity disease in man. However, more evidence is required to support this hypothesis.

Numerous other syndromes have been described with lesions which are histologically similar to the ones in the drug-induced form of hypersensitivity angiitis. The major differences involve the distribution and age of lesions as well as the size of vessels involved. In classic polyarteritis nodosum there are lesions of variable ages and stages of development primarily involving medium size muscular arteries, and causing frequent renal impairment. Similar syndromes have been described with predominant involvement of smaller vessels in such organs as the lungs, the central nervous system, skin, and gastrointestinal tract (Arkin, 1930; Churg and Strauss, 1951; Zeek, 1952, 1953). These distinctions are not without exceptions, however, since cases of polyarteritis nodosum have demonstrated capillary and venule lesions. Moreover, the acute vasculitis of all these diseases are histologically identical.

It would appear, therefore, that the events which caused the vascular damage in these other syndromes may also represent manifestations of hypersensitivity disease. If this assumption were to be proved correct, then the clinical and pathological differences would be a consequence of differences in the duration of antigenic stimulation, which would explain the varied stages of development of the vascular lesions and/or the localizations of the chemical damage to vessels, depending on the tissue involved.

The above points emphasize these factors.

(a) Local vascular phenomena may be important factors in these diseases. Localization of antigen-antibody complexes seems to be dependent on the release of vasoactive peptides (Henson and Cochrane, 1971; Koffler *et al.*, 1967), and also may be a function of differences in filtration coefficient of vessels (Kniker and Cochrane, 1968). The higher the coefficient, the higher the concentration of antigen-antibody complex in the interstitial aspect of the vessel. The more appropriate the ratio of the concentrations of antigen and antibody, the more complement activation, and the more severe the damage to the vessel. The filtration coefficient of the glomerular capillaries could explain the high incidence of glomerulitis in these diseases.

(b) Different antigens in combination with precipitating antibody will cause identical lesions in vessels. Once activation of complement and release of lysozymes is initiated, a common pathway is followed to vascular damage.

(c) Organ dysfunction is determined by the extent and outcome of the vascular damage. The immediate effect of the vascular lesion on the tissue has been demonstrated in sensitized rabbit ears observed *in vivo* (Abell and Schenck, 1938). Injection of the appropriate antigen causes an immediate constriction of the arterioles. This constriction diminishes circulation to the tissues. Vascular constriction is followed by adherence of leukocytes to the vessel wall and agglutination of white cells within the lumen, as well as interstitial edema. Hemorrhage and necrosis, associated with excessive complement activation, further reduces the circulation to the tissues. Once the vascular lesion is created, the effects on the surrounding tissue will depend on the extent to which the particular vessel involved supplied the area. This can be demonstrated by the careful study of biopsy samples from patients with these vasculidities (McCombs *et al.,* 1956; Sokoloff, 1961). The skin may show a great deal of edema, necrosis, hemorrhage, and deposition of fibrin, as well as infiltration with leukocytes; muscles may undergo ischemic degeneration, necrosis, and lysis; and the kidney may show focal glomerulitis. Other areas of the same biopsies, however, will not demonstrate vasculitis, and the tissue will appear normal. It follows, therefore, that the prognosis in these diseases will depend on the extent to which the function of the vital organs involved is permanently impaired.

B. Systemic Lupus Erythematosus

Systemic lupus erythematosus represents a disorder in which both vascular and extravascular disease are present. The initiating event may be dependent on injury to a tissue, with release into the circulation of free DNA or other nuclear material. The cause of the injury remains unknown. Antibodies are formed against the nuclear proteins as well as whole cells resulting in damage to vessels and tissues (Grisham and Churg, 1971; Klemperer *et al.*, 1941). The tissue pathology presumably is localized to those areas where the initial damage occurred. However, once antibodies against nuclear proteins or tissues are formed, these can combine with the appropriate tissue antigens and cause damage by complement activation. The evidence for this type of direct destruction is based on careful studies of involved areas which demonstrate tissue injury in the absence of any vascular pathology (Grishman and Churg, 1971). The vascular lesions, on the other hand, are determined by antigen-antibody complexes formed in the serum (Koffler *et al.*, 1967; Mellors *et al.*, 1957; Morse *et al.*, 1962; Robbins *et al.*, 1957; Schur and Sandson, 1968; Tan *et al.*, 1966; Vazquez and Dixon, 1957). These complexes are filtered across capillaries and venules, such as the glomerulus, and are deposited on the epithelial side. Complement is activated and the typical acute vasculitis is produced. Antinuclear antibodies and complement are found in the vessel wall (Koffler *et al.*, 1967; Vazquez and Dixon, 1957). Nuclear material is present in the fibrinoid necrosis of the lesion (Klemperer *et al.*, 1950).

The vascular lesions are at various stages of development, suggesting that they were produced at different times. This hypothesis is substantiated by the clinical pattern of the disease, which follows a chronic course highlighted by acute episodes. During these episodes, the serum and/or cerebrospinal fluid complement concentration falls (Morse *et al.*, 1962; Petz *et al.*, 1971; Schur and Sandson, 1968; Townes and Stewart, 1965). The organs involved include the kidneys, skin, brain, muscle, intestinal tract, pericardium, myocardium, and pleura. Based on these facts, it has been accepted that the nature of the vascular damage represents another example of the immune complex type of hypersensitivity reaction. The clinical manifestations, however, are more complex than those of the drug-induced hypersensitivity reaction. Tissue dysfunction is not merely dependent on vessel pathology that leads to ischemic damage, but also on direct damage to cells. The event which initiated cellular damage is unknown, though infectious and/or genetic factors may be involved. Once cellular damage is initiated, however, it may perpetuate the disease by liberating nuclear proteins and thus ensure a continuous source of antigen. The prognosis must be assessed, therefore, on the basis of the progressive, continued stimulus for tissue and vessel destruction.

C. Rheumatoid Arthritis

Rheumatoid arthritis represents an example of a disease in which both vascular and tissue pathology are found. The etiology of all the lesions are less well understood. Vasculitis is present, involving not only capillaries and venules, but also arterioles and small arteries (Kulka, 1959 a, b; Scott *et al.*, 1961; Sokoloff and Bunin, 1957; Sokoloff, 1961). The pathology is quite variable. The lesions are in different stages of development, from acute to healing (Cruickshank, 1954; Sokoloff, 1961), and the classic characteristics of vasculitis are present: necrosis of endothelium, elastica, and media, cellular infiltration, and fibrinoid necrosis. The fibrinoid necrosis contains depolymerized ground substance (Ziff *et al.*, 1953). The cellular infiltration in the acute necrotizing forms shows polymorphonuclear leukocytes (as in the acute necrotizing lesions of lupus erythematosus or drug-induced vasculitis). There is evidence that some of these lesions are initiated by antigen-antibody activation of the complement system. In the joint cavity, where damage is most prominent, the concentration of complement in the synovial fluid is decreased (Klemperer *et al.*, 1941). Immunoglobulins and complement are found in the synovial tissue itself (Brandt *et al.*, 1968; Fish *et al.*, 1966; Rodman *et al.*, 1967); moreover, as in lupus erythematosus, complement and gamma globulin are also found in many of the extrasynovial vascular lesions. These lesions then are morphologically similar to the vasculitis seen in the immune complex type of hypersensitivity reactions. The plasma may contain antigamma globulin antibodies complexed with the appropriate gamma globulin (rheumatoid factor). The concentration of rheumatoid factor is important since the frequency of arteritis and acute inflammation of capillaries and venules (the vascular inflammation involves not only the synovium, but also skeletal muscle, heart, skin, and peripheral nerves) is greater with elevated titers of rheumatoid factor (Cruickshank, 1954; Epstein and Engelman, 1959).

It is not certain if the disease itself is initiated by injury to some tissues, such as synovium, with subsequent release of an antigen into the circulation, as may occur in lupus erythematosus. Moreover, the explanation for the formation of antigamma globulin antibody remains a mystery. Knowledge of the origin of the rheumatoid factor is most important, since the complex itself may be expected to cause vascular damage through activation of the complement system independent of rheumatoid disease. As in lupus erythematosus, the tissue may serve to provide a continued supply of antigen from the synovial tissue and further the disease process. In favor of this possibility is the observation that some patients with rheumatoid arthritis may develop antinuclear antibodies, some found in the synovial tissues.

There are other vascular lesions in the synovium, however, which are histologically different from the lesions of the immune complex type of hypersensitivity. In these lesions there is cellular infiltration of the stroma which is primarily of the mononuclear type, as seen in lesions produced by the delayed type of hypersensitivity. Evidence for the role of delayed hypersensitivity in the pathogenesis of this disease, however, is not available.

A most intriguing peculiarity in this disease, which may have some bearing on the pathogenesis, is the relationship between the tissue pathology and the vascular damage. The pathology of tissues, such as skin, nerve, or muscle where acute necrotizing lesions exist, is similar to the vascular lesions of the Arthus type, as observed in drug-induced vasculitis or lupus erythematosus: focal vascular lesions associated with focal tissue pathology. Necrosis and fibrosis of synovium also occur in relation to focal vascular damage. However, one of the predominant aspects of the synovial pathology is proliferation in association with synovial vessels which appear morphologically normal. This finding suggests that this characteristic parenchymal pathology may not be a direct function of vessel damage. Tissue pathology, however, could be a consequence of events occurring in the interstitial fluid phase. It has been suggested that damage to synovium and cartilage can follow activation of the complement system in the joint fluid, independent of any vascular damage (Ruddy and Austen, 1970). This hypothesis is based principally on observations of the destructive effect on bone culture of presumed activation of complement and lysozymes in the extracellular medium (Fell and Weiss, 1965). This mechanism, however, could explain the synovial and cartilage destruction only after the appropriate stimuli for complement fixation were present, i.e., after the disease process had been initiated and antigen-antibody complexes had been formed. The initiating event in the tissue disorder, therefore, must be the result of direct insult to the cells themselves, perhaps by a virus. Direct cellular insult could lead to proliferation, damage, and release of antigens into the circulation and interstitial fluid. Release of antigen, with subsequent antibody formation, could account for some of the lesions which resemble immune complex-induced vasculitis. No single mechanism, however, can account for the varied pathology in this disease.

IV. Tissue–Circulatory Imbalance

Thus far, the pathology of tissues or vessels has been described primarily in terms of the histological and immuno-chemical aspects of the lesions. In the present section, I will attempt to present data on the extent to which one of the functional aspects of vascular physiology presented in Section I has been affected in rheumatoid arthritis. Focal or segmental lesions are not necessarily associated with whole tissue disease, since a great number of vessels supply a unit volume of tissue. This situation makes it possible to quantitatively diminish the microcirculation to a tissue without rendering it hypoxic and affecting its function. Therefore, vessel damage is clinically significant only if it causes malfunction by sufficiently disturbing the balance between blood supply and cellular requirement. This imbalance can be caused not only by vessel damage, but also can result from an increase in cellular demand above the potential compensatory capabilities of the microcirculation. The proliferative synovium in rheumatoid arthritis, which is known to possess an increased demand for oxygen (Dingle and Page Thomas, 1956), can also be shown to have an abnormal functional relationship to its blood supply (Falchuk *et al.*, 1970). Therefore, although rheumatoid arthritis may not be representative of diseases where vascular damage is the primary event, a definition of an abnormality in the functional aspects of vascular physiology in this disease may serve to focus attention on the need for similar definitions in the other diseases.

The joint represents an ideal experimental cavity in which to define the relationship between tissue demand and blood supply. It can be assumed that the synovial fluid is in equilibrium with joint regional mixed venous blood (Falchuk *et al.*, 1970), thus making it possible to use the Fick equation to study the relative tissue perfusion.

The relationship between the blood flow to a tissue and the oxygen consumption of that tissue determines the arterial–venous oxygen content difference. This concept was defined by Fick:

$$\dot{Q} = \dot{V}_{O_2}/Ca_{O_2} - C\bar{v}_{O_2}$$

where
$\dot{Q}$ = blood flow/min
$\dot{V}_{O_2}$ = oxygen consumption/min
Ca_{O_2} = arterial oxygen content in volumes percent
$C\bar{v}_{O_2}$ = mixed regional venous oxygen content

By rearranging one can obtain

$$\dot{Q}/\dot{V}_{O_2} = 1/Ca_{O_2} - C\bar{v}_{O_2}$$

This rearrangement gives a term which can be interpreted as representing a ratio of flow $\dot{Q}$, to demand for oxygen $\dot{V}_{O_2}$. The terms, Ca_{O_2} and $C\bar{v}_{O_2}$ were obtained by taking a constant arterial content and assuming equilibrium of synovial fluid oxygen partial pressures with that of regional mixed venous, respectively. Once values for arterial and venous oxygen contents were determined, the ratio of supply of blood to metabolic demand $\dot{Q}/\dot{V}_{O_2}$ can be calculated for different joints (Falchuk *et al.*, 1970). Table II shows the values for synovial fluid P_{O_2} in two groups of patients. The values in the control group are from patients with osteoarthritis, whereas the values in the second group are from patients with rheumatoid arthritis. The table also shows the calculated ratios $\dot{Q}/\dot{V}_{O_2}$ derived from $1/A - V$. The joints from patients with rheumatoid arthritis have lower ratios than those from patients with osteoarthritis. Based on *in vitro* studies comparing oxygen consumption of synovium from patients with osteoarthritis and rheumatoid arthritis per milligram of tissue nitrogen (Dingle and Page Thomas, 1956), it is possible to calculate a relative value for $\dot{Q}$, as shown in the table. The calculated effective blood flow, $\dot{Q}$, is greater for the joints of the patients with rheumatoid arthritis. This increase in both oxygen consumption and effective blood flow has recently been confirmed by *in vivo* studies in man (Dick *et al.*, 1970; Goetzl *et al.*, 1971; St. Onge *et al.*, 1968). In the presence of an increased oxygen consumption, one would predict an increase in blood flow to maintain a constant tissue oxygenation. An absolute increase in blood flow was confirmed. If the assumptions concerning the equality of synovial fluid P_{O_2}

TABLE II

METABOLIC–CIRCULATORY IMBALANCE IN RHEUMATOID ARTHRITIS

	P_{O_2} (mm Hg)	$\frac{1}{A - V}$	$\dot{V}_{O_2}$ [a]	Calculated[a] $\dot{Q}$	Measured[a] $\dot{Q}$
Control (osteoarthritis)	Above 37	0.2 — 0.6	1	1	1
Rheumatoid arthritis	Below 27	Less than 0.1	20[b]	4[c]	3[c], 2[d]

[a] Values are relative to *control*.
[b] From Dingle and Page (1956).
[c] From Dick *et al.* (1970).
[d] From Goetzl *et al.* (1971).

with that of regional blood are correct, however, then the decrease in synovial fluid P_{O_2} in the joint fluid from patients with rheumatoid arthritis would indicate that blood flow does not increase proportionately to oxygen consumption. The overall increase in blood flow, therefore, is insufficient to meet the demand for oxygen of the diseased tissues. The effect of the abnormal relationship between effective blood flow and tissue requirement on the disease process is not known. The high synovial fluid hydrogen ion concentration which is found in this disorder, and which is partially accounted for by the imbalance of flow (Falchuk *et al.*, 1970), may affect tissue activity and be harmful to the cells.

The local tissue environment has not been defined in the other syndromes discussed in this chapter. It is assumed, on the basis of the pathology, that the end result of the vascular damage is a decrease in either the removal or delivery of important metabolites from cells. The failure to perform this function leads to cellular dysfunction and disease. Techniques to study the functional relationship between vessel and tissue are primitive, making it difficult to examine this assumption. Since treatment, theoretically, might be directed at the reestablishment of an adequate circulatory tissue relationship, the importance of developing techniques to study microcirculatory function in disease needs to be emphasized.

References

Abell, R. G., and Schenck, H. P. (1938). Microscopic observations on the behavior of living blood vessels of the rabbit during the reaction of anaphylaxis. *J. Immunol.* **34,** 195–213.

Arkin, A. (1930). A clinical and pathological study of pericarditis nodosa. *Amer J. Pathol.* **6,** 401–426.

Arthus, M. (1903). Injections répétees de sérum de cheval chez le lapin. *C. R. Soc. Biol.* **55,** 817–820.

Austen, K. F. (1971). Inborn and acquired abnormalities of the complement system of man. *Johns Hopkins Med. J.* **128,** 57–74.

Brandt, K. D., Cathcart, E. S., and Cohen, A. S. (1968). Studies of immune deposits in synovial membranes and corresponding synovial fluids. *J. Lab. Clin. Med.* **72,** 631–647.

Churg, J., and Strauss, L. (1951). Allergic granulomatosis allergic angiitis and periarteritis nodosa. *Amer. J. Pathol.* **27,** 277–302.

Clark, E., and Kaplan, B. I. (1937). Endocardial arterial and other mesenchymal alterations associated with serum disease in man. *Arch. Pathol.* **24,** 458–475.

Cochrane, C. G., and Müller-Eberhard, H. J. (1968). The derivation of two distinct anaphylatoxin activities from the third and fifth components of human complement. *J. Exp. Med.* **127,** 371–386.

Cruickshank, B. (1954). The arteries of rheumatoid arthritis. *Ann. Rheum. Dis.* **13,** 136–146.

Dias da Silva, W., and Lepow, I. H. (1967). Complement as a mediator of inflammation. II. Biological properties of anaphylatoxin prepared with purified components of human complement. *J. Exp. Med.* **125,** 921–946.

Dick, W. C., Whaley, K., St. Onge, R. A., Downie, W. W., Boyle, J. A., Nuki, G., Gillespie, F. C., and Buchanan, W. W. (1970). Clinical studies on inflammation in human knee joints: Xenon (^{133} Xe) clearances correlated with clinical assessment in various arthritis and studies on the effect of intra-articular administered hydrocortisone in rheumatoid arthritis. *Clin. Sci.* **38,** 123–133.

Dingle, J. T. M., and Page Thomas, D. P. (1956). *In vitro* studies of human synovial membrane. A metabolic comparison of normal and rheumatoid tissue. *Brit. J. Exp. Pathol.* **37,** 318–323.

Epstein, W. V., and Engleman, E. P. (1959). The relation of rheumatoid factor content of serum to clinical nervous manifestations. *Arthritis Rheum.* **2,** 250–258.

Falchuk, K. H., Goetzl, E. J., and Kulka, J. P. (1970). Respiratory gases of synovial fluids; an approach to synovial tissue circulatory-metabolic imbalance in rheumatoid arthritis. *Amer. J. Med.* **49,** 223–231.

Fell, H. B., and Dingle, J. T. (1963). Studies on the mode of action of excess of vitamins A6, lysosomal protease and the degeneration of cartilage matrix. *Biochem. J.* **87,** 403–408.

Fell, H. B., and Weiss, L. (1965). The effect of antiserum, alone and with hydrocortisone on foetal mouse bones in culture. *J. Exp. Med.* **121,** 551–560.

Fish, A. J., Michael, A. F., Gewirz, H., and Gord, R. A. (1966). Immunopathologic changes in rheumatoid arthritis synovium. *Arthritis Rheum.* **9,** 267–280.

Goetzl, E. J., Falchuk, K. H., Zeiger, L. S., Sullivan, A. L., Hebert, C. L., Adams, J. P., and Decker, J. L. (1971). A physiological approach to the assessment of disease activity in rheumatoid arthritis. *J. Clin. Invest.* **50,** 1167–1180

Grisham, E., and Churg, J. (1971). Connective tissue in systemic lupus erythematosus. Demonstration of disseminated vascular and extravascular "wire loop" deposits. *Arch. Pathol.* **19,** 156–166.

Hawn, C. V., and Janeway, C. A. (1947). Histological and serological sequences in experimental hypersensitivity. *J. Exp. Med.* **85,** 571–590.

Henson, P. M., and Cochrane, C. G. (1971). Acute immune complex disease in rabbits. The role of complement and of a leukocyte-dependent release of vasoactive amines from platelets. *J. Exp. Med.* **133,** 554–571.

Jensen, J. (1967). Anaphylatoxin in its relation to the complement system. *Science* **155,** 1122–1123.

Klemperer, P., Gueft, B., Lee, S. L., Lenchtenberger, C., and Pollester, A. W. (1950). Cytochemical changes of acute lupus erythematosus *A. M. A. Arch. Pathol.* **49,** 503–516.

Klemperer, P. L., Pollock, A. D., and Boehr, G. (1941). Pathology of disseminated lupus erythematosus. *Arch. Pathol.* **32,** 569-631.

Kniker, W. T., and Cochrane, C. G. (1968). The localization of circulating immune complexes in experimental serum sickness. The role of vasoactive amines and hydrodynamic forces. *J. Exp. Med.* **127,** 119–136.

Koffler, D., Schur, P. H., and Kunkel, H. G. (1967). Immunological studies concerning the nephritis of systemic lupus erythematosus. *J. Exp. Med.* **126,** 607–624.

Kulka, J. P. (1959a). The pathogenesis of rheumatoid arthritis. *J. Chronic Dis.* **10,** 388–408.

Kulka, J. P. (1959b). The vascular lesions associated with rheumatoid arthritis. *Bull. Rheum. Dis.* **10,** 201–202.

McCombs, R. P., Patterson, J. F., and MacMahon, H. E. (1956). Syndromes associated with "allergic" vasculitis. *N. Engl. J. Med.* **255,** 251–261.

Mellors, N. C., Ortega, L. G., and Holman, H. R. (1957). Role of gamma globulins in pathogenesis of renal lesions in systemic lupus erythematosus and chronic membranous glomerulonephritis with an observation on the lupus erythematosus cell reaction. *J. Exp. Med.* **106,** 191–202.

Morse, J. H., Müller-Eberhard, H. J., and Kunkel, H. G. (1962). Antinuclear factors and serum complement in systemic lupus erythematosus. *Bull. N. Y. Acad. Med.* [2] **38,** 641–651.

Movat, H. Z., and More, R. H. (1957). The nature and origin of fibrinoid. *Amer. J. Clin. Pathol.* **28,** 331–353.

Opie, E. L. (1924). Pathogenesis of specific inflammatory reaction of immunized animals (Arthus phenomenon). The relation of local "sensitization" to immunity. *J. Immunol.* **9,** 259–268.

Petz, L. D., Sharp, G. C., Cooper, N. R., and Irvin, W. S. (1971). Serum and cerebral spinal fluid complement and serum autoantibodies in systemic lupus erythematosus. *Medicine Baltimore* **50,** 259–276.

Rich, A. R. (1946–1947). Hypersensitivity in disease with special reference to periarteritis nodosa, rheumatic fever, disseminated lupus erythematosus and rheumatoid arthritis. *Harvey Lect.* **42,** 106–147.

Rich, A. R., and Follis, R. H. (1940). Study of the site of sensitivity of the Arthus phenomenon. *Bull. Johns Hopkins Hosp.* **66,** 106–122.

Robbins, W. C., Holman, H. R., Dercher, H. R., and Kunkel, H. G. (1957). Complement fixation with cell nuclei and DNA in lupus erythematosus. *Proc. Soc. Exp. Biol. Med.* **96,** 575–579.

Rodman, W. S., Williams, R. C., Jr., Bilka, P. J., and Müller-Eberhard, H. J. (1967). Immunofluorescent localization of the third and the fourth component of complement in synovial tissue from patients with rheumatoid arthritis. *J. Lab. Clin. Med.* **64,** 141–150.

Ruddy, S., and Austen, K. F. (1970). The complement system in rheumatoid synovitis. An analysis of complement component activities in rheumatoid synovial fluids. *Arthritis Rheum.* 13, 713–723.

Schur, P. H., and Sandson, J. (1968). Immunologic factors and clinical activity in systemic lupus erythematosus. *N. Engl. J. Med.* **278,** 533–538.

Scott, J. J., Hourihane, D. D., Doyle, F. H., Steiner, R. E., Laws, J. W., Dixon, A., and Bywaters, E. G. L. (1961). Digital arteries in rheumatoid disease. *Ann. Rheum. Dis.* **20,** 224–234.

Sokoloff, L. (1961). Biopsy in rheumatic diseases. *Med. Clin. N. Amer.* **45,** 1171–1180.

Sokoloff, L., and Bunin, J. J. (1957). Vascular lesions in rheumatoid arthritis. *J. Chronic Dis.* **5,** 668–687.

Stelos, P., and Talmage, D. W. (1957). The separation by starch electrophoresis of two antibodies to sheep red cells differing in hemolytic efficiency. *J. Infec. Dis.* **100,** 126–135.

Stetson, C. A. (1951). Similarities in the mechanisms determining the Arthus and Schwartzman phenomena. *J. Exp. Med.* **94,** 347–358.

St. Onge, R. A., Dick, W. C., Bell, G., and Boyle, J. A. (1968). Radioactive xenon (^{133}Xe) disappearance rates from the synovial cavity of the human knee joint in normal and arthritic subjects. *Ann. Rheum. Dis.* **27,** 163–166.

Talmage, D. W., Freter, G. G., and Taliafferro, W. H. (1956). Two antibodies of related specificity but different hemolytic efficiency separated by centrifugation. *J. Infec. Dis.* **98,** 300–305.

Tan, E. M., Schur, P. H., Carr, R. I., and Kunkel, H. G. (1966). Deoxyribonucleic acid (DNA) and antibodies to DNA in the serum of patients with systemic lupus erythematosus. *J. Clin. Invest.* **45,** 1732–1740.

Townes, A. S., and Stewart, C. R. (1965). Methods for the estimation of the second component and third component complex of complement in the serum of patients with systemic lupus erythematosus. *Bull. Johns Hopkins Hosp.* **117,** 331–347.

Uhr, J. W. (1966). Delayed hypersensitivity. *Physiol. Rev.* **46,** 359–419.

Vazquez, J. J., and Dixon, J. F. (1957). Immunohistochemical study of lesions in rheumatic fever, systemic lupus erythematosus and rheumatic arthritis. *Lab. Invest.* **6,** 205–217.

Waksman, B. H. (1960). *Cell. Aspects Immunity, Ciba Fund. Symp., 1959* pp. 280–322.

Waksman, B. H. (1961). *In* "Mechanism of Cell and Tissue Damage Produced by Immune Reactions" (P. Grabar and P. Miescher, eds.), pp. 147–160. Schwabe, Basel.

Ward, P. A., and Cochrane, C. G. (1965). Bound complement and immunologic injury of blood vessels. *J. Exp. Med.* **131,** 215–234.

Ward, P. A., and Newman, L. J. (1969). A neutrophil chemotactic factor from human C′5. *J. Immunol.* **102,** 93–99.

Ward, P. A., Cochrane, C. G., and Müller-Eberhard, H. J. (1966). Further studies on the chemotactic factor of complement and its formation *in vivo. Immunology* **11,** 141–153.

Zeek, P. M. (1952). Periarteritis nodosa: A critical review. *Amer. J. Clin. Pathol.* **22,** 777–796.

Zeek, P. M. (1953). Periarteritis nodosa and other forms of necrotizing angiitis. *N. Engl. J. Med.* **248,** 764–772.

Ziff, M., Kantor, T., Bien, E., and Smith, A. (1953). Study on the composition of fibrinoid material of the subcutaneous nodule of rheumatoid arthritis. *J. Clin. Invest.* **32,** 1253–1259.

8 MICROCIRCULATION IN PERIPHERAL ARTERIAL ISCHEMIC DISEASE

ROBERT L. DILTS, M.D.

I. Introduction

A valuable relationship between the microcirculation and the function of living human cells becomes apparent since these variously combined cells depend on the microvasculature for their metabolism. Guyton (1971) states that a functional cell of the body is rarely more than 20 to 30 μm from a capillary. Peripheral vascular diseases result primarily from functional cellular loss in the extremities. Resulting diseases of arterial branches and venous tributaries of the vascular system are described in several texts available today (Abramson, 1962; Allen *et al.*, 1962; Burch and Phillips, 1963; Winsor, 1959). The more commonly encountered ischemic diseases include atherosclerotic arterial occlusive disease, thromboangiitis obliterans, Raynaud's phenomenon, diabetes mellitus, scleroderma, and frostbite. Collectively referring to these diseases, the term ischemic disease is preferable to arterial occlusive disease, since the latter term should be employed only after arteriography has substantiated the presence and location of a stenotic lesion. Ischemia refers to a reduced amount of blood in an area due to functional vasoconstriction or to obstruction of a supply vessel. Although peripheral ischemic disease refers to conditions of both upper and lower extremities, the preponderance of ischemic limb disease occurs in the lower extremity.

II. Anatomical Studies

Dible (1954) investigated limbs amputated as a result of severe ischemia or gangrene. He examined them by high pressure arteriography at 15 lb/in^2. (Dible, 1967) and revealed in limbs from atherosclerotic patients "an abundance of potential vascular supply" in the foot where the arteries were anatomically preserved. Patent digital vessels were demonstrated in limbs where major arteries had been occluded. This patency was most frequently observed in limbs which had been associated clinically with long-standing intermittent claudication and pathologically with occlusive lesions and gangrene. He concluded that only the vessel function was lost since the vessels were preserved in the digits.

Thromboangiitis obliterans delineates thrombosis and obliteration of the small- and medium-sized vessels. In the acute stage, the exudative reaction may be more prominent in small veins than in arteries. The microvasculature is involved at the outset of the disease. The obstructive effects produce ischemia and usually tissue loss (McMillan, 1962).

Scleroderma is identified by a hyperplasia and thickening of the intimal cells of the skin arterioles along with a thickening of the fibrous tissue of the wall. These changes may cause intermittent (Raynaud's phenomenon) or persistent vasospasm (Allen *et al.*, 1962, pp. 149–150).

Raynaud's phenomenon occurs as an intermittent partial or complete vasoconstrictive occlusion of the arterioles in the skin, fingers, or toes. It usually occurs secondary to an associated disease such as lupus erythematosis, scleroderma, multiple myeloma (Morris, 1968), rheumatoid arthritis (Gifford, 1970), lymphosarcoma, ergot poisoning, and scalenus anticus syndrome (McMillan *et al.*, 1962).

The microangiopathic study of the limbs in diabetes mellitus has centered around the nonspecific thickening of the basement membrane of capillaries in skeletal muscle and fat (Siperstein *et al.*, 1966). The angiopathy of the diabetic has been related to the reduction in function associated with atherosclerosis (Bloodworth, 1967). However, "glomerulus" lesions of toe nail bed capillaries have been reported with coinvolvement of the large vessels of the lower extremities and thus may be evidence of diabetic microangiopathy (Chazan *et al.*, 1970). The foregoing forms of ischemic limb disease relate to metabolic and hereditary influence. The ischemia from these diseases frequently progresses to gangrene.

Frostbite presents a form of ischemia initiated environmentally. The involvement of the microvasculature here is in the form of thrombosis, direct cellular dehydration, enzymatic effects, or the effect of ice crystals. The extent of vascular damage may be the deciding factor in tissue survival. Cells frequently recover if the blood supply to them is adequate (Sumner *et al.*, 1971).

Trauma may cause ischemia affecting the small vessels, resulting in thrombosis. Nerve damage may contribute to vasospasm. Nonpenetrating, repeated injury may occlude the microvasculature in the hands as in pneumatic hammer disease (Horwitz, 1971). Posttraumatic reflex sympathetic dystrophy (Sudeck's atrophy) may be related to vasospastic disturbances of the bone blood supply. In the later stages of the disease, the blood supply diminishes though it may or may not be initiated by trauma (Domb and Fried, 1959).

Ischemia may be the result of inflammatory conditions such as ischemic thrombophlebitis. The ischemic phase is in the form of an obstruction to the arterial flow and is not directly due to an alteration in the microvasculature (Haimovici, 1966).

Thyroid function and its relationship to atherosclerosis has been recounted extensively by Fisher (1967). Hyperlipidemia has been investigated for its part in the development of atherosclerosis. Type IV familial hyperlipoproteinemia generally does not have the microangiopathy of diabetes mellitus as a complication (Sanbar, 1969). Nail fold venule dilatation has been reported in Types III and IV hyperlipoproteinemia (Kuo *et al.*, 1970). Buchanan and Humpston (1968) suggest that a high correlation exists between collagen diseases and the presence of hemorrhages from the tips of nail fold capillaries with greater than 28 μm loop diameter.

III. Pathophysiology

The microvasculature of the body and particularly that related to the peripheral vasculature has a regulatory function in controlling the flow of blood from the arterial supply to the venous return. As the arteriolar pressure drops, the percentage of functioning capillary beds reduces to an amount unable to maintain the metabolism of the tissue supplied—the point of critical minimal function. In chronic arterial insufficiency, the blood may flow through shunting vessels when shunt systems are available, such as the arteriovenous anastomoses. If there is sufficient rise in arteriolar pressure, blood would again be available to the capillary network (Harpuder *et al.*, 1940). In diabetic gangrene, the first evidence of primary degeneration is in the intima of preglomic arterioles, while the intima of the afferent artery remains intact (Popoff, 1934).

There has been much controversy regarding the etiology of diabetic mononeuropathy. Occlusion of nutrient vessels to the involved nerve remains the most likely cause. Polyneuropathy involves the distal portions of many nerves, relating to varied clinical manifestations. Pregnancy and the taking of oral contraceptives have been implicated as a possible cause of recurrent symmetrical polyneuropathy (Calderón-González *et al.,* 1970). The symmetrical polyneuropathy of the diabetic has been suggested to have a metabolic etiology as determined from clinical and pathological evaluation (Dreyfus, 1967). Lundborg and Brånemark (1968) have revealed that, experimentally, the microcirculation of a peripheral nerve has an extrinsic and an intrinsic system of vessels. Although these systems are independent, they are also integrated. As a result, with the loss of all but one nutrient supply artery, the nerve can still function and regeneration of a traumatized nerve may, therefore, be a possibility. Total nutrient vessel destruction was necessary to stop blood flow in the intrinsic system. It may be that the explanation for the development of diabetic neuropathy lies in the fact that ischemia of the vasa nervorum develops slowly. Dible (1967, p. 94) reports advanced nerve atrophy is absent in less than one-fourth of his series with atherosclerotic ischemia. The greatest incidence of the most severe atrophic lesions was among diabetic subjects. This lesion appeared more often in the digital nerves compared to the posterior and plantar nerves. It would appear that, possibly, loss of pressure in nutrient vessels to the microcirculation of digital nerves whether in a diabetic or arteriosclerotic nondiabetic may be a contributing factor in the development of neuropathies.

Precapillary sphincters respond to sufficient pressure by opening (Johnson, 1968). However, we have every reason to believe all of the sphincters do not normally open to the exact same pressure since a varying number of capillary systems will be functioning from time to time in the same area (Rushmer, 1970). The hypotension associated with ischemia of the skin causes a diversion of blood from the capillary network through arcades to arteriovenous shunts (Zweifach, 1961). If the hypotension drops far enough the arteriovenous shunts close and, unless the critical perfusion is reestablished, degeneration of the area will occur.

Not all tissues of the extremities are supplied with precapillary sphincters. However, intraluminal pressure is necessary to maintain the functioning lumen of any vessel which does not have sufficient wall rigidity to withstand the transmural pressure of extravascular tissues. It is conceivable this could be a negative pressure if the supplied tissue is under negative pressure. This does not occur normally in the extremities. When these concepts are applied to peripheral ischemic diseases the deterioration of a given tissue depends upon (a) the rate of lowering of the pressure to the extremity and (b) the efficiency of the shunt systems. It should be noted that intraluminal pressure measurement of human ischemic tissues is impractical to obtain at this time due to the potential deleterious effects of trauma to such tissue.

It is obvious that the way to open the active flow channels is to increase the arterial systolic pressure. Thoma (1884) intimated this when he showed that the growth of collaterals was in ratio to the blood flow through them. Strandness (1969a) was of similar thinking when he observed that the development of collateral circulation might be encouraged if the systemic blood pressure were elevated. Maximal hyperemia has been measured in calf muscles after walking. The results lend support to the concept that new and/or larger collaterals may develop. By walking, a slight rise in the systemic blood pressure was conveyed repeatedly to a distal region of "pathologically" low pressure and thus improved the collateral circulation in the calf muscle (Alpert *et al.*, 1969). Rubor of the dependent foot in occlusive arterial disease is further evidence of increased pressure. This deep red color is considered to be due to the fact that the shunt systems of the foot permit the standing venous pressure to be added to the much reduced arterial pressure in sufficient amount to open the capillary networks. The effect is reversed in the elevated limb. Venous pressure is not added. The arterial pressure is ineffective against gravity and the blood drains, resulting in foot pallor.

There is much controversy concerning the cause of peripheral arterial occlusive disease. The known variables involved include hyperlipidemia (Sanbar, 1969), diabetes mellitus (Albrink *et al.*, 1963), hypothyroidism (Guyton, 1971, p. 912), smoking (Lord, 1965), genetic factors (Kuo, 1971), and the deficiency of several trace mineral elements, potassium, copper, and chromium (Schroeder, 1971). Nevertheless, there is one factor common to all peripheral vascular disease. Sooner or later, unless brought under control, there will be eventual tissue loss. The correction of the metabolic factor alone may be sufficient to sustain the recovery process in the individual with adequate cardiac output, if the recovery process can occur faster than the rate of tissue deterioration. However, in the patient where the reverse is true and where advanced years have permitted extensive atherosclerosis, correction of the metabolic factors is usually not sufficient to reverse the process or to bring it under control.

IV. Clinical Evaluation of Peripheral Ischemic Disease

The ideal approach to the diagnosis and treatment of a disease involves objectively collecting evidence of the disease state and monitoring the patient's progress to recovery. Clinically, the availability of the skin for observation is of utmost importance in the diagnosis of peripheral ischemic disease. Because of the poor recovery nature of ischemic tissue, atraumatic, nonintrusive methods of diagnosis are suggested.

A. Skin as a Monitor of Function

The skin, particularly that of the finger and toe pads, has an abundant supply of arteriovenous shunts (Grant and Bland, 1931), capillary loops, and subpapillary venous plexuses (Greenfield, 1963). Vessels of the digit pads best reflect the function of the vascular system upstream. The principle physical effect of reduced function is a pressure drop from (1) occlusive disease, (2) reduced cardiac output, and (3) vasoconstrictive agents, such as adrenaline, noradrenaline (Edholm *et al.*, 1956), and vasopressin (Kitchin, 1957).

B. Clinical Observations

Clinical observation of the skin is extremely valuable with regard to microcirculatory function in peripheral ischemic disease and involves: (1) color in the dependent, horizontal, and elevated positions, (2) discoloration due to arterial infarct, embolism, or necrosis, (3) presence of hair and its extent of growth, (4) dryness of the skin of the foot and ankle, (5) condition of nails, including an evaluation of the rate of growth, (6) presence of ischemia-related processes, such as delayed recovery of traumatized skin, and (7) temperature of the distal portions of the extremities, particularly of the digit pads. These clinical features should be monitored during the course of treatment. The function of the microvasculature may also be monitored at the digit pads by examination of the volume pulse utilizing a photocell and light source sensor (Hertzman, 1938). By this technique the extent of the opacity or volume pulse in the highly microvascular digit pad may be observed and recorded for evaluation.

C. Additional Methods of Flow Evaluation

Plethysmography involves the recording of volume variations in a portion of the limb due to modification of the circulation. The mercury-in-silastic strain gauge method of plethysmography uses a mercury-filled silastic tube to facilitate recording variations in the composite volume change of the tissue beneath it (Strandness and Bell, 1965).

Another method of digital plethysmography uses a 4-ml volume of the distal phalanx to determine the pulse volume changes of the digit. An air-filled acetate cup is applied to this finger volume. Recordings are made of direct volume change per pulse beat. Venous occlusion plethysmography, in addition to the air-filled cup, uses the application of a venous occluding cuff just proximal to the compartment. Recordings from the air-filled cup can be calibrated to measure pulse volume (Winsor, 1959, p. 181).

Impedance plethysmography employs the use of an instrument designed to record variations in resistive impedance to the flow of alternating current through living tissue. Nyboer (1959) made volume pulse recordings using the impedance and direct compartment methods simultaneously from the same area of a digit. The curves on both records are remarkably similar, indicating their volume changes are proportional.

The three systems of plethysmography have these two facts in common: (1) their records are influenced by the volume pulse of the digital arteries and (2) the application of the sensing devices is next to impossible in the severely painful digit. They are of little value in determining the efficiency of the microvasculature of the ischemic digit.

The use of the Doppler principle to detect blood velocity ultrasonically is limited to larger vessels where flow velocity is at least 6 cm/sec (Strandness, 1969a, pp. 368–404). The velocity of blood in the microvasculature is less than 1 cm/sec (Winsor, 1959, p. 59). The Doppler ultrasonic method has limited value in evaluating the microvascular flow because of the low velocity of blood through the microvessels.

Isotopes of sodium (Kety, 1948), iodine (Bauer *et al.*, 1956; Brakkee and Vendrik, 1969), and xenon (Lassen, 1964) have been used to measure blood flow and volume of shunt vessels and capillary systems. Xenon has been used as an indicator of vascular flow in muscles (Lassen, 1964). Use of radioisotopes has not proved valuable in the determination of flow volumes in human ischemic microvasculature.

Arteriography is of greatest benefit to the vascular surgeon, since it pinpoints the location of vascular occlusion (Coran and Warren, 1966). Equipment and methods have been improved to permit arteriograms of very small vessels. Use of magnification techniques and the availability of 0.1 to 0.3 mm focal spot x-ray targets make possible the viewing of the microvessels (Isard and Cullinan, 1967). However, the inherent discomfort, risks, and added radiation do not make it a desirable technique for frequent studies in monitoring the progress of treatment.

Indicator–dilution studies are useful in determining limb blood flow, but are not particularly so in the study of the microcirculation of an ischemic limb. Again, this method is limited in its frequency of safe use because of the placement of needles in the femoral vein and artery (Rushmer, 1970).

Postexercise hyperemia is a useful test relating to the extent of the ischemia produced by a stenotic lesion upstream. Blood pressure is determined at the ankle before and after exercise. Digit volume pulse changes correlate with the ankle blood pressure reduction as the blood is shunted from the foot to the calf in arterial occlusive disease. If the equipment is available, this test is valuable in determining the capacity of the collaterals to supply calf muscles and the foot during exercise (Strandness, 1969a, pp. 368–404). It does not directly relate to microvascular flow in a particular digit.

The use of thermography has been suggested to substantiate the distribution of skin temperature variation in Raynaud's disease, thromboangiitis obliterans, atherosclerosis, and embolism (Buwalda, 1969). Skin temperature relates to the microvascular flow and lends validity to this method of evaluating the microcirculation. However, the instrumentation involved is available at this time only in large medical centers.

No information is available which describes an easily applied atraumatic, nonintrusive method of determining accurately calibrated flow in the microvascular network from the arterioles through the shunts and capillaries to the venules of ischemic digits.

D. Tests of Proprioceptive Sense

The degree of peripheral neuropathy, as pertains to the vibratory sense, may be measured by a device which determines the percent of vibratory sense loss (Vibrometer)* (Winsor, 1959, p. 337). The loss of this proprioceptive sense (pallanesthesia) occurs bilaterally in pernicious anemia, diabetic neuritis (Winsor, 1959, p. 337), and hypothyroidism (DeJong, 1967) and unilaterally in ischemic neuritis from poor blood flow or trauma to nerves (Winsor, 1959, p. 337). The vibratory sense should be evaluated at the ulnar styloid processes and the medial malleoli.

* Electro-Medical Engineering Company, Burbank, California.

Ability of the patient to discriminate between smooth and rough surfaces is another valuable test of proprioception. A ⅜-in. diameter carriage bolt 3 in. long is an ideal instrument for this purpose. When the bolt is gently but firmly drawn across the digit pad, inability to distinguish the threads indicates loss of tactile sense. Long nerve fibers are nourished by intrafascicular microvessels supplied by adjacent arteries (Lundborg and Brånemark, 1968). Since the arterial supply relates to nerve function, the neuropathies also relate to small vessel failure (Burch and Phillips, 1963, p. 1218).

E. Practical Microvascular Monitoring

It is evident from clinical experience that skin color, temperature, and the opacity pulse are the three most rewarding indicators over the course of time. Improvement in these qualities is immediately discernible and the opacity pulse is recordable.

1. *Color Variation*

The variation in the color quality of the skin ranges from pallor through normal tint to rubor and cyanosis. Pallor results from the shutdown of the capillaries as a consequence of (a) vasoconstriction from a cold environment (Henry and Meehan, 1971), drug, or nerve function and (b) drainage due to the lack of arterial pressure in the elevated limb with arterial occlusive disease (Ross, 1965). Normal color skin under the influence of relatively normal blood pressure has a balance between functioning arterioles, capillary networks, arteriovenous shunts, subpapillary venous plexuses, and venules. When rubor-colored skin is present, all of the capillaries and venous plexuses are dilated (Henry and Meehan, 1971). Dependent rubor of the skin occurs in the presence of peripheral arterial occlusive disease with the lower leg in the pendent position. The arterial pressure is reduced to the extent that the venous flow cannot overcome gravity. The orthostatic venous pressure added via the shunts to the reduced arteriolar pressure is sufficient to open the capillary networks and venous plexuses. As pressures drop further, the acute stasis can become chronic. Oxyhemoglobin is reduced and the color of the skin appears blue. A single cyanotic toe may indicate an embolus producing stenotic lesion upstream (Strandness, 1969b, pp. 231–234).

2. *Temperature*

Temperature correlates with skin color as an indicator of microvascular flow. Generally, the redder the skin, the warmer it is, and conversely, the less red, the colder. The red, warm skin has increased flow (Guyton, 1971, p. 376) and the cool, pale skin has a decreased blood flow, particularly in the sudden vasoconstriction of frostbite. However, if blood flow through the capillaries is slow due to an obstructed venous return, deoxygenated blood flow gives the skin a bluish color (Guyton, 1971, p. 376). Acute arterial obstruction produces a sudden temperature drop. Inability to regulate temperature causes the skin surface to approach room temperature rapidly. A refrigeration effect may develop from evaporation of moisture from the skin. A skin surface temperature several degrees lower than room temperature has been observed following frostbite. The loss of temperature regulation following cold injury may persist many weeks. The temperature of a finger pad may drop 3.7°C below room temperature of 24°C (author's patient). Normal temperature of the finger skin ranges between 30° and 35°C and that of the toe skin between 28° and 35° in a 23°C environment (Winsor, 1959, p. 309). Ideally, temperature studies should be made in a constant temperature room. However, if there is good air diffusion without draft and the room is not too small, the air temperature may be sufficiently constant. Distinct changes in skin color are not always apparent in ischemia. Temperature levels are more reliable. Here, too, direct recording may be in error since the skin is constantly losing heat in a cooler environment. The thermal index of Burton (1955) is considered to be more accurate comparatively than actual skin temperature, but the index is not applicable when the skin temperature is below room temperature.

In using temperature monitoring as a guide of treatment progress, one should remember that cold hands and feet have long been associated with emotional stress. The extremity that is cold and clammy to touch, which we find approaching or below room temperature, without an associated generalized diaphoresis should alert the clinician to the possibility of poor microvascular flow. The patient who has hot moist hands and/or feet may be undergoing an autosympathectomy from diabetes mellitus (Coffman, 1971).

3. *Opacity Pulse Recording*

The third indicator and monitor of microcirculation function in the digit pads is the opacity or volume pulse recording. Opacity pulse recordings have been used by many authors since the first reports of Hertzman (1937) and Goetz (1940). Standardization of the opacity pulse wave obtained electronically has to this day eluded investigators in their effort to calibrate a volume change in the recorded wave form. Hertzman (1938) used a glass filter in an effort to quantitate his photoelectric plethysmo-

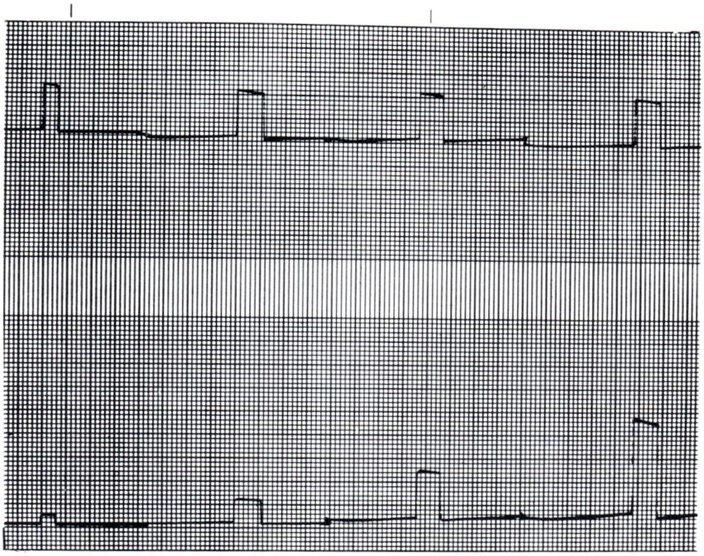

Fig. 1. Standardization record using 1 mV. Upper channel standardized for ECG. Lower channel standardized for opacity pulse recording left to right: 2 mm at $\times 50$, 5 mm at $\times 20$, 10 mm at $\times 10$, and 20 mm at $\times 5$ attenuation (see text).

grams. The method was an arbitrary one subject to controversy. An attempt to standardize the recording method was initiated in our laboratory as follows.

A Sanborn* 350 series 2 channel recorder was used to trace the ECG on the upper channel and the opacity pulse on the lower. The pulse channel incorporates an attenuation system of $\times 50$, $\times 20$, $\times 10$, $\times 5$, $\times 2$, and $\times 1$. The sensitivity of the pulse channel was adjusted to create a 1-cm amplitude trace at $\times 10$ attenuation when the 1-mV signal from the ECG channel output was used as a standard. The amplitude of the standard (Fig. 1) is 2 mm at $\times 50$, 5 mm at $\times 20$, 10 mm at $\times 10$, and 20 mm at $\times 5$. This method was devised to keep the records continuously comparable and to make restandardization relatively easy.

The lower channel recorded the opacity signal from a Scopette.† The digit sensor of this unit uses a noise-free light source and photocell which

* Hewlett–Packard Company, Waltham Division, 175 Wyman Street, Waltham, Massachusetts 02154.

† Gould, Inc., C–S Medical Division, 3400 Hillview Ave., P. O. Box 11577, Palo Alto, California 94306.

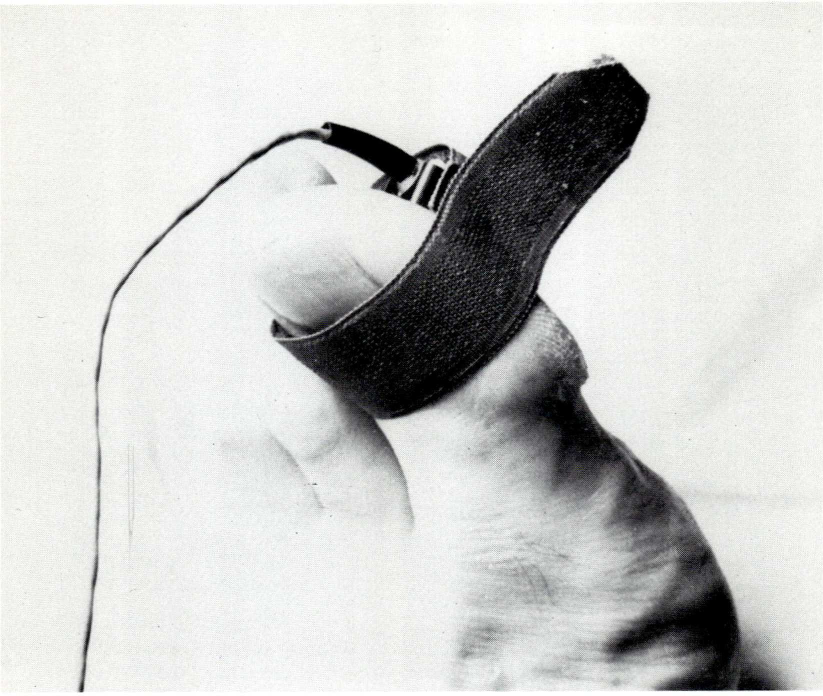

Fig. 2. Scopette micromodule sensor attached to great toe pad.

are micromoduled for ease of application to the digit pad (Fig. 2). The amplitude of the recorded opacity pulse of the finger pads has been shown not to be influenced by callouses or heavy racial pigmentation (Hertzman, 1938). The use of the digit sensor is not practical on the skin of the arms and legs due to reduced arterial supply in these areas (Hertzman, 1938). The microvascular pulse variations are of greatest value in determining the extent of degradation of the systemic pressure measured from the brachial and popliteal arteries. The nailbed transillumination type of photoelectric plethysmograph described by Hertzman (1937) is not practical for use with painful ischemic toes. Also, it is not able to discriminate between the pulse of the large vessels and that of the microvasculature (Hertzman, 1938). However, this method does take advantage of the extremely high vascularity of the nailbed (Grant and Bland, 1931). The present device is a solid state modification of the side-by-side type described by Hertzman (1938).

The fact that cells die when the microcirculation fails is impetus enough to determine the earliest possible sign of microvascular shut down. The skin presents the first visible signs of ischemia and microcirculation loss. The mercury strain gauge, impedance, and compartment methods of plethysmography were evaluated and compared with the opacity pulse for sensitivity to microvessel changes. The opacity pulse method was adopted because it does not include an appreciable influence from the composite arterial pulse volume and represents the highest percentage of microvascular function.

The control group of subjects, free from symptoms or signs of peripheral arterial ischemic disease, ranged from 19 to 86 years of age. "Normal" opacity pulse recordings were taken from the finger and toe pads and averaged to determine: (a) the range of normal amplitude, (b) the character of a normal wave form, smooth or notched, and (c) the length of a normal travel time from the R wave of the ECG to the peak of the related pulse wave. The records of the group below age 56 years were evaluated to determine maximum normal pulse travel time. Amplitude of the finger and toe recordings varied from 12 to 40 mm. All had smooth wave forms (Fig. 3). The upper limit for normal pulse travel time (time from the peak of the R wave to the peak of the opacity pulse wave) was 0.48 sec on the finger pads and 0.52 sec on the toe pads. These travel times compare favorably with those recorded by Gross (1960) using a photoelectric plethysmographic method.

4. *Interpretation of the Opacity Pulse Recording*

Each of the three characteristics, wave form, amplitude, and opacity pulse travel time, has a different interpretation. These are best explained by examples. The patient with a slightly elevated femoral blood pressure and a notched recorded wave form with an amplitude of 10 to 12 mm and 0.52 sec travel time to the toe pad has the minimal variation from normal. The first pathophysiological development in the microvasculature is the shut down of some of the capillary networks, due to reduced pressure (Zweifach, 1961).

Any high frequency notching of the opacity pulse wave suggests the pressure pulse may have undergone an alteration as recorded from the digit pad at $\times 50$ attenuation. The dicrotic notch is not present with peripheral arterial disease (Strandness, 1969b; Winsor, 1959, p. 157). Notching of the wave form has not been seen in patients with femoral blood pressures within 10 mm Hg of their normal brachial pressures. The explanation of the notching is open to conjecture. The opacity pulse wave recorded from an ischemic toe pad shows a ½ to 1 mm notching at 25 to 30 Hz which appears to be a reflected light variant. The notching is not related to an electronic or mechanical failure of the recorder since a similar wave

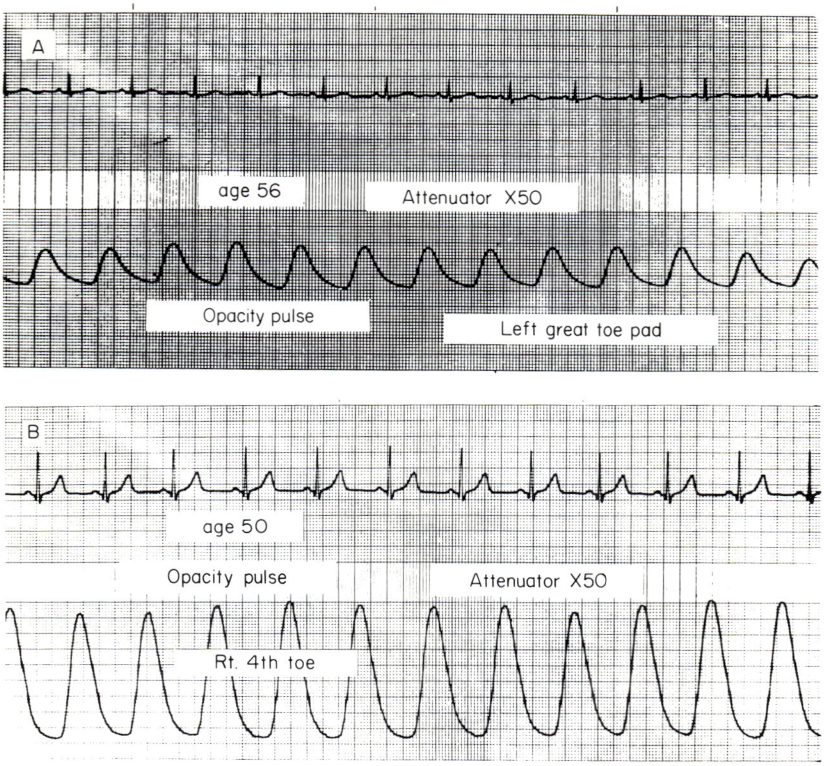

Fig. 3. Range of normal recordings. (A) Upper record is a minimal recording showing smooth wave form of average 12 mm amplitude and 0.52 sec pulse travel time. (B) Lower record is the maximum extent of normal amplitude showing smooth wave form.

form is seen on the monitoring oscilloscope of the Scopette. The sawtooth appearance of the wave form is the first indication of ischemia observed in the opacity pulse (Fig. 4). The notching does not change frequently with increased attenuation or reduced pulse amplitude. Only the depth of the notches diminishes as the pulse amplitude reduces toward a pulseless state and disappears completely near terminal ischemia. The frequency of function in the pulsatile portion of the microvasculature may be reduced permitting a recordable variation between the groups of functioning and nonfunctioning pulse carrying microvessels. Lower arteriolar pressure may affect the rate of vasomotor activity and increase the contrast between dilated and constrictive phases of the involved vessels (Chambers and Zweifach, 1946).

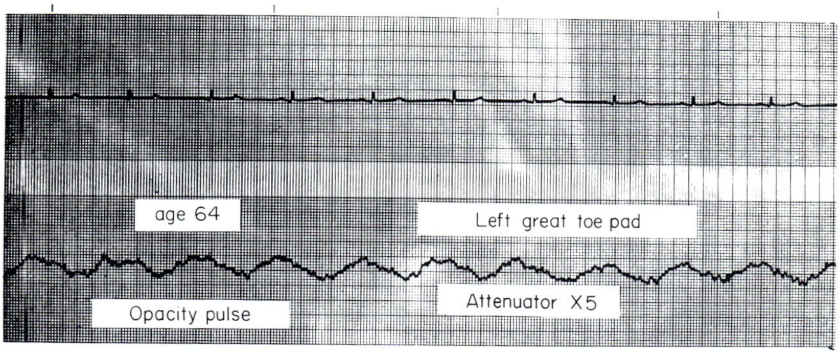

Fig. 4. Extremely long pulse travel time showing extensive use of collaterals.

The pulse wave recorded from the toe pad relates to the pressure wave which has traversed the long vessels of the limb and the rapid narrowing of the channels from the named vessels. This pressure wave, in the case of obstructed arteries, may not have enough pressure remaining to keep the digit arterioles open (Burton, 1965). The opacity pulse recorded from ischemic toe pads may vary in amplitude from 10 to 0 mm depending on (a) the elevation of the femoral blood pressure and how much energy is lost passing down the long vessels, (b) the number, length, density, and location of any stenotic lesions, and (c) any vasocontrictive effects, such as from a cold environment (Burton, 1939). Stenotic lesions may develop slowly and permit growth of collateral pathways (Liebow, 1963). The pulse may travel through several collateral vessels and arrive at the toe pad as much as 0.96 sec after being initiated by the heart (Fig. 4).

Experience has shown emotional stress to have some influence on the recordings. This is apparent when the recordings lack stability. A reassuring explanation of the procedure and a few moments relaxation will usually condition the patient for a stable recording.

The atraumatic, nonintrusive method of attachment of the sensor is repeatable (Fig. 2). Successive application at approximately the same location produced recordings identical to within 1 mm amplitude. The sensor is maintained in position by a Velcro strap which facilitates gentle application to painful ischemic toes. The effect of heat from the lamp is minimized by a clear plastic guard which covers the photocell and lamp assembly.

F. Relative Femoral Hypertension

Relative femoral hypertension refers to the relationship between brachial and femoral systolic blood pressures. The femoral systolic blood pressure shows relative hypertension when it is more than 10 mm Hg above the normal brachial systolic blood pressure, the diastolic pressures being similar. Systolic blood pressure in the thigh may be 10 to 40 mm Hg higher than the brachial pressure and accepted to be normal (Sapp *et al.*, 1955). In the author's series, pressure differences of over 10 mm Hg were associated with the opacity pulse alterations noted.

Symptoms of peripheral arterial ischemic disease occur when the process responsible for the ischemia is well advanced. A technique is needed with which the clinician may become aware of the impending disease process in the peripheral vessels (Strandness, 1969b). Several procedures have been suggested (cf. Section IV, B and C), but none of these is practical in the course of the usual physical examination. Alterations in blood flow have been associated with elevated femoral systolic blood pressure compared with the brachial systolic pressure. This relationship suggests the use of supine 4-limb blood pressures may be a method of early detection of the presence of lumen encroachment.

The blood pressures of the four limbs are taken with the patient in the supine position during the vascular examination. The patient should be allowed to rest in this position 20–30 min before the examination to permit stabilization of the body hemodynamics. The prone position may be difficult for patients with painful ischemic limbs. The author uses a double bladder cuff (Comparatif)* which gives a wider area of compression than a single bladder cuff of the same width. The double bladder cuff is 13 cm wide and gives readings comparable to a single bladder cuff of 18-cm width when applied to the thigh. The double bladder cuff has an inextensible backing which reflects the pressure centripetally.

An atherosclerotic limb may have a stenosis of the distal portion of the superficial femoral artery producing an elevation of the blood pressure immediately proximal to the lesion (Strandness, 1969a, pp. 368–404). Atherosclerotic patients with normal brachial blood pressure may have elevated blood pressure of the femoral artery without a blocking stenosis of a distal named vessel. The toe pad opacity pulse from this type of vasculature displays an amplitude of 2 to 3 mm (normal minimum, 12 mm). The palpable pulses are present with diminished intensity, and one of the pedal pulses is usually absent.

Brachial and femoral hypertension of short duration measured in the supine position is associated with relatively normal toe pad opacity pulse recordings. Systemic hypertension of long duration in 80-year-old patients may show only a minimal amplitude wave form with no notching and

*Siemens Corporation, 186 Wood Ave. So., Iselin, New Jersey 08830.

slightly extended travel time. An unusual finding incident to the routine taking of 4-limb pressures is that of brachial hypertension and femoral hypotension which suggests coarctation of the aorta or an obstruction of the aorta or the iliac or common femoral arteries.

Where the brachial and femoral systolic pressures have been equal (less than 10 mm Hg difference) and normal, the opacity pulse recordings from the toe pads have also been normal, that is, smooth at $\times 50$ attenuation, over 12 mm amplitude and under 0.52 sec pulse travel time. Many patients exhibit minimal femoral hypertension, and these have the notched wave form at $\times 50$ attenuation. A larger group show a slightly reduced amplitude and lengthened travel time. Almost all of these two groups have pedal pulses. Universally, they have a greater than normal vibratory sense loss (pallanesthesia) at the medial maleoli. The accepted usual loss of vibratory sense is up to 10% using the Vibrometer. Because of this small vessel involvement, tests for glucose tolerance and thyroid function are indicated as well as routine serology and hematologic studies for pernicious anemia (DeJong, 1967). In some patients the minimum 10 mm difference between the brachial and femoral blood pressures is accompanied by severe microvascular depression.

V. Therapy

"To improve" and adequately maintain "perfusion pressure" through the microcirculation is the aim of all treatment methods (De Takats, 1966).

The surgical approach to improving the microcirculation in peripheral ischemic disease includes bilateral sympathectomy, scalenotomy, reconstructive vessel surgery, embolectomy, thrombendarterectomy, and the repair of aneurysms when possible. There is a controversy at this time concerning the value of the sympathectomy approach to ischemic disease. A sympathetic nerve block is used to indicate the possible effectiveness of the sympathectomy. Sympathectomy is frequently performed in conjunction with arterial reconstruction. Postsympathectomy gangrene may complicate the procedure. Dilatation of the digit arterioles and shunts may reduce the microvascular pressure enough to permit closure of the capillary networks and promote gangrene of the toes. If all other methods of therapy have failed to encourage sufficient collateral development, arterial surgery is usually indicated as the last resort in treatment.

Observations of the physical functions of the microcirculation in peripheral arterial ischemic disease are more valuable when evaluated during the course of therapy. The ischemic process begins with pressure at the arteriolar level reducing sufficiently to permit closing of some capillary networks but not enough to close the arteriovenous shunts. There is still a supply of blood in the area to support the metabolic processes. Dible (1954) reported vessels of the toes were "generally healthy" as evidenced by postmortem angiographic studies. He thought severe ischemia was from "stagnant circulation" which he attributed to blood supplied at "low pressure."

Pressure is initiated by cardiac contraction (Rushmer, 1964) and transmitted to the peripheral vessels by the pressure pulse. To increase the pressure at the small vessel level, the pressure of the pulse must be increased. Thus, a physiological approach to the treatment of peripheral arterial ischemic disease is considered in terms of microvascular perfusion.

Maurice Fuchs (1945a) introduced the principle of Syncardial Massage. This is a method by which the pressure of the pulse may be increased. The pressure pulse is augmented by the compression of a cuff as the pulse passes under the cuff. Compression is indexed by the R wave of the ECG, giving the process the descriptive name of Heart Synchronized Pulse Compression or HSPC, and more correctly Heart Synchronized Pulse Augmentation by Compression. The Syncardon,* the invention of Fuchs (1945b), employs electronic circuitry which uses self-contained ECG electrodes and permits the determination of the arrival time of the pulse beneath the cuff (Fig. 5). The cuff can be placed on the extremity as determined by the operator. The timing of the compression and the amount and duration of pressure are all accurately controlled.

Figure 6 graphically explains the process of pulse augmentation. The pulse has just passed under the cuff. The pulse, for this illustration, has a pressure of 150 mm Hg systolic. Since the cuff is proximal to the peak of the pulse, the cuff pressure of 20 mm Hg will not be applied at the 150 mm level, but instead, will be applied at a pressure of, possibly, 140 mm. The pulse wave, to which the pressure is applied, will have a systolic pressure of 160 mm immediately beyond the cuff. For this illustration the extremity exhibits ischemia. The 150 mm systolic wave without augmentation degrades to an amount less than the critical closing pressure (Burton, 1965) to permit ischemia. The pressure delivered to the small vessels may be only a few millimeters of mercury shy of the required opening pressure. The complementary augmented pressure is able to arrive at the ischemic level and cause capillary perfusion because of the added 10 mm pressure.

* Jaquet, Ltd., 19–25 Thannerstrasse, Basel, Switzerland. Not in production.

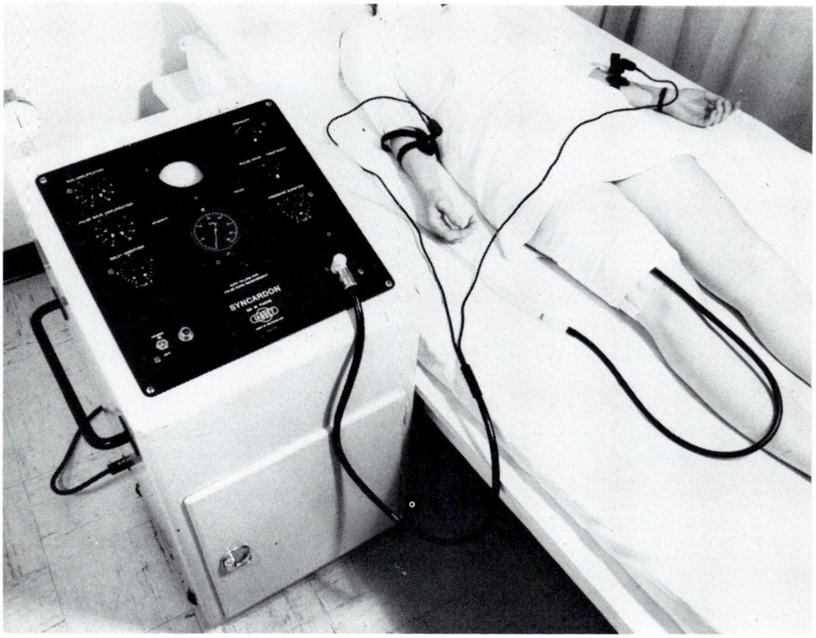

Fig. 5. Attachment of Syncardon to the patient. ECG electrodes placed on the arms and pressure cuff on the thigh.

Several concepts of mechanical massage therapy for peripheral vascular diseases have been promoted over the past 40 years (Licht, 1960). As a group they have included application of positive pressure to the entire limb or sections of it, application of negative pressure, and even sequential use of these pressures. However, only the method described here uses the R wave to index the compression of the pulse.

VI. Case Reports

The following five cases are presented to show the effectiveness of the monitoring concepts and treatment in a variety of peripheral arterial ischemic diseases.

Heart Synchronized Pulse Compression is presented as a valuable adjunctive therapy in the treatment of peripheral arterial ischemic disease except for rapidly spreading gangrene. It is not indicated for and is not to be used in the presence of aortic insufficiency, acute thrombophlebitis,

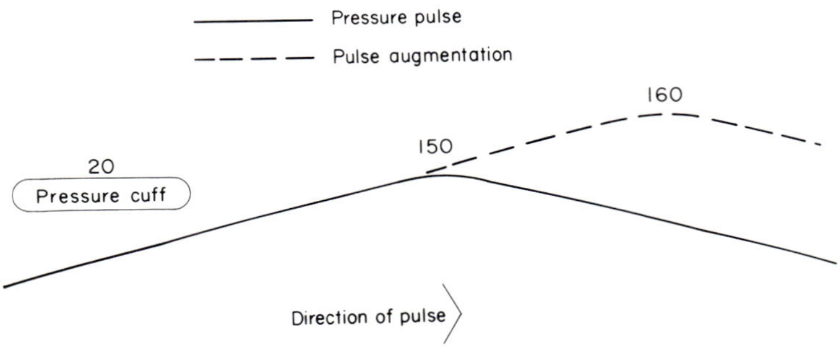

Fig. 6. Graphic representation of Heart Synchronized Pulse Compression (HSPC).

severe cachexia, latent syphilis, or acute inflamed conditions, such as severe respiratory conditions, because any of these conditions may be aggravated by the slight increase in pressure created (Fuchs, 1960).

The presentation of this method of treatment in this chapter is not designed as a critical appraisal of the method, but has been provided for completeness. However, the method of monitoring the effect of HSPC adds evidence to the value of this treatment in peripheral arterial ischemic disease.

The effects of HSPC were monitored by the photoelectric sensor (Fig. 2) placed on the digit pad in all cases to be presented. The Syncardon instrument was applied and adjusted according to the manufacturer's instructions (Fuchs, 1955).

Case 1. An amputation was imminent for this 61-year-old diabetic, according to his diabetologist. There were no palpable pulses distal to the femoral canal. He had extreme rest pain in the right foot and cyanotic discoloration of the toes. Arteriograms were not done. Segmental blood pressures were undeterminable. The recording in Fig. 7 was made on the day of the first visit. The Syncardon cuff in this case was applied to the right thigh, and the recording was made from the right great toe pad. Initially there was no pulse wave recorded until the HSPC was applied. A pronounced wave form was produced, which, when the HSPC was discontinued, returned to its nonpulsatile character. This pulse wave indicated the toe pad had pulse-carrying capability. The temperature of the toe pad was taken with a Barnes Infrared Thermometer* (as in all of these cases) before the HSPC therapy and again after a 20-min treatment. The second

* Barnes Engineering Company, Stamford, Connecticut.

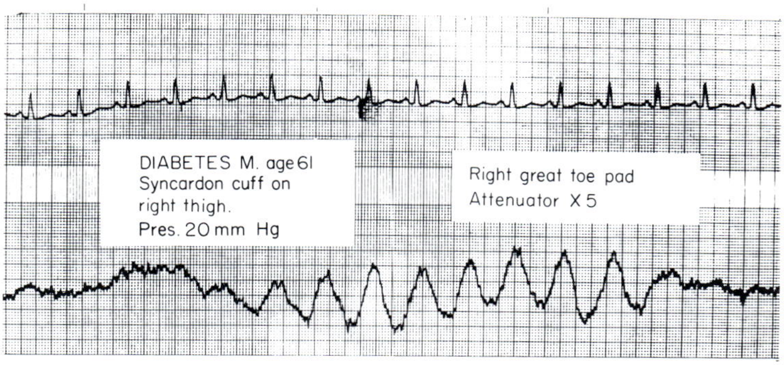

Fig. 7. Opacity wave form of patient with diabetes mellitus and atherosclerosis shows the effect of Heart Synchronized Pulse Compression (HSPC). Pulse travel time 0.72 sec. Note: The pulse wave arrives after the next R wave. Increased attenuation (×5) is necessary to obtain the effect; this demonstrates the extreme sensitivity available.

temperature reading was taken while the treatment was in progress. There was an increase on the right great toe pad of 5.5°F (3.0°C). The temperatures of the digits are shown in Fig. 8. From this result one may conclude that blood did indeed flow through the microvessels to warm the skin. Amputation was not necessary with continuing treatment.

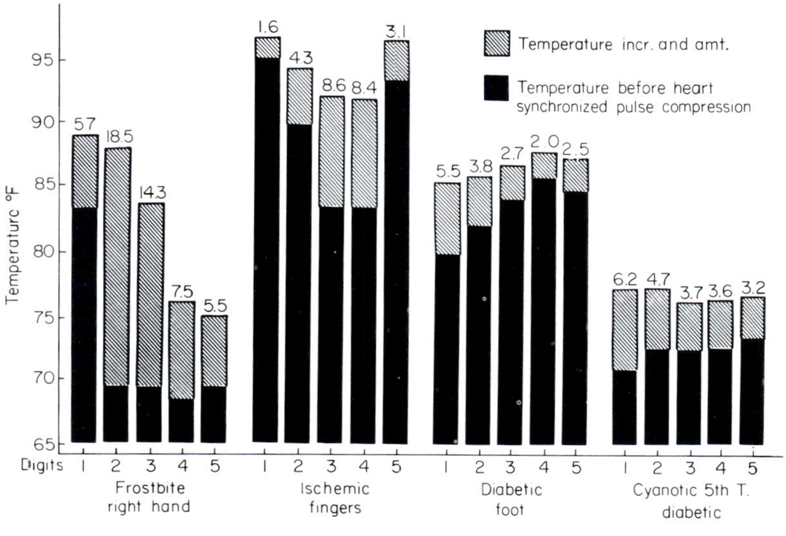

Fig. 8. Temperature increase due to Heart Synchronized Pulse Compression (HSPC).

Case 2. This 103-year-old man had a typical picture of occlusive arterial disease: severe rest pain for several months, dependent rubor, nocturnal rest pain, intermittent claudication, no pedal pulses, no ankle vibratory sense, and cool extremities. He also had no opacity pulse recorded from the left great toe pad at $\times 50$, $\times 20$, or $\times 10$ attenuation (Fig. 9). He did have a trophic ulcer proximal to the left external maleolus (Fig. 10). He also had a decubitus ulcer of the left heel and a small infarct at the tip of the left great toe. HSPC was applied to the left calf and produced a pulse where there was none (Fig. 11). After a period of 21 weeks of daily therapy, the three lesions recovered, the trophic scar is shown in Fig. 10. There was also a return of the opacity pulse to the skin of the left great toe pad, recorded at $\times 50$, $\times 20$, and $\times 10$ attenuation (Fig. 12). It is important to note here, though the amplitude was greater, the pulse travel time produced by HSPC on the first visit (Fig. 11) was shorter than that recorded in the patient's unaugmented pulse wave at the later date (Fig. 12). This indicates that the collateral channels used by the augmented pulse probably were not the same used at the time of the later recording which demonstrates a longer travel time. Apparently new channels are now available to supply an unaugmented opacity pulse to the toe pad. Another observation is that the wave form on the earlier recording is of greater amplitude and smoother, indicating that more pressure was transmitted to the area to open a larger number of pulse-carrying systems. This case is further evidence of the concept of critical minimal function which is a clinical adaptation of Burton's (1951) critical closing pressure of blood vessels. After 10 months of maintenance therapy of one treatment a week, the foot remains intact though still without pedal pulses and without rest pain.

Case 3. This 41-year-old man suffered frostbite of the right hand four weeks before the first picture was taken (Fig. 13). Note the gray nature of the nail bed of the ring finger. Temperatures were taken from the finger pads with the Infrared Thermometer and are recorded in the frostbite case of Fig. 8. The other picture was taken after 20 min of HSPC was applied to the hand and shows a lighter shading of the ring finger nail bed indicating improvement with less cyanosis. The original color slides show distinct color improvement. Note that the involved areas of frostbite were as follows: the distal half of the third phalanx of the index finger, the third phalanx of the middle finger, and distal two phalanges of both the ring and little fingers. The extreme rise in the temperature of the distal half of the third phalanx of the index finger is explained by the fact the mass of blood from the hand through the finger was available to supply the small volume required.

Case 4. A 52-year-old man came to me with two cold fingers, the middle and ring fingers, on the left hand. Figure 14 shows the $\times 10$ attenuated

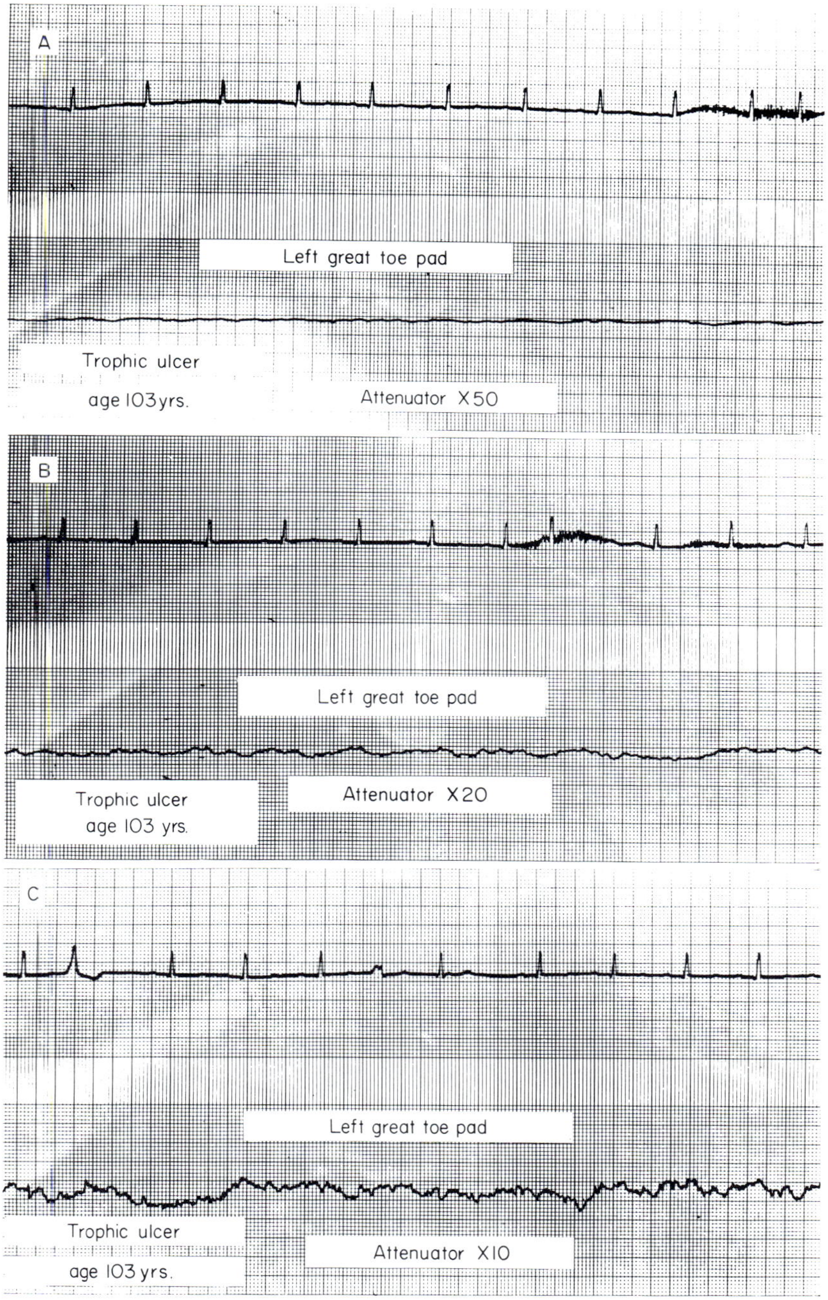

Fig. 9. A 103-year-old man with no opacity pulse wave at ×50, ×20, or ×10 attenuation. This patient had the trophic ulcer shown in Fig. 10.

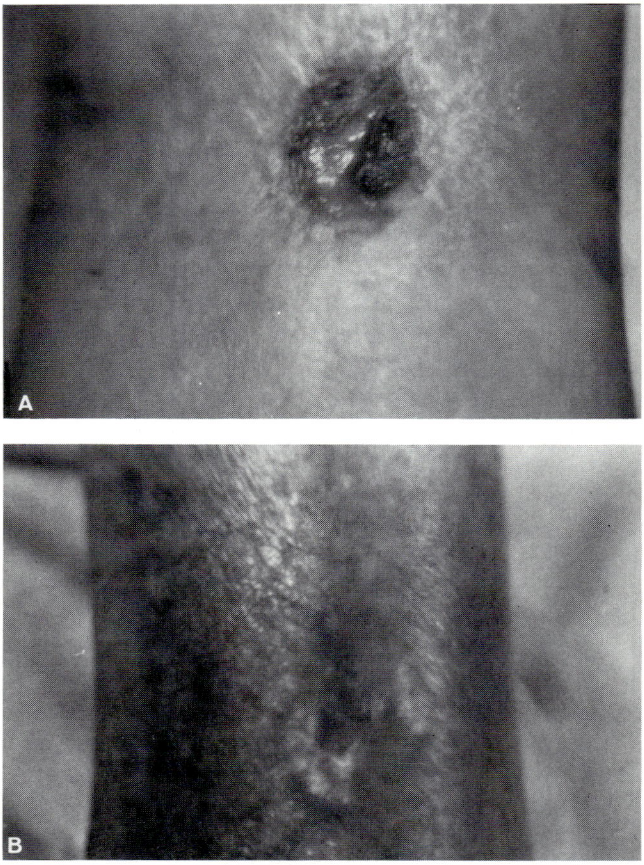

Fig. 10. (A) Trophic ulcer proximal to left external malleolus in the 103-year-old patient. (B) Ulcer scar, recovery after 21 weeks of treatment.

opacity pulse recording from the pad of the left middle finger. Note that the Syncardon was turned on before the last unaugmented wave but after the preceding R wave. The next R wave triggered the instrument to produce the first augmented wave by HSPC. Also notice the pulse travel time here, as in other cases of severe ischemia, is longer during augmentation due, I suspect, to an increased use of collaterals. The temperature rise of all fingers is displayed in the ischemic fingers group in Fig. 8.

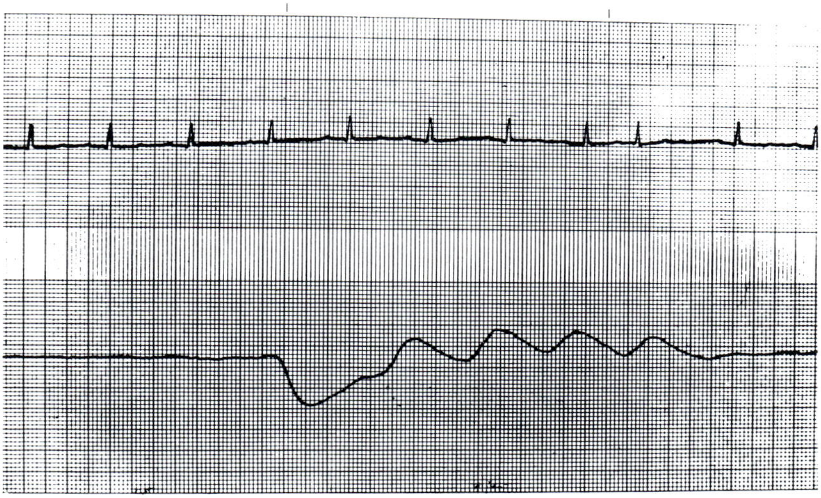

Fig. 11. Pulse wave produced by Heart Synchronized Pulse Compression in the same patient as Fig. 9. Recorded at $\times 50$ attenuation from the left great toe pad.

Case 5. This 59-year-old controlled diabetic had a cyanotic fifth toe of the right foot. After 20 min therapy by HSPC, the toe responded with an increase in the amplitude of the opacity pulse, a normal color, and a definite temperature increase not only in the fifth toe, but also in the other toes. The temperature bars are in Fig. 8. After several weeks treatment and continued control of the diabetes, the toe retained normal color.

VII. Other Observations

The only work similar to the foregoing found in the literature was that of Gross (1960). He used transmitted light in a manner similar to Hertzman's (1937) early work. The micromodule, using reflected light, has improved the ease of application to ischemic toes. Gross made observations of the effects of various amounts of applied pressure to the upper arm of healthy persons. He made recordings from patients with arteriosclerosis, diabetic angiopathy, M. Raynaud (he did not differentiate Raynaud's disease from Raynaud's phenomenon), traumatic angiopathy, M. Sudeck (atrophy), and endoangiitis obliterans. Gross found "light plethysmography" a "qualified method" for observing the effect of Syncardon, while controlling peripheral vascular therapy.

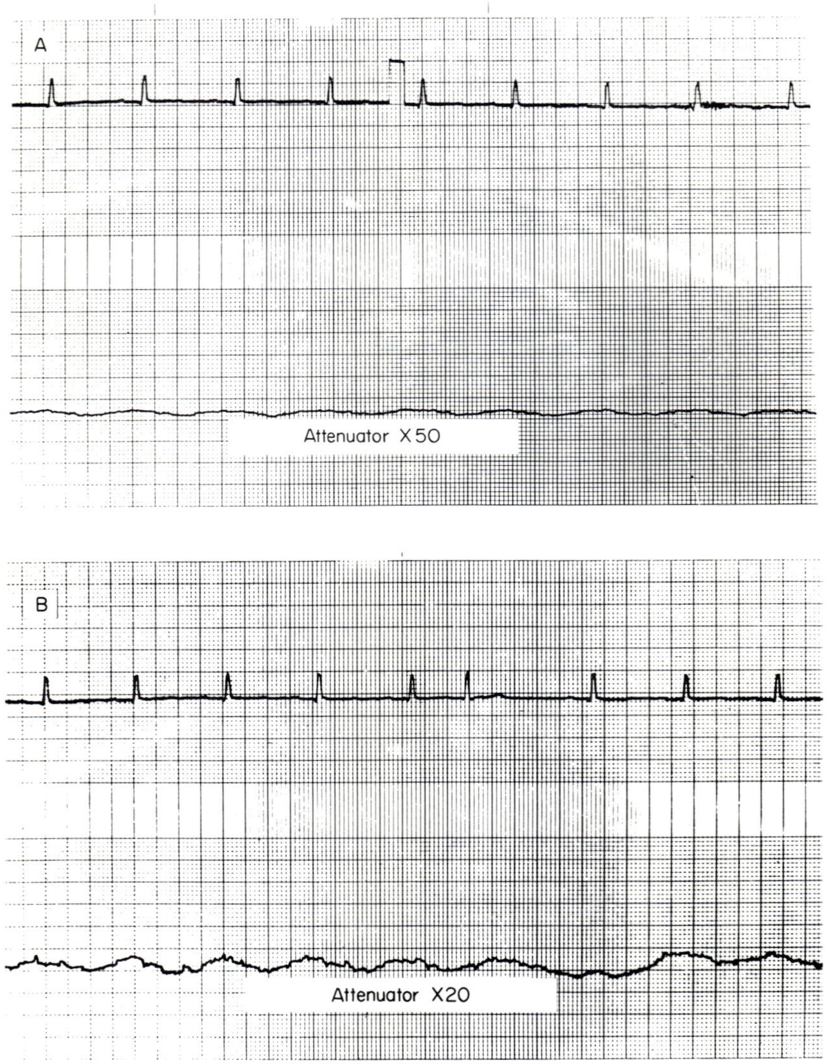

Fig. 12. Unaugmented wave form developed after 21 weeks of treatment. The three records of the opacity pulse from the left great toe demonstrate the advantage of attenuation.

Another method of observing the effect of HSPC is intraarterial catheterization. However, because of the hazards involved with trauma in ischemic tissues, catheterization for pressure effects by Syncardon in humans is not practical. This work has been done in the laboratory animal. Sonnen *et al.* (1970), by the use of intrafemoral artery catheters placed 5–6 cm above and below a pressure cuff in dogs, were able to record increased pressure proximally as well as distally when the cuff was augmenting by compression synchronized with the R wave.

VIII. Summary

The approach here has been to show the inherent relationship of the microcirculation to the diagnosis and treatment of peripheral arterial ischemic disease. The anatomical and physiological basis for this presentation has been documented. The living vessels of the digits are healthy and capable of functioning if the pressure necessary to open them is available. In patients with adequate cardiac output and minimal peripheral ischemia, correction of associated states may be sufficient to sustain the recovery from peripheral vascular disease.

Three main areas emerge as the most valuable in the monitoring of peripheral arterial ischemic disease: color, temperature, and the opacity pulse. The critical minimal function concept evolves from a clinical ap-

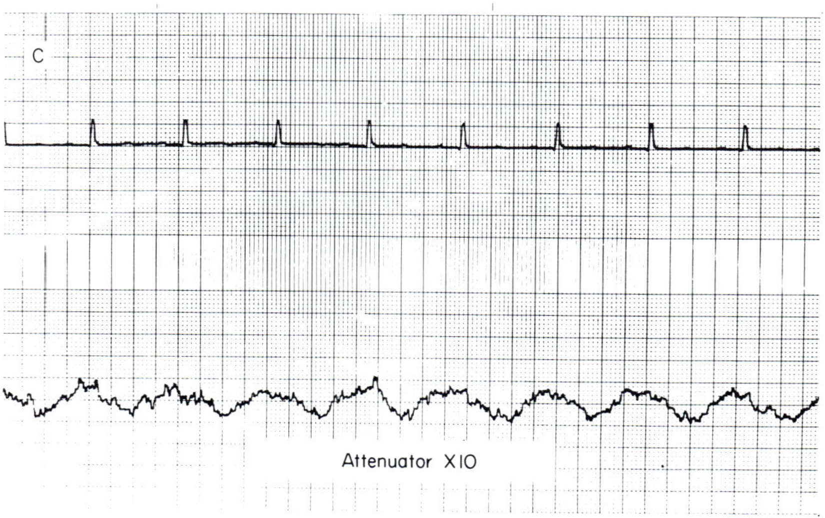

Fig. 12 (*continued*)

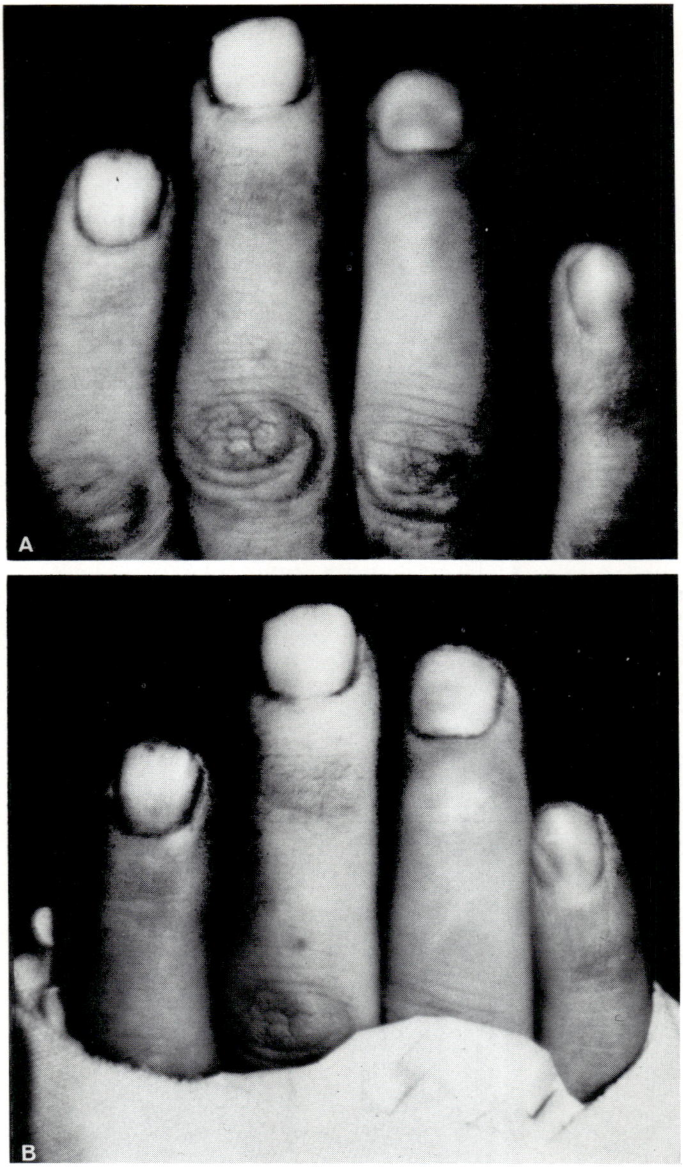

Fig. 13. (A) Note the ring finger (second from right) has a gray nail bed from frostbite 4 weeks before. (Color slide is blue from cyanosis.) (B) After 20 min of Heart Synchronized Pulse Compression (HSPC) the nail bed is less dark. (Color slide showed a pink tinge on the nail bed.)

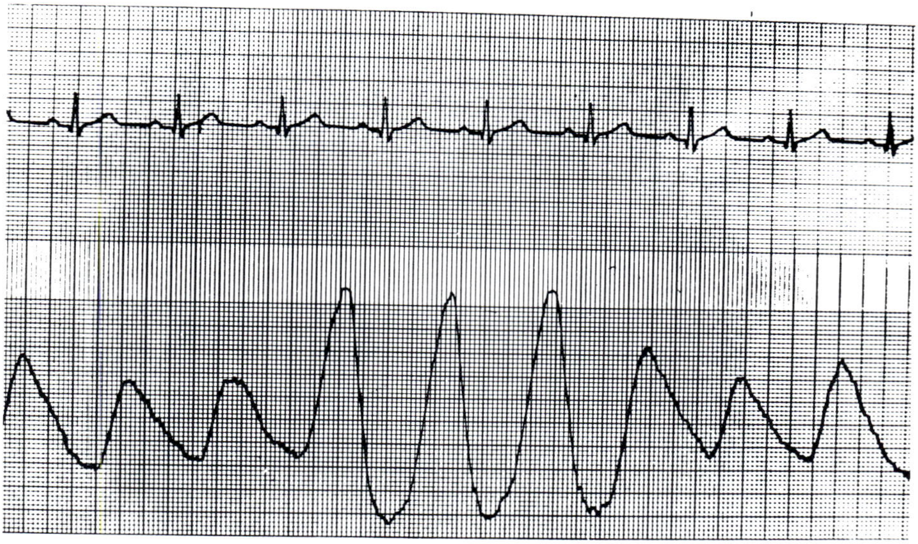

Fig. 14. Effect of Heart Synchronized Pulse Compression (HSPC) on the left hand and recorded at ×10 from the pad of the left middle finger. Note that the indicator bar at the bottom of the recording shows that the Syncardon was turned on after the R wave and before the last unaugmented wave form. The augmented form was produced when the instrument was triggered by the R wave immediately before it, indicating definite heart synchronization.

praisal of the gradual functional loss of tissue. The value of a rise in systolic pressure has been recognized by several authors (Thoma, 1884; Harpuder *et al.,* 1940; Johnson, 1968; Strandness, 1969a; Alpert *et al.,* 1969).

Importance of standardization of the recording method, determination of "normals," and interpretation of the opacity pulse recordings have also been very valuable. The use of routine 4-limb blood pressures in the supine position to determine the presence of relative femoral hypertension was stressed because of its influence on the modification of the opacity pulse and its value in detecting minimal arterial ischemia.

Heart Synchronized Pulse Compression is presented as a physiological treatment of peripheral arterial ischemic disease. Case reports are presented to illustrate the value of the monitoring methods and the effect of treatment.

References

Abramson, D. I., ed. (1962). "Blood Vessels and Lymphatics." Academic Press, New York.

Albrink, M. J., Lavietes, P. H., and Man, E. B. (1963). Vascular disease and serum lipids in diabetes mellitus. Observations over 30 years (1931–1961). *Ann. Intern. Med.* **58,** 305–323.

Allen, E. V., Barker, N. W., and Hines, E. A., Jr. (1962). "Peripheral Vascular Diseases." Saunders, Philadelphia, Pennsylvania.

Alpert, J. S., Larsen, O. A., and Lassen, N. A. (1969). Exercise and intermittent claudication. Blood flow in the calf muscle during walking studied by the xenon–133 clearance method. *Circulation* **39,** 353–359.

Bauer, F. K., Mugle, F. R., Jr., Lieberman, V. W., and Westergart, J. P. (1956). Clearance of radioactive iodine from the lower extremities of patients with myocardial infarction. *Amer. J. Med. Sci.* **232,** 44–49.

Bloodworth, J. M. B., Jr. (1967). *In* "Diabetes Mellitus: Diagnosis and Treatment" (G. J. Hamwi and T. S. Danowski, eds.), Vol. II, Chapter 5, p. 25. Amer. Diabetes Ass., New York.

Brakkee, A. J. M., and Vendrik, A. J. H. (1969). 5th European Conference on Microcirculation, Gothenburg 1968. *Bibl. Anat.* **10,** 528–531.

Buchanan, I. S., and Humpston, D. J. (1968). Nail-fold capillaries in connective tissue disorders. *Lancet* **1,** 845–847.

Burch, G. E., and Phillips, J. (1963); *In* "Handbook of Physiology" (Amer. Physiol. Soc., J. Field, ed.), Sect 2, Vol. II, Chapter 36, p. 1215. Williams & Wilkins, Baltimore, Maryland.

Burton, A. C. (1939). The range and variability of the blood flow in the human fingers and the vasomotor regulation of body temperature. *Amer. J. Physiol.* **127,** 437–453.

Burton, A. C. (1951). On physical equilibrium of small blood vessels. *Amer. J. Physiol.* **164,** 319–329.

Burton, A. C. (1955). "Man in a Cold Environment," p. 82. Arnold, London.

Burton, A. C. (1965). "Physiology and Biophysics of the Circulation," p. 81. Yearbook Publ., Chicago, Illinois.

Buwalda, G. (1969). *In* "Medical Thermography" (S. F. C. Heerma van Voss and P. Thomas, eds.), Bibl. Radiol. No. 5, pp. 123–124. Karger, Basel.

Calderón-González, R., González-Cantu, N., and Rizzi-Hernandez, H. (1970). Recurrent polyneuropathy with pregnancy and oral contraceptives. *N. Engl. J. Med.* **282,** 1307–1308.

Chambers, R., and Zweifach, B. W. (1946). Functional activity of the blood capillary bed with special reference to visceral tissue. *Ann. N. Y. Acad. Sci.* **46,** 683–695.

Chazan, B. I., Balodimos, M. C., Lavine, R. L., and Koncz, L. (1970). Capillaries of the nailfold of the toe in diabetes mellitus. *Microvasc. Res.* **2,** 504–507.

Coffman, J. D. (1971). *In* "Management of Arterial Occlusive Disease" (W. A. Dale, ed.), Chapter 4, p. 53. Yearbook Publ., Chicago, Illinois.

Coran, A. G., and Warren, R. (1966). Arteriographic changes in femors popliteal arteriosclerosis obliterans. A five year follow-up study. *N. Engl. J. Med.* **274,** 643–647.

DeJong, R. N. (1967). "The Neurologic Examination," 3rd ed., pp. 88–90. Harper (Hoeber), New York.

De Takats, G. (1966). Microcirculation: The last frontier. *J. Cardiovas. Surg., Suppl.* **1,** 13–42.

Dible, J. H. (1954). *In* "Peripheral Circulation in Man" (G. E. W. Wolstenholme and J. S. Freeman, eds.), pp. 173–184. Little, Brown, Boston, Massachusetts.

Dible, J. H. (1967). "The Pathology of Limb Ischemia," p. 39. Green, St. Louis, Missouri.

Domb, H., and Fried, A. (1959). Reflex sympathetic dystrophy: Treatment by synocardial compression. *Angiology* **10,** 109–114.

Dreyfus, P. M. (1967). *In* "Diabetes Mellitus: Diagnosis and Treatment" (G. J. Hamwi and T. S. Danowski, eds.), Vol. II, Chapter 39, p. 211. Amer. Diabetes Ass., New York.

Edholm, O. G., Fox, R. H., and MacPherson, R. K. (1956). The affect of body heating on the circulation in skin and muscle. *J. Physiol. (London)* **134,** 612–619.

Fisher, E. R. (1967). *In* "Atherosclerotic Vascular Disease" (A. N. Brest and J. H. Moyer, eds.), Chapter 16, p. 194. Appleton, New York.

Fuchs, M. (1945a). Neue Methode zur Förderung der lokalen Blutzirkulation: "Synkardiale Massage." *Schwiez. Med. Wochenschr.* **26,** 542–543.

Fuchs, M. (1945b). Das Prinzip der synkardialen Massage und seine Anwendung. *Schweiz. Med. Wochenschr.* **26,** 971–973.

Fuchs, M. (1955). "Syncardon Instruction Manual Type 55." Jaquet, Ltd., Basel.

Fuchs, M. (1960). *In* "Massage, Manipulation and Traction" (S. Licht, ed.), p. 97. Licht, New Haven, Connecticut.

Gifford, R. W., Jr. (1970). Raynaud's Disease. *Hosp. Med.* **6,** 37–43.

Goetz, R. H. (1940). Plethysmography of the skin in the investigation of peripheral vascular disease. *Brit. J. Surg.* **27,** 506–520.

Grant, R. T., and Bland, E. F. (1931). Observations on arteriovenous anastomoses in human skin and in the bird's foot with special reference to the reaction to cold. *Heart* **15,** 385–411.

Greenfield, A. D. M. (1963). *In* "Handbook of Physiology" (Amer. Physiol. Soc., J. Field, ed.), Sect. 2, Vol. II, pp. 1325–1351. Williams & Wilkins, Baltimore, Maryland.

Gross, D. (1960). On light plethysmographic studies in syncardial massage. *Z. Kreislaufforsch.* **49,** 550–558.

Guyton, A. C. (1971). "Textbook of Medical Physiology," 4th ed., p. 230. Saunders, Philadelphia, Pennsylvania.

Haimovici, H. (1966). The ischemic forms of venous thrombosis. 1) Phlegmasia cerulea doleus. 2) Venous gangrene. *J. Cardiovasc. Surg., Suppl.* **1,** 164–173.

Harpuder, K., Stein, I. D., and Byer, J. (1940). The role after arteriovenous anastomosis in peripheral vascular disease. *Amer. Heart J.* **20,** 539–545.

Henry, J. P., and Meehan, J. P. (1971). "The Circulation," pp. 136–137. Yearbook Publ., Chicago, Illinois.

Hertzman, A. B. (1937). Photoelectric plethysmography of the fingers and toes in man. *Proc. Soc. Exp. Biol. Med.* **37,** 529–534.

Hertzman, A. B. (1938). The blood supply of various skin areas as estimated by the photoelectric plethysmograph. *Amer. J. Physiol.* **124,** 328–340.

Horwitz, O. (1971). *In* "Cardiac and Vascular Diseases" (H. L. Conn, Jr. and O. Horwitz, eds.), p. 1517. Lea & Febiger, Philadelphia, Pennsylvania.

Isard, H. J., and Cullinan, J. E., Jr. (1967). Roentgenographic enlargement techniques. *J. Albert Einstein Med. Cent.* **15,** 201–205.

Johnson, P. C. (1968). The splanchnic microcirculation in shock and hypotension. *In* "Microcirculation as Related to Shock" (D. Shepro and G. P. Fulton, eds.), p. 16. Academic Press, New York.

Kety, S. S. (1948). Quantitative measurement of regional circulation by the clearance of radioactive sodium. *Amer. J. Med. Sci.* **215,** 352–353.

Kitchin, A. H. (1957). The effect of Pitressin on hand and forearm blood flow. *Clin. Sci.* **16,** 639–644.

Kuo, P. T. (1971). *In* "Cardiac and Vascular Diseases" (H. L. Conn, Jr. and O. Horwitz, eds.), p. 978. Lea & Febiger, Philadelphia, Pennsylvania.

Kuo, P. T., Feng, L. Y., and Pamintaun, J. (1970). Study of nail-fold capillaries in hypertriglyceridemia (types 3 and 4 hyperlipoproteinemia. *Circulation* **41,** 309–315.

Lassen, N. A. (1964). Muscle blood flow in normal man and in patients with intermittent claudication evaluated by simultaneous Xe-133 and Na-24 clearances. *J. Clin. Invest.* **43,** 1805–1812.

Licht, S., ed. (1960). "Massage, Manipulation and Traction," p. 86. Licht, New Haven, Connecticut.

Liebow, A. A. (1963). *In* "Handbook of Physiology" (Amer. Physiol. Soc., J. Field, ed.), Sect. 2, Vol. II, pp. 1251–1276. Williams & Wilkins, Baltimore, Maryland.

Lord, J. W., Jr. (1965). Cigarette smoking and peripheral atherosclerotic occlusive disease. *J. Amer. Med. Ass.* **191,** 249–251.

Lundborg, G., and Brånemark, P. I. (1968). *In* "Advances in Microcirculation" (H. Harders, ed.), Vol. 1, p. 66. Karger, Basel.

McMillan, G. C. (1962). *In* "Blood Vessels and Lymphatics" (D. I. Abramson, ed.), p. 648. Academic Press, New York.

McMillan, G. C., Melville, K. I., and Shister, H. E. (1962). *In* "Blood Vessels and Lymphatics" (D. I. Abramson, ed.), p. 670. Academic Press, New York.

Morris, L. E. (1968). Diagnosis and treatment for Raynaud's Phenomenon. *Heart Bull.* **17,** 81–85.

Nyboer, J. (1959). "Electrical Impedance Plethysmography," pp. 77–90. Thomas, Springfield, Illinois.

Popoff, N. F. (1934). The digital vascular system with reference to the state of glomus in inflammation, arterio-sclerotic gangrene, diabetic gangrene, thromboangitis obliterans and supernumerary digits in man. *Arch. Pathol.* **18,** 295–330.

Ross, J. V. (1965). Color changes in the extremities as they relate to peripheral vascular disease. *Angiology* **16,** 514–520.

Rushmer, R. F. (1964). *In* "Pulsatile Blood Flow" (E. O. Attinger, ed.), pp. 221–235. McGraw-Hill (Blakiston), New York.

Rushmer, R. F., ed. (1970). "Cardiovascular Dynamics," p. 115. Saunders, Philadelphia, Pennsylvania.

Sanbar, S. S. (1969). "Hyperlipidemia and Hyperlipoproteinemia," p. 115. Little, Brown, Boston, Massachusetts.

Sapp, O. L., Arney, G. V., and Marringly, T. W. (1955). Determination of arterial blood pressure in the lower extremities. Use of an eighteen centimeter sphygmomanometer thigh cuff. *J. Amer. Med. Ass.* **159,** 1727–1730.

Schroeder, H. A. (1971). *In* "Cardiac and Vascular Diseases" (H. L. Conn, Jr. and O. Horwitz, eds.), pp. 973–977. Lea & Febiger, Philadelphia, Pennsylvania.

Siperstein, M. D., Norton, W., Unger, R. H., and Madison, L. L. (1966). Muscle capillary basement membrane width in normal diabetic and prediabetic patients. *Clin. Res.* **14,** 101.

Sonnen, V. G., Link, M. S., and Hammer, L. G. (1970). An experimental and clinical appraisal of "syncardial" compression. *Arch. Phys. Med. Rehabil.* **51,** 656–666.

Strandness, D. E., Jr., ed. (1969a). "Collateral Circulation in Clinical Surgery," pp. 22–23, 368–404. Saunders, Philadelphia. Pennsylvania.

Strandness, D. E., Jr. (1969b). "Peripheral Arterial Disease," pp. 92–94, 231–234. Little, Brown, Boston, Massachusetts.

Strandness, D. E., Jr., and Bell, J. W. (1965). Peripheral vascular disease: Diagnosis and objective evaluation using a mercury strain gauge. *Ann. Surg.* **161,** Suppl., 3–35.

Sumner, D. S., Boswick, J. A., Jr., Criblez, T. I., and Doolittle, W. H. (1971). Prediction of tissue loss in human frostbite with xenon-133. *Surgery* **69,** 899–903.

Thoma, R. (1884). Ueber die Abhängigkeit der Bindegewebsneubildung in der Arterienintima von der mechanischen Bedingungen des Blutumlaufes. *Virchows Arch. Pathol. Anat. Physiol. Klin. Med.* **95,** 294–336.

Winsor, T. (1959). "Peripheral Vascular Diseases." Thomas, Springfield, Illinois.

Zweifach, B. W. (1961). "Functional Behavior of the Microcirculation," p. 34. Thomas, Springfield, Illinois.

9 DISEASES OF SMALL CORONARY ARTERIES

GEORGE K. MASSING, M.D. and
*THOMAS N. JAMES, M.D.**

I. Introduction

Abnormalities of small coronary arteries are more frequent than is generally recognized by either clinicians or pathologists. Narrowing of these vessels may be the sole cause of cardiac disease, or may occur concomitant with and adversely affect other forms of heart disease. Because the diagnosis of small coronary artery disease can be made at the bedside in certain distinctive syndromes (James, 1967b), greater awareness of this possibility may obviate the need for many expensive and uncomfortable diagnostic tests. In this review we will present first the pathophysiology that is common to all these diseases and then the etiology and histopathology of each, emphasizing the clinical clues for the diagnosis of important pathology in small coronary arteries.

*Work on which this chapter is based was supported in part by grants from the National Heart and Lung Institute, U. S. Public Health Service.

II. Pathophysiology

The pathophysiology resulting from small coronary artery diseases depends primarily on the prevalence and rapidity of luminal narrowing, as well as on the involvement of certain crucially important arteries, rather than upon the specific etiology. The small coronary arteries (defined in this chapter as those 40 to 1000 μm in diameter) can be divided into three functional (but obviously overlapping) groups: the nutrient arteries to the conduction system; the arteries supplying the working myocardium; and the coronary anastomoses. Although disease almost never involves only one of these groups selectively, the clinical features may reflect predominant dysfunction of a single group.

A. Nutrient Arteries to the Conduction System of the Heart

Although several arteries perfuse different parts of the human conduction system, the sinus node and atrioventricular (AV) node arteries are unquestionably the two most important because of the critical electrophysiological functions of the structures they perfuse. These two small arteries are unique in that their course can be followed in every human heart (James, 1961a), and the structures they perfuse are known and identifiable. Therefore, lesions in these arteries can be correlated with structural alterations of specific tissues, and compared from one heart to the next.

The *sinus node artery* (the largest atrial artery—usually about 1 mm in diameter) perfuses the sinus node, most of the internodal pathways, and a large part of both the left and right atrial working myocardium (James, 1961a, 1963). An acute occlusion of this artery (e.g., by an embolus) will usually produce a characteristic acute infarction at the junction of sinus node with right atrium (James, 1961b), resulting in profound alterations of sinus impulse formation and propagation, and often causing rapid supraventricular arrhythmias. Gradual narrowing of the sinus node artery usually produces chronic ischemia and focal degeneration of the sinus node. Because of the chronicity of the process, collateral circulation may permit normal sinus rhythm for long periods of time. Persistent atrial bradyarrhythmias usually mean severe structural damage of the sinus node and its connections, whereas transient or intermittent sinus node dysfunction suggests lesser damage to these structures. The consequences of nodal disease are additionally modified by variations in vagal and sympathetic tone, effective coronary perfusion pressure, degree of cardiac compensation, arterial blood pH and pO_2, and the adequacy of collateral circulation.

The clinical manifestations resulting from these rhythm disturbances range all the way from no cardiac symptoms to angina, congestive failure, syncope, or sudden death. The more serious of these consequences do not usually result from these arrhythmias alone, but from their complex hemodynamic and electrophysiological effects on an impaired myocardium.

The *AV node artery* perfuses the AV node and proximal His bundle, and to a lesser degree the distal portion of His bundle and proximal bundle branches. The primary blood supply to these latter regions comes more often from the proximal right or left coronary arteries, or from septal branches of the left anterior descending artery. Narrowing of the AV node artery therefore can produce all degrees of AV block and (less often) bundle branch block by causing ischemic damage of these critical areas. Impaired AV conduction and a slow and unreliable AV junctional or idioventricular pacemaker, plus ischemia of the ventricular myocardium, all combine to create an ideal milieu for the development of serious ventricular arrhythmias (Han *et al.*, 1966; Han, 1969a,b). Most of the same factors which may modify the consequences of disease in the sinus node artery also apply in AV node artery disease.

B. Small Arteries Supplying the Working Myocardium

It is more difficult to evaluate the functional significance of lesions of small coronary arteries in the ventricles. There are several facets to this problem: (1) Only a few small coronary arteries have a readily identifiable course and constant anatomical distribution which might permit correlation of myocardial changes with specific vascular lesions. (2) Small coronary artery diseases are characteristically focal in distribution, so that a vessel may be widely patent a few hundred micrometers from a severely affected segment; therefore, a small number of narrowed arteries per histologic section may connote a much greater anatomical and functional involvement. (3) Small coronary artery abnormalities are not uniform in distribution throughout the heart, the free wall of the left ventricle often being the site of least involvement. The tendency to sample either primarily or only from this region may help explain why the true prevalence of small coronary artery diseases is often underestimated. (4) Medial fibrosis, a common abnormality of small coronary arteries, may cause no luminal narrowing but may alter the distensibility and tone of the vessel, distorting dilatation and other normal responses during periods of increased cardiac work. (5) With the narrowing of many small arteries the remaining channels may dilate, giving the false impression of a widely patent arterial tree (More and Sommers, 1962).

Clinically, patients with disease primarily of the small arteries perfusing the working myocardium most often present with unexplained cardiac enlargement (Plaut and Kramer, 1936; Okada *et al.*, 1960; James, 1964; Varnauskas *et al.*, 1967; Hamby *et al.*, 1970). Chest pain may be present but is not characteristic of angina pectoris, although nitroglycerin may inconsistently provide relief. The most frequent electrocardiographic abnormality is generalized inversion of T waves, but left, right, or combined ventricular hypertrophy and atrial enlargement or conduction defects often occur. Electrocardiographic evidence of myocardial infarction is rare, but may occur by the coalescence of many microinfarcts.

In the absence of any other significant primary cardiac pathology, such as valvular disease, the cause and effect relationship of small coronary artery narrowing to multifocal areas of myocardial ischemia, necrosis, and fibrosis is straightforward. The small coronary artery pathology which may compound myocardial dysfunction in large coronary atherosclerosis or valvular heart disease (including infective endocarditis), however, is very often overlooked, yet may be a crucially important factor limiting the success of a coronary revascularization operation or of a valve replacement (Grismer *et al.*, 1967).

C. Coronary Anastomoses

Coronary anastomoses, ranging in size up to several hundred micrometers in diameter, exist in every normal human heart. Normally there is no net flow through these channels, primarily, because there is no transanastomotic pressure gradient (James, 1970). Narrowing of a large coronary artery sufficient to lower the arterial pressure distally creates a transanastomotic pressure gradient, resulting in a net collateral flow from the unoccluded artery through the coronary anastomoses into the distal segment of the narrowed artery. This important compensatory mechanism functions to limit the volume of ischemic myocardium caused by large coronary artery narrowing. Intrinsic narrowing of these coronary anastomoses, which is a distinct feature of any form of small coronary disease, increases their resistance to collateral blood flow, and inevitably impairs the effectiveness of this compensatory process.

The importance of the coronary collateral circulation is most apparent following an occlusion of the parent artery proximal to the origin of the AV node artery. The resulting AV junctional ischemia is usually only transient, because of the collateral blood supply to this region [frequently through Kugel's artery or arteries (Kugel, 1927)], but if these collateral channels are diseased, prolonged AV block may result. Viewed in this

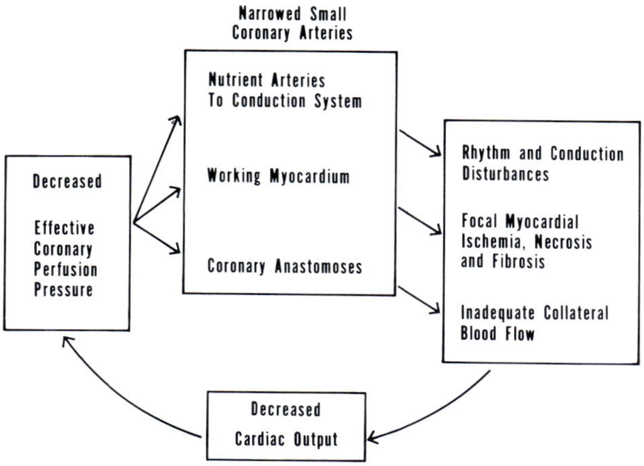

Fig. 1. Pathophysiology of small coronary artery diseases.

light, the adequacy of the coronary collateral circulation, which depends on patency of the anastomoses, may mean the difference between survival and death following occlusion of a large coronary artery (James, 1969a,b).

D. Summary of Pathophysiology

Figure 1 schematically presents the principles discussed in the preceding section and demonstrates the self-perpetuating decline in cardiac performance caused by small coronary artery diseases. Narrowing of small arteries may cause rhythm and conduction disturbances, focal ischemia, necrosis and fibrosis of the working myocardium, and decreased collateral blood flow. All these factors combine to decrease cardiac output, resulting in decreased effective coronary perfusion pressure (James, 1961c). In the presence of a high and fixed resistance due to narrowing of small coronary arteries, the lowering of effective coronary perfusion pressure must result in a further decrease in coronary blood flow and greater deterioration of cardiac performance. The vicious cycle is set.

III. Etiology and Histopathology

A general framework for the discussion of the individual small coronary artery abnormalities is presented in Table I. Some of these processes may involve both large and small coronary arteries, as well as capillaries and

TABLE I
SMALL CORONARY ARTERY DISEASES

Intraluminal
Embolic
In situ platelet aggregation and thrombosis
Intramural
Inflammatory
Collagen diseases
Infectious
Degenerative
Hereditary medial necrosis
Aging
Diabetes
Amyloidosis
Metabolic
Alcohol
Hypomagnesemia
Pheochromocytoma

veins, but discussion will be limited to their effects on small coronary arteries.

A. INTRALUMINAL

1. *Embolic*

There are a number of possible sources for embolization to the coronary arteries: mural thrombus from the left side of the heart (Fig. 2); left atrial or ventricular myxoma fragments; septic or bland vegetations discharged from infected heart valves; calcified valvular tissue broken off during surgical replacement or valvulotomy; air and nonspecific debris during cardiopulmonary bypass (Fig. 3); granular components of contrast medium used for coronary angiography; atheromatous material from a ruptured coronary atheroma or from an ulcerated plaque in the proximal aorta; or platelet aggregates formed upstream on a complicated atheroma.

Embolic occlusions abruptly cause myocardial ischemia, requiring an efficient collateral circulation to prevent infarction. Unfortunately, as can be seen from the examples cited, in most circumstances in which coronary embolization occurs there is an associated significant underlying disease already taxing the myocardial reserve.

2. *In Situ Platelet Aggregation and Thrombosis*

Platelet aggregation in the coronary microcirculation has been recognized as a potentially important factor contributing to myocardial ischemia,

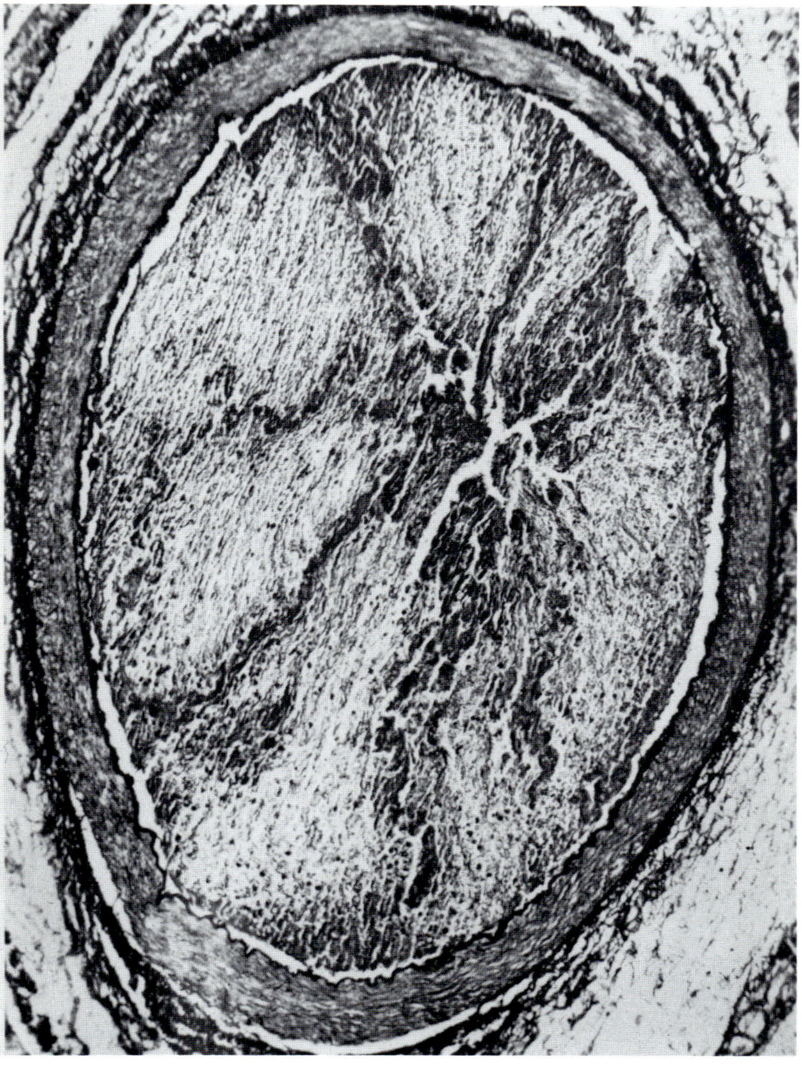

Fig. 2. The sinus node artery is occluded by an embolus. Atrial fibrillation began shortly prior to the death of this patient with mitral stenosis. 160×, Verhoeff elastic stain. Reproduced from James (1967b) with the permission of the publisher.

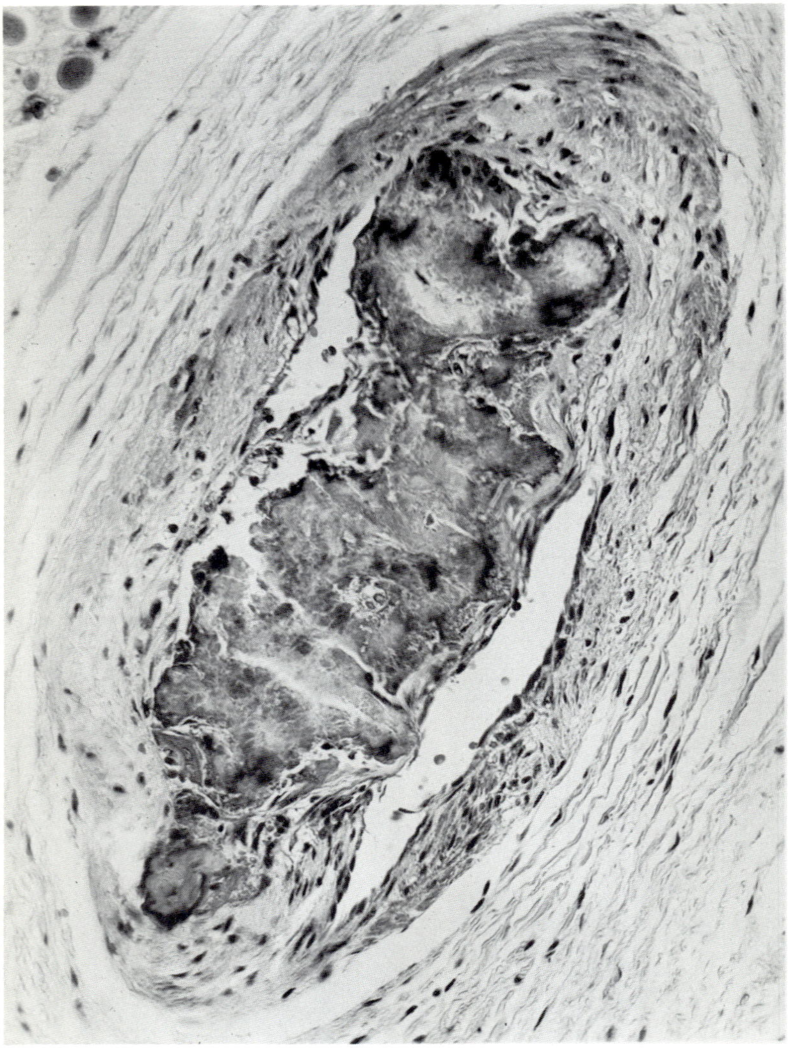

Fig. 3. Embolic debris almost completely occludes this left ventricular artery. The patient died shortly after open heart surgery to replace the aortic valve. 300×, Goldner trichrome stain. Reproduced from James (1967b) with the permission of the publisher.

but documentation of its frequency has been difficult because of the known propensity of these clumps to disaggregate and be inapparent at postmortem examination. Platelet aggregation may be initiated or enhanced by abnormalities of the arterial intima that expose underlying collagen or basement membrane, by local release of adenosine diphosphate and other nucleotides from injured myocardial cells, and by increased levels of circulating catecholamines or free fatty acids (both of which are frequently elevated in the early postmyocardial infarction period) (Mustard and Packham, 1969). Thrombotic thrombocytopenic purpura causes widespead platelet aggregation which may cause fatal cardiac rhythm and conduction disturbances by occluding the nutrient arteries to the conduction system (James and Monto, 1966).

The cardiac enlargement commonly observed in patients with sickle cell disease (SS hemoglobin) may be due to either chronic anemia or multiple small coronary artery sickle cell thromboses, or both. A pure example of the effects of coronary intravascular sickling has been demonstrated in several *nonanemic* patients with sickle trait (Oliveira and Gomez–Patino, 1963; Fleischer and Rubler, 1968; Jones *et al.*, 1970). Some of these patients during life were thought to have an idiopathic cardiomyopathy, while others were previously healthy and died suddenly after extreme exertion. The cause of death in the latter patients was multiple sickle cell thromboses in the small vessels of the heart and other organs, resulting from the metabolic effects of extreme exertion on S hemoglobin. In these same hearts, and in the group with known cardiomegaly, there was diffuse, patchy myocardial fibrosis, presumably the result of previous episodes of small artery occlusion.

B. Intramural

1. *Inflammatory*

a. *Collagen Diseases.* Clinically significant involvement of the small coronary arteries has been documented in systemic lupus erythematosus (James *et al.,* 1965), polyarteritis nodosa (James and Birk, 1966), rheumatoid arthritis (Cruickshank, 1953; Sobin and Hagstrom, 1962), rheumatic fever (Karsner and Bayless, 1934; Gross *et al.*, 1935), and scleroderma (Lev *et al.*, 1966). The histologic changes in the arteries vary with the stage of the disease—acute lesions demonstrating transmural or perivascular inflammation, with or without medial hyperplasia, reactive endothelial proliferation, or luminal thrombosis (Fig. 4); chronic lesions may demonstrate a few residual perivascular plasma cells or lymphocytes, medial hyperplasia, and fibrosis of any or all of the vascular coats, with or without

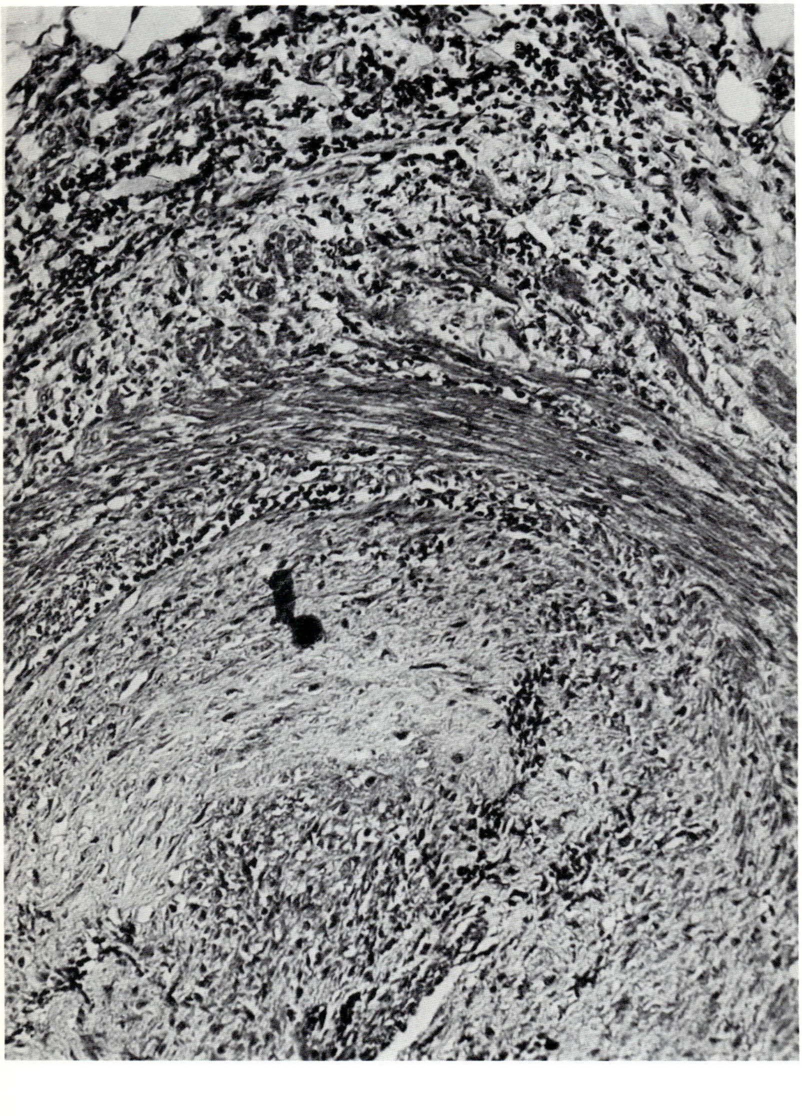

Fig. 4. The AV node artery shows transmural inflammation and endothelial proliferation in a patient with polyarteritis nodosa. Inflammatory reaction is present in the AV node to the right. 175×, Goldner trichrome stain. Reproduced from James and Birk (1966) with the permission of the publisher.

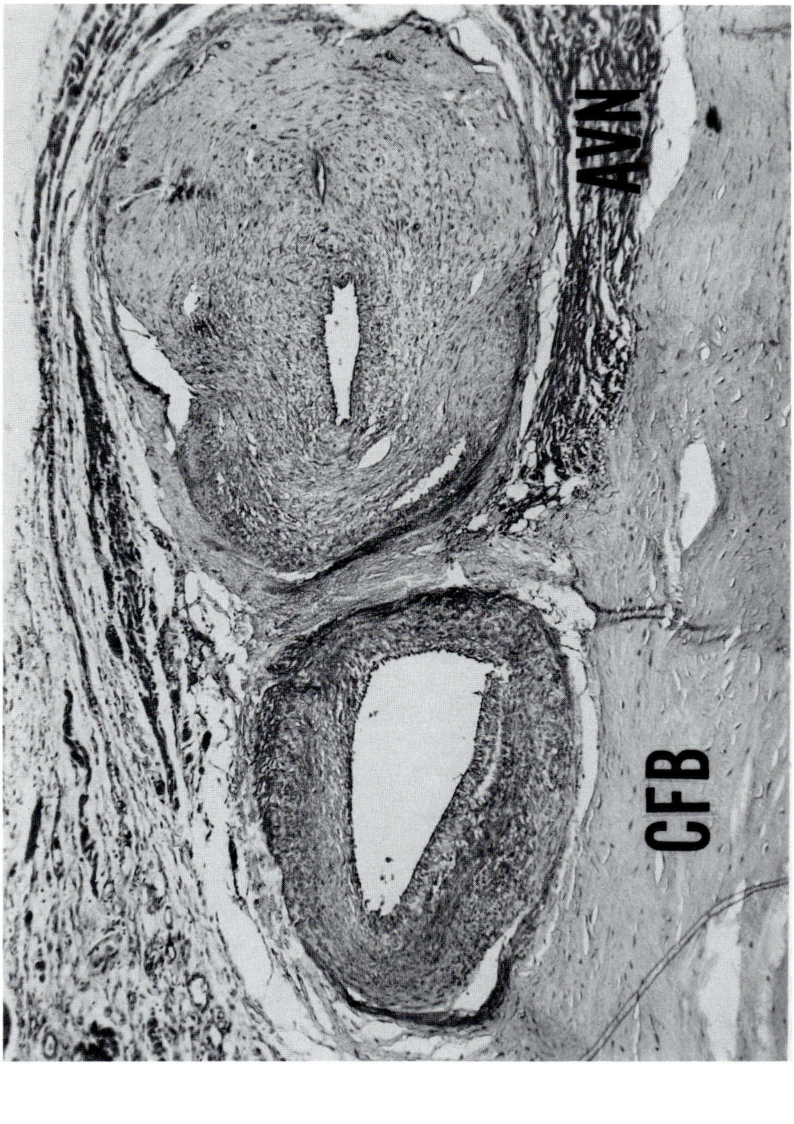

Fig. 5. Photomicrograph of the AV node showing marked narrowing of the AV node artery (right) and minimal narrowing of one of its branches. These lesions represent the healed stage of arteritis in a patient with polyarteritis nodosa. CFB, central fibrous body; AVN, AV node. 63×; Goldner trichrome stain.

luminal stenosis (Fig. 5). The chronic lesions frequently cannot be differentiated from those seen in noninflammatory diseases of the small coronary arteries. The sinus node, being a periarterial and subepicardial structure, tends to be severely and frequently affected by the combination of ischemia due to stenosis of the sinus node artery, direct extension of the arteritis into the surrounding nodal tissue, and pericarditis (James, 1962a) which is a frequent accompaniment of these disorders. The cardiac involvement in these diseases may be clinically insignificant or may be the major cause of disability and death.

b. *Infectious*. Relatively little is known about the effects of the common infectious diseases on small coronary arteries. Endothelial proliferation and medial smooth muscle swelling have been reported (Cowan, 1904; Gross *et al.*, 1935), but the role of these lesions in the subsequent development of permanent small coronary artery narrowing is unknown. The literature on myocarditis contributes little data on this subject.

2. *Degenerative*

a. *Hereditary Medial Necrosis*. Marfan's syndrome (James *et al.*, 1964), Friedreich's ataxia (Nadas *et al.*, 1951; James and Fisch, 1963; Ivemark and Thoren, 1964), and progressive muscular dystrophy (James, 1962b; Thomson, 1968; Demany and Zimmerman, 1969) comprise a group of distinctive, hereditary neuromusculoskeletal syndromes in which young patients may have seemingly unexplained cardiomegaly and disturbances of cardiac rhythm and conduction. A cause of cardiac disease in these patients has been demonstrated to be a characteristic abnormality of small coronary arteries. We believe that the basic defect in these arteries is a heritable necrosis of smooth muscle cells of the tunica media resulting in focal medial weakness and partial collapse (Fig. 6). Disorderly medial smooth muscle hyperplasia, medial fibrosis, and endothelial proliferation are frequent reparative or reactive changes (Fig. 7). Inflammatory reaction in these vessels is conspicuously absent. An inflammatory response to focal myocardial necrosis frequently occurs, however, and has been misleadingly termed a myocarditis (Russell, 1946).

In the same patients, the small pulmonary arteries may be affected by the identical process. Although pulmonary disease occurring in these disorders has classically been attributed to thoracic skeletal deformities or to weakness of respiratory muscles, it is possible that medial necrosis of the small pulmonary arteries may play an important role. There is, thus, an interesting link between this group of disorders and certain patients with primary pulmonary hypertension. In patients with so-called primary

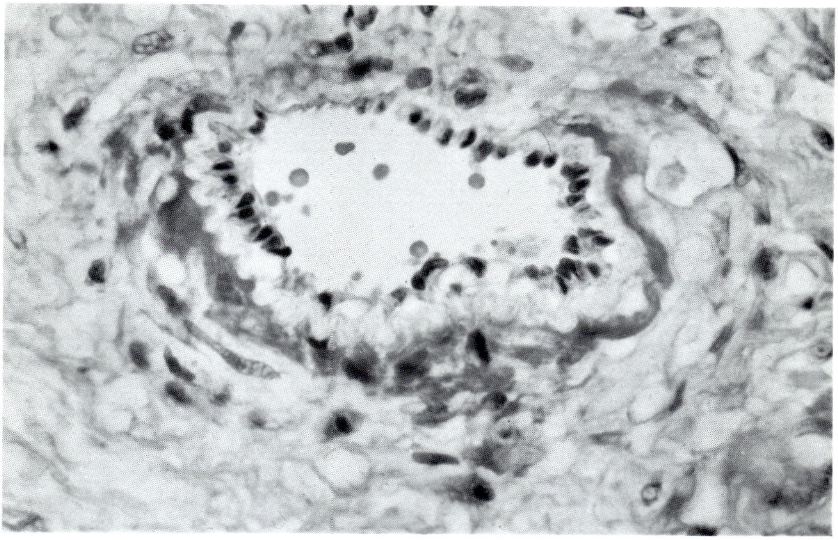

Fig. 6. This sinus node artery of a patient with progressive muscular dystrophy demonstrates marked vacuolar degeneration of the smooth muscle cells of the tunica media. 480×; Goldner trichrome stain.

pulmonary hypertension and a history of syncope and sudden death, medial necrosis has been demonstrated in small pulmonary and systemic arteries, including the small coronary arteries (Fig. 8) (James, 1961d, 1962c). The presence of medial necrosis in small arteries of both the pulmonary and systemic circulation weakens the argument that the small artery changes in the lung are secondary to the pulmonary hypertension and strengthens the concept that a primary abnormality of small pulmonary arteries (Bredt, 1932; Evans *et al.*, 1957) causes the pulmonary hypertension. We do not imply that all patients with Marfan's syndrome, Friedreich's ataxia, progressive muscular dystrophy, or primary pulmonary hypertension have concomitant small coronary and pulmonary artery medial necrosis, but those patients with otherwise unexplained rhythm and conduction abnormalities and cardiomegaly probably do. Family members of patients with one of these syndromes who have no neuromusculoskeletal manifestations may have isolated medial necrosis of small coronary arteries.

A small number of young patients with the heritable syndrome of congenital deafness, electrocardiographic QT prolongation, and sudden death have been demonstrated to have hereditary medial necrosis of small coronary arteries (Fraser *et al.,* 1964; James, 1967a). The precise relationship between

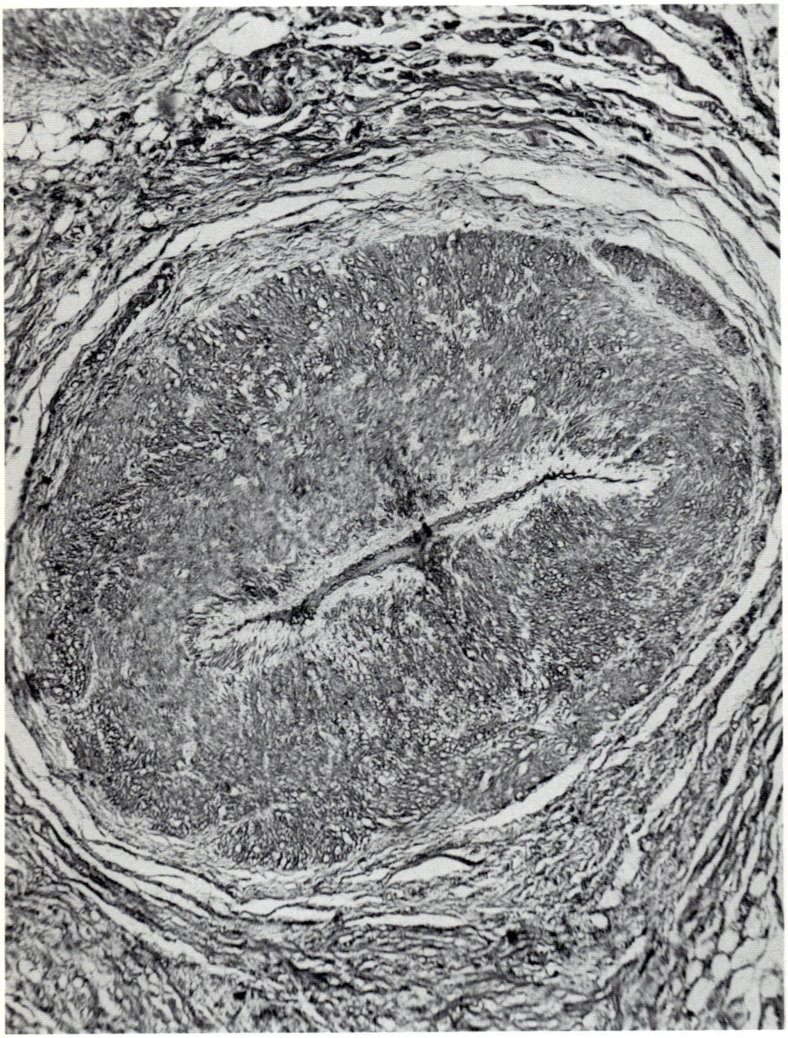

Fig. 7. This sinus node artery of a patient with Marfan's syndrome demonstrates disorderly medial smooth muscle hyperplasia, a reactive response to medial smooth muscle necrosis. 118×, Goldner trichrome stain. Reproduced from James (1967b) with the permission of the publisher.

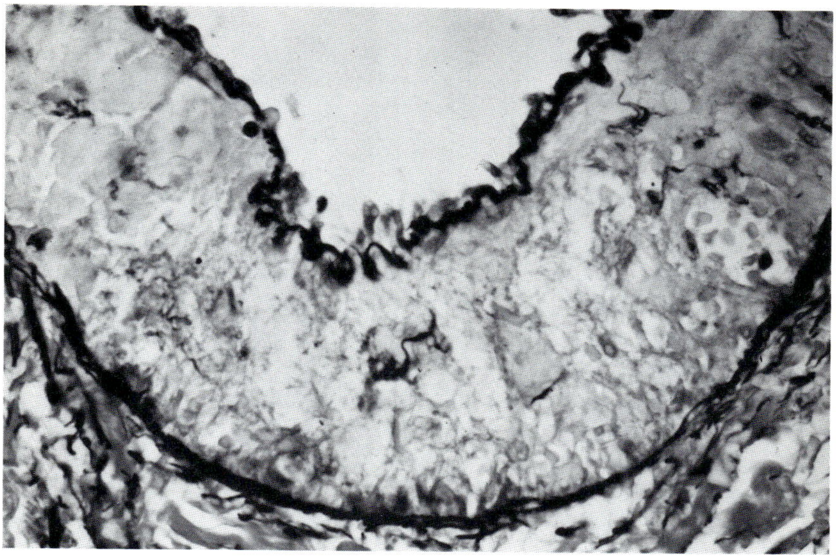

Fig. 8. Marked medial degeneration can be seen in this sinus node artery from a patient with primary pulmonary hypertension. 480×, Verhoeff's elastic stain.

the hereditary medial necrosis and QT prolongation has not been clearly established. Finally, there are rare instances of the same hereditary abnormality of small coronary arteries without any of the previously described syndromes, and idiopathic familial cardiomyopathy may be a specific example.

b. *Aging Changes.* Although a detailed discussion of aging changes in small coronary arteries is not appropriate here, several facts should be stressed. In studying normal hearts in all age groups, Gross and his colleagues (1934) described an age-related change in small coronary arteries, characterized by elastification of the media and intima with subsequent fibrosis and fusion of these layers, a process they termed fibroelastic metamorphosis. Several other studies (Blumenthal *et al.*, 1960; Ledet, 1968) have confirmed that endothelial proliferation, subendothelial deposition of PAS-positive material, and medial hypertrophy and hyperplasia of small coronary arteries occur with advancing age. Laubry *et al.* (1948) noted a functional correlate of these observations—septal anastomoses can be demonstrated less frequently in patients over 70 years of age.

Just as large coronary atherosclerosis may be considered an aging change, the progress of which may be accelerated by known or unknown factors, so it is for the aging changes in small coronary arteries. Diabetes can accelerate all of the histologic components of aging in small coronary arteries, particularly the endothelial proliferation and subendothelial PAS deposits (Blumenthal *et al.,* 1960; Ledet, 1968; Saphir *et al.,* 1956), and it may do so without concomitant large coronary atherosclerosis (Hamby *et al.*, 1970). Whereas hypertension might also be expected to exaggerate these small artery changes in the heart, the evidence in humans, paradoxically, is to the contrary (Moritz and Oldt, 1937; Donomae *et al.*, 1962; Naeye, 1967).

The histologic features of all other small coronary artery abnormalities must be viewed on the background of these aging changes. The lesions seen in hereditary medial necrosis can be differentiated histologically from those due to aging by the presence of prominent medial smooth muscle degeneration in the former. Endothelial proliferation and medial hyperplasia and fibrosis are common to both.

The interaction between large coronary atherosclerosis and small coronary artery aging changes is poorly understood, perhaps, in part, because coronary atherosclerosis is almost certainly not the unitary process so often assumed. In a given patient, the large coronary arteries may be badly diseased and the small ones normal (and the reverse). Arteries of both sizes may display accelerated aging changes due to a known predisposing factor such as diabetes or due to totally unknown influences. The possibility that large coronary atherosclerosis may cause structural alterations of small coronary arteries must be considered. Platelets or atheromatous debris may embolize downstream and incite various reactive changes in the distal vessel wall, leaving no identifiable evidence of the preceding embolic event. Conversely, abnormalities of small arteries may include the vasa vasorum and thus damage the walls of the larger coronary branches. How often either of these processes occurs is uncertain.

c. *Amyloidosis.* Amyloid deposits have been found in the hearts of many older patients (Pomerance, 1965; Schwartz and Kurucy, 1965; Wright *et al.*, 1969), directly infiltrating the myocardium and cardiac nerves, as well as in the arteries and veins, both large and small (Fig. 9). All layers of these vessels may be affected. The sinus node may be extensively damaged, usually more than the AV node or His bundle, possibly due to the periarterial structure of the sinus node (James, 1966). Amyloidosis causes marked sinus node dysfunction in the elderly more often than is currently recognized.

d. *Metabolic.* Alcohol may affect the heart in many ways, one of which is via an influence on small coronary arteries. Whether this effect is a toxic one, or related to hypomagnesemia, or to intense, prolonged vaso-

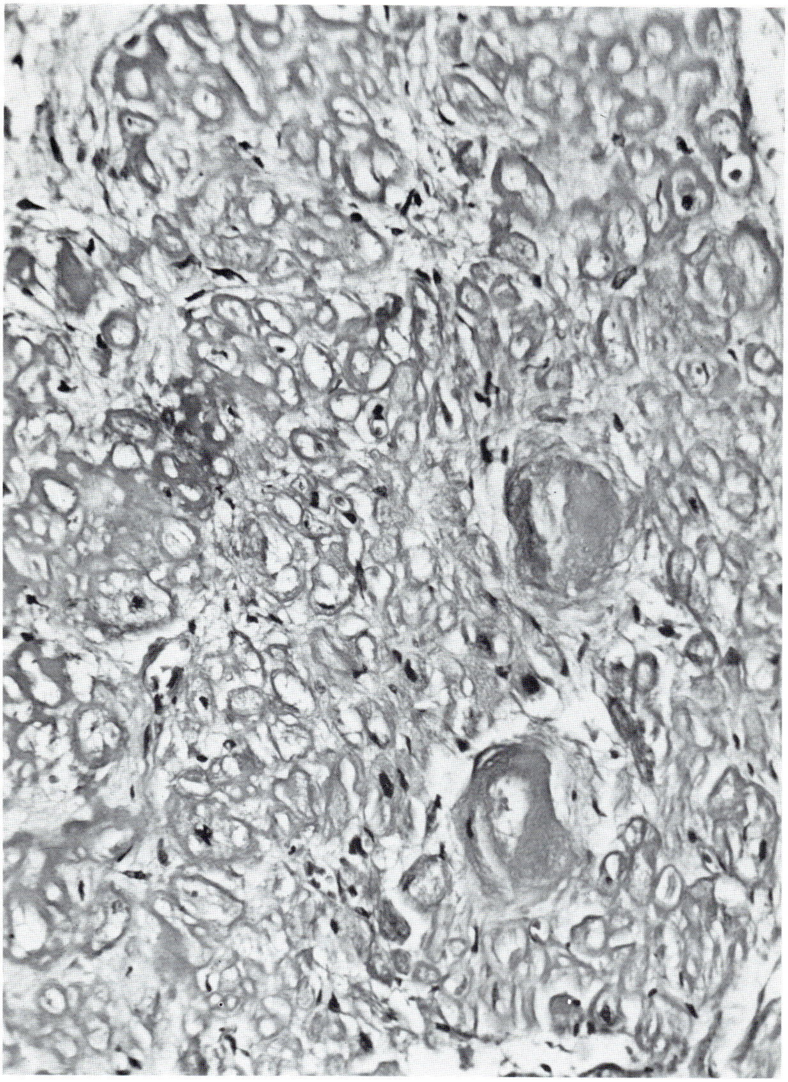

Fig. 9. This photomicrograph demonstrates marked amyloid infiltration of the sinus node and several small branches of the sinus node artery. 80×, Goldner trichrome stain.

constriction due to chronic release of catecholamines by acetaldehyde (the first breakdown product of ethanol) (James and Bear, 1967), or to other mechanisms is uncertain. In alcoholic cardiomyopathy, Pintar *et al.* (1965) described disorganization of the media of small coronary arteries by edema and degeneration, with subintimal PAS-positive homogeneous deposits causing luminal narrowing. They suggested that alcoholic intoxication caused increase vascular permeability leading to plasma infiltration into the vessel wall. They likened these changes to the degeneration and vacuolization of smooth muscle cells and edema of the media of small coronary arteries in hypomagnesemic young dogs (Wener *et al.,* 1964), and reiterated the well-known observation that alcoholics frequently are hypomagnesemic.

The pathology described in these alcoholic patients and hypomagnesemic young dogs strongly resembles that of hereditary medial necrosis. The possibility that hereditary medial necrosis may be due to a genetic abnormality of magnesium metabolism is purely speculative, but worthwhile investigating, especially in the absence of more promising possibilities.

Some patients with pheochromocytoma have been reported as having edema and fibrosis of small coronary arteries (Van Vleit *et al.*, 1966). It is not known whether the effect of catecholamines on small coronary arteries is a direct chemical one, or due to intense vasoconstriction, or to increased compression of intramyocardial and subendocardial arteries because of the positive inotropic action.

C. Summary of Etiology and Histopathology

Unexplained disturbances of cardiac rhythm and conduction and idiopathic cardiomegaly in patients with one of several hereditary syndromes or collagen diseases are the surest hallmarks for the presence of small coronary artery abnormalities. Elderly patients are not only likely to have some degree of coronary atherosclerosis, but nonspecific small artery aging changes and cardiac amyloidosis as well. Diabetics are more prone to disease of both large and small coronary arteries, but disease of the small branches may occur alone. The clinical diagnosis of small coronary artery disease sometimes can clarify otherwise puzzling aspects of a patient's illness, not only giving the physician a more precise data base, but also obviating certain costly, uncomfortable, and dangerous investigative procedures.

References

Blumenthal, H. T., Alex, M., and Goldenberg, S. (1960). Study of lesions of the intramural coronary artery branches in diabetes mellitus. *Arch. Pathol.* **70,** 13–28.

Bredt, H. (1932). Die primare erkrankung der lungenschlagader in ihren verschiedenen formen. *Virchows Arch. Pathol. Anat. Physiol.* **284,** 126–153.

Cowan, J. M. (1904). The heart in acute disease. *J. Pathol. Bacteriol.* **9,** 87–109.

Cruickshank, B. (1953). The arteritis of rheumatoid arthritis. *Ann. Rheum. Dis.* **12,** 136–139.

Demany, M. A., and Zimmerman, H. A. (1969). Progressive muscular dystrophy: Hemodynamic, angiographic and pathologic study of a patient with myocardial involvement. *Circulation* **40,** 377–384.

Donomae, I., Matsumoto, Y., Kokubu, T., Koide, R., Kobayashi, R., Ikegami H., Ueda, E., Fujisawa, T., and Fujimoto, S. (1962). Pathological studies of coronary atherosclerosis: Especially of sclerosis of intramural coronary arteries. *Jap. Heart J.* **3,** 423–441.

Evans, W., Short, D. S., and Bedford, E. (1957). Solitary pulmonary hypertension. *Brit. Heart J.* **19,** 93–116.

Fleischer, R. A., and Rubler, S. (1968). Primary cardiomyopathy in nonanemic patients. Association with sickle trait. *Amer. J. Cardiol.* **22,** 532–537.

Fraser, G. R., Froggatt, P., and James, T. N. (1964). Congenital deafness associated with electrocardiographic abnormalities, fainting attacks and sudden death. A recessive syndrome. *Quart. J. Med.* **33,** 361–385.

Grismer, J. T., Anderson, W. R., and Weiss, L. (1967). Chronic occlusive rheumatic coronary vasculitis: A potential cause of postoperative mortality in mitral valve surgery. *Amer. J. Cardiol.* **19,** 132 (abstr.).

Gross, L., Epstein, E. Z., and Kugel, M. A. (1934). Histology of the coronary arteries and their branches in the human heart. *Amer. J. Pathol.* **10,** 253–274.

Gross, L., Kugel, M. A., and Epstein, E. Z. (1935). Lesions of the coronary arteries and their branches in rheumatic fever. *Amer. J. Pathol.* **11,** 253–280.

Hamby, R. I., Zonereich, S., and Sherman, L. (1970). Primary myocardial disease and diabetes. *Circulation* **42,** III–44 (abstr.).

Han, J. (1969a). Mechanisms of ventricular arrhythmias associated with myocardial infarction. *Amer. J. Cardiol.* **24,** 800–813.

Han, J. (1969b). Ventricular vulnerability during acute coronary occlusion. *Amer. J. Cardiol.* **24,** 857–864.

Han, J., DeTraglia, J., Millet, D., and Moe, G. K. (1966). Incidence of ectopic beats as a function of basic rate in the ventricle. *Amer. Heart J.* **72,** 632–639.

Ivemark, B., and Thoren, C. (1964). The pathology of the heart in Friedreich's ataxia. *Acta Med. scand.* **175,** 227–237.

James, T. N. (1961a). "Anatomy of the Coronary Arteries." Harper (Hoeber), New York.

James, T. N. (1961b). Myocardial infarction and atrial arrhythmias. *Circulation* **24,** 761–776.

James, T. N. (1961c). Effective coronary perfusion pressure. *Amer. Heart J.* **62,** 427–429.

James, T. N. (1961d). Degenerative arteriopathy with pulmonary hypertension. A revised concept of so-called primary pulmonary hypertension. *Henry Ford Hosp. Med. Bull.* **9,** 271–311.

James, T. N. (1962a). Pericarditis and the sinus node. *Arch. Intern. Med.* **110,** 305–311.

James, T. N. (1962b). Observations on the cardiovascular involvement, including the cardiac conduction system, in progressive muscular dystrophy. *Amer. Heart J.* **63,** 48–56.

James, T. N. (1962c). On the cause of syncope and sudden death in primary pulmonary hypertension. *Ann. Intern. Med.* **56,** 252–264.

James, T. N. (1963). The connecting pathways between the sinus node and AV node and between the right and left atrium in the human heart. *Amer. Heart J.* **66,** 498–508.

James, T. N. (1964). An etiologic concept concerning the obscure myocardiopathies. *Progr. Cardiov. Dis.* **7,** 43–64.

James, T. N. (1966). Pathology of the cardiac conduction system in amyloidosis. *Ann. Intern. Med.* **65,** 28–36.

James, T. N. (1967a). Congenital deafness and cardiac arrhythmias. *Amer. J. Cardiol.* **19,** 627–643.

James, T. N. (1967b). Pathology of the small coronary arteries. *Amer. J. Cardiol.* **20,** 679–691.

James, T. N. (1969a). Pathogenesis of arrhythmias in acute myocardial infarction. *Amer. J. Cardiol.* **24,** 791–799.

James, T. N. (1969b). The role of small vessel disease in myocardial infarction. *Circulation* **39/40,** IV–13–19.

James, T. N. (1970). The delivery and distribution of coronary collateral circulation. *Chest* **58,** 183–203.

James, T. N., and Bear, E. S. (1967). Effects of ethanol and acetaldehyde on the heart. *Amer. Heart J.* **74,** 243–255.

James, T. N., and Birk, R. E. (1966). Pathology of the cardiac conduction system in polyarteritis nodosa. *Arch. Intern. Med.* **117,** 561–567.

James, T. N., and Fisch, C. (1963). Observations on the cardiovascular involvement in Friedreich's ataxia. *Amer. Heart J.* **66,** 164–175.

James, T. N., and Monto, R. W. (1966). Pathology of the cardiac conduction system in thrombotic thrombocytopenic purpura. *Ann. Intern. Med.* **65,** 37–43.

James, T. N., Frame, B., and Schatz, I. J. (1964). Pathology of the cardiac conduction system in Marfan's syndrome. *Arch. Intern. Med.* **114,** 339–343.

James, T. N., Rupe, C. E., and Monto, R. W. (1965). Pathology of the cardiac conduction system in systemic lupus erythematosus. *Ann. Intern. Med.* **63,** 402–410.

Jones, S. R., Binder, R. A., and Donowho, E. M., Jr. (1970). Sudden death in sickle-cell trait. *N. Engl. J. Med.* **282,** 323–325.

Karsner, H. T., and Bayless, F. (1934). Coronary arteries in rheumatic fever. *Amer. Heart J.* **9,** 557–585.

Kugel, M. A. (1927). Anatomical studies on the coronary arteries and their branches. I. Arteria anastomotica auricularis magna. *Amer. Heart J.* **3,** 260–270.

Laubry, C., Soulie, P., and Thys, H. (1948). Les anastomoses septales. *Arch. Mal. Coeur Vaiss.* **41,** 1–24.

Ledet, T. (1968). Histological and histochemical changes in the coronary arteries of old diabetic patients. *Diabetologia* **4,** 268–272.

Lev, M., Landowne, M., Matchar, J. C., and Wagner, J. A. (1966). Systemic scleroderma with complete heart block. Report of a case with comprehensive study of the conduction system. *Amer. Heart J.* **72,** 13–24.

More, B. M., and Sommers, S. C. (1962). The status of the myocardial arterioles in angina pectoris. *Amer. Heart J.* **64,** 323–333.

Moritz, A. R., and Oldt, M. R. (1937). Arteriolar sclerosis in hypertensive and nonhypertensive individuals. *Amer. J. Pathol.* **13,** 679–728.

Mustard, J. F., and Packham, M. A. (1969). Platelet function and myocardial infarction. *Circulation* **39/40,** IV–20–28.

Nadas, A. S., Alimurung, M. M., and Sieracki, L. A. (1951). Cardiac manifestations of Friedreich's ataxia. *N. Engl. J. Med.* **244,** 239–244.

Naeye, R. L. (1967). Arteriolar abnormalities with chronic systemic hypertension. A quantitative study. *Circulation* **35,** 662–670.

Okada, R., Harumi, K., Nomura, M., and Murao, S. (1960). Case of coronary sclerosis in small arteries associated with diffuse myocardial fibrosis. *Jap. Heart J.* **1,** 348–356.

Oliveira, E., and Gomez-Patino, N. (1963). Falcemic cardiopathy. Report of a case. *Amer. J. Cardiol.* **11,** 686–688.

Pintar, K., Wolanskyj, B. M., and Gubbay, E. R. (1965). Alcoholic cardiomyopathy. *Can. Med. Ass. J.* **93,** 103–107.

Plaut, A., and Kramer, M. L. (1936). Arteriolar disease of the heart: Associated with severe myomalacia; coronary arteries intact. *Arch. Pathol.* **22,** 393–397.

Pomerance, A. (1965). Senile cardiac amyloidosis. *Brit. Heart J.* **27,** 711–718.

Russell, D. S. (1946). Myocarditis in Friedreich's ataxia. *J. Pathol. Bacteriol.* **58,** 739–748.

Saphir, O., Ohringer, L., and Wong, R. (1956). Changes in the intramural coronary branches in coronary arteriosclerosis. *Arch. Pathol.* **62,** 159–170.

Schwartz, P., and Kurucy, J. (1965). Amyloid deposits in the hearts of aged persons. New aspects of cardiovascular disease. *J. Amer. Geriat. Soc.* **13,** 718–722.

Sobin, L. H., and Hagstrom, J. W. C. (1962). Lesions of cardiac conduction tissue in rheumatoid aortitis. *J. Amer. Med. Ass.* **180,** 1–5.

Thomson, A. M. P. (1968). Dystrophia cordis myotonica studied by serial histology of the pacemaker and conducting system. *J. Pathol. Bacteriol.* **96,** 285–295.

Van Vliet, P. D., Burchell, H. B., and Titus, J. L. (1966). Focal myocarditis associated with pheochromocytoma. *N. Engl. J. Med.* **274,** 1102–1108.

Varnauskas, E., Ivemark, B., Paulin, S., and Ryden, B. (1967). Obscure cardiomyopathies with coronary artery changes. *Amer. J. Cardiol.* **19,** 531–541.

Wener, J., Pintar, K., Simon, M. A., Motola, R., Friedman, R., Mayman, A., and Schucher, R. (1964). The effects of prolonged hypomagnesemia on the cardiovascular system in young dogs. *Amer. Heart J.* **67,** 221–231.

Wright, J. R., Calkins, E., Breen, W. J., Stolte, G., and Schultz, R. T. (1969). Relationship of amyloid to aging. Review of the literature and systematic study of 83 patients derived from a general hospital population. *Medicine* (*Baltimore*) **48,** 39–60.

10 PULMONARY DISEASE AND THE MICROCIRCULATION

JAMES W. WILSON, Ph.D., M.D.

I. Introduction

The lung is the largest unsupported vascular bed in the body, and if all of its vessels were opened and measured, the surface area would be larger than a tennis court. Unsupported in this context implies no solid organ support such as is found in the liver or spleen. The microvasculature of the lung is unique in many respects. The wall of the pulmonary capillary is a membrane 0.15 to 0.3 μm in thickness that separates the internal fluids of the body from the atmosphere. Any serious change in the thickness or character of this microvascular wall often results in pulmonary failure and death. Recently, research has conclusively demonstrated that each individual respiratory unit, or alveolus, is not isolated with its own set of capillaries where gaseous exchange occurs. Anatomic reconstruction of these alveoli with their capillary-covered walls has demonstrated that many of the capillaries penetrate the thin alveolar septae and extend into adjacent alveoli by anastomotic connections. Frequently these connections occur through as many as 15 to 25 single alveoli before the cellular elements of the blood are returned to the venous side of the pulmonary circulation. This anatomic finding has enlightened us to the fact that mean red cell transit time through the lung's vasculature is highly variable, depending on the route which blood flow may take. Flow across these capillary beds may be altered by regulatory mechanisms of seemingly various types, which have not been precisely defined. Figure 1 demonstrates the complexity of this arrangement and the number of channels found in a small unit area of the alveolus.

As blood traverses the lumen of the two main pulmonary arteries, it enters an arborizing network of dividing right angle pulmonary arterioles which taper into conelike structures terminating in blind end or blunt arterioles (Fig. 2). These unusual anatomic passages lie proximal to the capillary beds of the alveolus. At this precise location in the distal pulmonary arterioles, precapillary sphincters have been shown to regulate blood flow across the complex capillary network of the alveolus. Smooth muscle in these sphincters is under control of the X cranial or vagus nerve, and the closure of these arteriole regulatory sentries can be stimulated in a variety of conditions which alter flow patterns through the lung. The "shunting" of blood through alternate channels, when it occurs, permits blood to return to the venous side of the pulmonary circulation in a more direct manner. The pulmonary venous pO_2 falls as the result of less oxygen exchange in the lung when flow is bypassing the alveoli. Blood flow may be through arteriovenous shunts (particularly in the fetal and newborn lung), physiologic shunts, or simply deviation pathways from long to short routes by closure of the sphincters. At times, blood flow in any given lobular unit may cease for short intervals and resume as pathways reopen in the normal physiologic situation. The importance of these regulatory sphincters has been emphasized by energetic researchers, but little noted by the clinicians. "Pulmonary shunting" is becoming a more frequently used term for the clinician, and knowledge of the microvasculature and its basic mechanisms is important in understanding such a clinical entity. By using many modern techniques for isotope and opaque dye injection, shunting can be quantitated in human lungs. In some institutions, sophisticated research equipment will also demonstrate shunting by variations in oxygen saturation from venous to arterial systemic blood.

Injury to the cellular components of the pulmonary vascular network (Fig. 3) is initiated by a variety of insulting agents and disease states. Some of these are primary intravascular or blood cell injuries. Others involve the structure of the pulmonary vessels and the third category includes injury to the parenchyma of the lung lying outside the vascular network. Some of these insulting agents are produced in the peripheral vascular network and ultimately are transmitted to the pulmonary capillary network via the microcirculation.

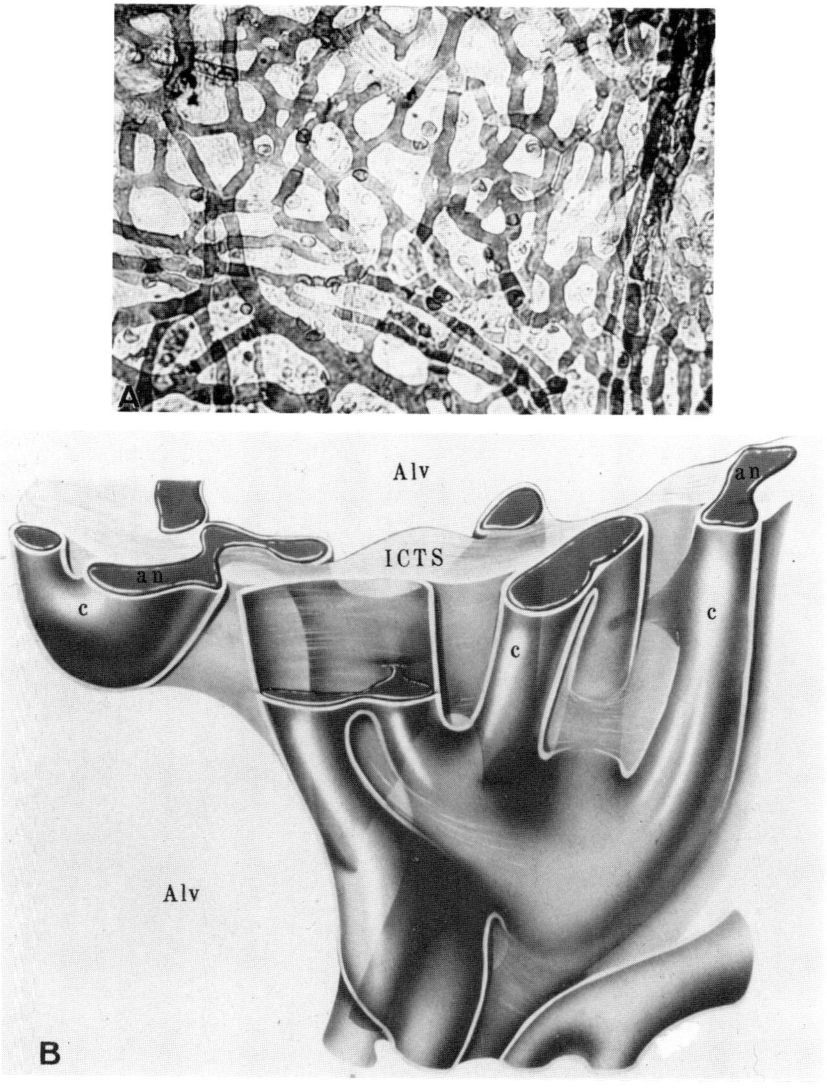

Fig. 1. (A) Photograph of a single alveolar septum showing the extensive anastomosing capillary network. Two distinct layers of capillaries are visible and clearly lie in two different planes. These layers connect via penetrating capillaries shown in B. (Courtesy of Dr. Steve Ryan, St. Luke's Hospital, New York City.) (B) Diagrammatic reconstruction of penetrating anastomotic capillaries interconnecting two alveoli. ICTS, Interstitial connective tissue septum; c, capillary lumen; an, anastomoses; Alv, alveolus. (Courtesy of Dr. Steve Ryan.)

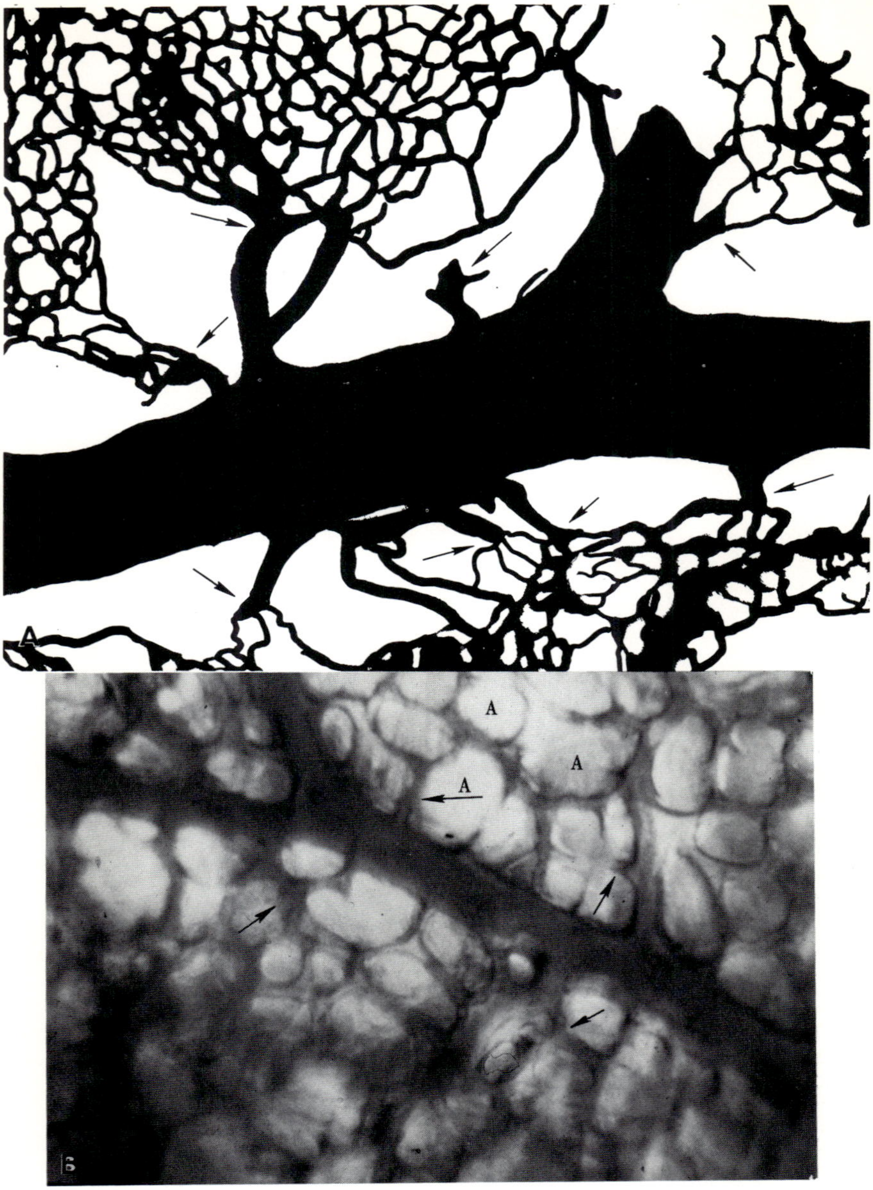

Fig. 2. (A) Schematic drawing from a vascular injection preparation of human lung. The blind end, blunt, precapillary arterioles (arrows) contain sphincters which regulate blood flow across the alveolar capillary network. These arterioles are under control of the X cranial nerve. (B) *In vivo* photograph from a 16-mm movie frame of a normal dog lung demonstrating the location of these precapillary arteriole sphincters which guard the entrance to the alveolar capillary beds. This low-power photograph does not show the capillaries running across the thin septal walls as in (A), but demonstrates the larger feeding vessels. A, Alveolus. (550×.)

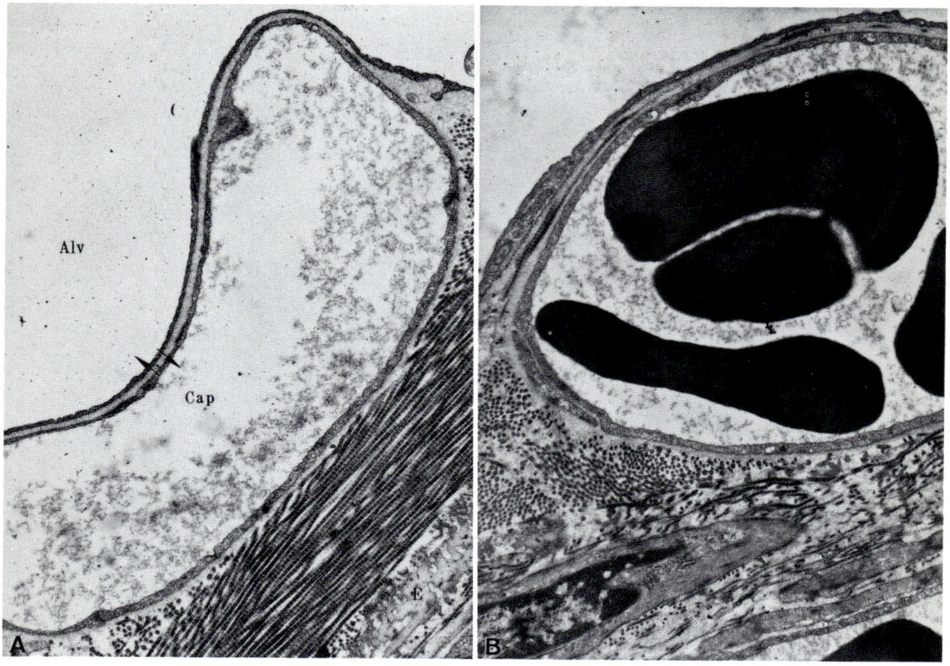

Fig. 3. (A) Electron photomicrograph of an alveolar capillary in the dog lung. Normal lung shows collagen fibrils in the lower right, giving the septal areas support. This capillary is not collapsed, but demonstrates plasma skimming with no cellular elements in the lumen. The air-blood barrier, so-called, should probably be called the air-blood pathway (arrows). It is composed of an endothelial cell, interstitial ground substance, and an alveolar epithelial cell or type I pneumocyte. E, Elastic tissue; Alv, alveolus; Cap, capillary. (10,000×.) (B) The photomicrograph from this normal dog lung shows the ovoid or rounded appearance seen when the capillary lumen contains erythrocytes or other blood elements. A few collagen fibrils extend into the thin part of the air-blood pathway. (10,000×.)

II. Lymphatics

In the conventional sense, the pulmonary parenchyma is thought of as having two separate vascular supplies. One is through the pulmonary vascular network which operates under low pressure and the second through the bronchial vessels which receive systemic blood under a much higher pressure. In reality, it possesses a third vascular network which is frequently overlooked but currently receiving renewed interest. The pulmonary lymphatic system is still relatively unexplored. Lymphatic channels were first seen and described by Herophilus in 300 B.C., but were rediscovered in the 1600's. The name lymphatics was first used by Bartholin in 1653. Lymph channels on the pleural surface as well as the deep lymphatics of the lung were described by Mascagni during that same period. Only recently have the valves in the main lymph trunks near the hilum been described. Lauweryns and Boussauw have reconstructed these valves by using camera lucida techniques and found them to be of an unusual structural configuration. Not only are the valves in these small lymphatic channels not the classic bicuspid type, but they are also extremely resistant to retrograde flow when pressure increases in any given vessel segment. They are tapering, funnel-shaped cones which compartmentalize the lymphatics into an orderly system of locks and dams (Fig. 4). Like the lymphatics of the extremities, they are stimulated to flow by force applied from outside their lumen. Vigorous ventilation with positive pres-

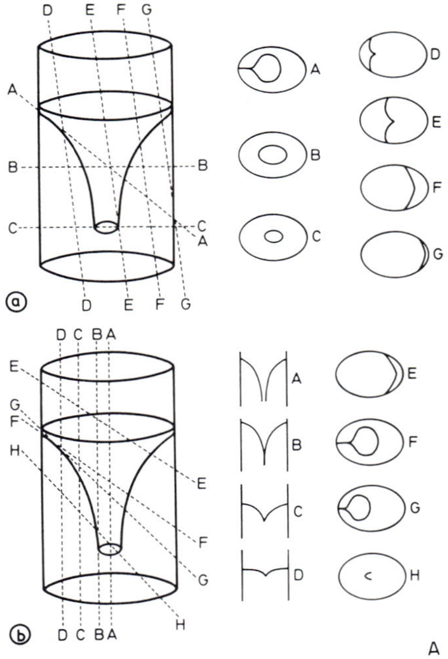

Fig. 4. (A) Diagrams of the funnel-shaped lymphatic valves which are interposed in the lymphatic channels. These valves, when cut on 6-μm sections, showed all the configurations shown in planes A through H in both drawings (a and b). Many of these can falsely mimic the classic bicuspid valves or produce rather unusual formations which would be difficult to recognize if the work had not been done with serial

sure at the end of expiration will produce flow in this system (PEEP). Positive End Expiratory Pressure is a current topic for debate and is in the forefront of respiratory therapy.

In the embryo, lymphatics invade the hilar region of the lung during the second month of life. By the end of the third month, lymphatics have extended along the bronchopulmonary artery and pulmonary veins to the pleural plexus. Valves also appear around the hilum about the same time.

The larger lymph vessels resemble veins in structure. Their diameters vary greatly within a short distance, becoming narrow and then widening almost immediately. There are three distinct layers in the larger lymphatics, the tunica intima, the tunica media, and the tunica adventitia. The tunica adventitia is made of connective and fibroelastic tissue. The tunica media consists of smooth muscle fibers running longitudinally and obliquely. The tunica intima is mainly endothelium.

Lymphatic capillaries of the lung differ from the larger lymph vessels in structure. The lymph capillaries are made of a thin, single layer of endothelium. Some of the vessels' most prominent ultrastructural characteristics are irregular lumina, basement membranes that are poorly defined or sometimes absent, and the absence of red blood cells. The lymphatic endothelial cells form innumerable irregular projections into the lumen of the

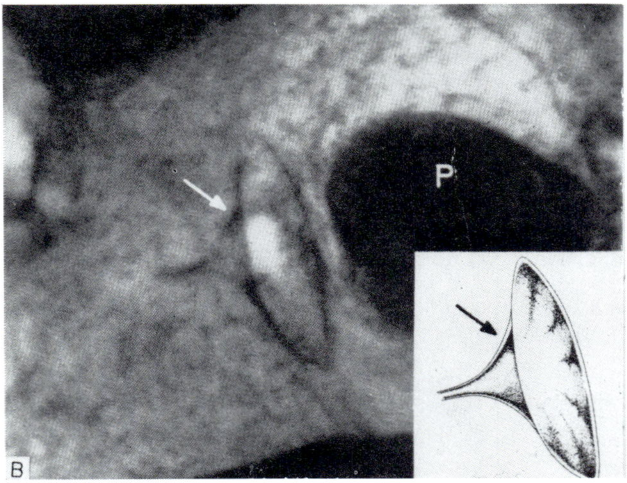

sectioning techniques, (courtesy of Dr. J. M. Lauweryns, University of Leuven, Belgium.) (B) Stereomicroscopic funnellike architecture of the pulmonary lymphatic valves is shown in an interlobular connective tissue space, around a pulmonary vein (P). This photo was made in human infant lung thick sections. (97×.) (Courtesy Dr. J. M. Lauweryns.)

surrounding vessels and connective tissue. Contact between these cells varies from the regular end-to-end connection to more complex junctions with various kinds of attachments. The cytoplasm of the endothelial cells contain dense bodies, coated vesicles, and a few irregular smooth surface vacuoles. All these factors suggest an intense transport of fluid. The lung exhibits an extraordinary, profuse network of lymphatics. In fact, this network is much larger than the lymphatics of other body organs.

Three main groups of pulmonary lymphatics occur in man's lung. These three types are distinguished not only by site, but also by origin. The first group begins at the periphery of the lung lobules. This includes the lymphatics lying in the pleura. These drain into trunks which give rise to the perivenous and periarterial channels. The second group originates as blind-ended tubes in the center of saclike dilatations around the alveolar ducts. Only a few sparse lymph capillaries lie in the walls of the alveoli. These tubes give rise to the peribronchial lymphatics which create a network around the bronchoarterial bundle that goes to the hilum. The third group lies in the interlobular septa deep in the lung. These anastomose with the peribronchial and perivenous groups.

Some investigators feel that the abundant and profuse supply of lymphatics is divided into a superficial and deep set. The superficial set is the pleura pulmonalis. The deep set consists of the areas of the bronchi, pulmonary artery, pulmonary veins, and the connective tissue septae between the lobules. These two sets of lymphatics are in connection with each other only within the pleura and at the hilum of the lung.

In the larger bronchi, the cartilage that covers them is enclosed by two sets of lymphatics. These are connected by anastomosing vessels which pass between the cartilages. In the smaller bronchi and their subsequent divisions, only one plexus of lymphatics is found. These become smaller and smaller until they terminate at the distal end of the ductuli alveolares, or alveolar ducts.

The branches of the pulmonary artery are accompanied by two or three lymph trunks so arranged that one trunk lies between the artery and accompanying bronchus all of the time. These trunks are connected by numerous loops. The bronchial lymph and arterial lymph are in communication at the divisions of the bronchi.

Pulmonary veins arise from the pleura, from the distal ends of the sacculi alveolares, and where bronchi divide. The smaller veins are accompanied by one or two lymphatics. As the veins increase in size, the lymphatics form a network which increases in complexity.

A single plexus of lymphatics is found in the pleura of the lungs. Pleural lymphatics are much more prominent over the lower lobes of the lungs.

These lymphatics lie within the confines of the visceral pleura and not in the subpleural plane. Trunks drain into the lymph nodes at the hilum of the lung. The lymphatics in this area of the lung are somewhat different in that they seem to form irregular polyhedral rings with either fewer or more unequal sides than those in other areas.

For several years there have been experiments and research on the question of whether there were any lymphatics in or about the alveoli. The work of J. M. Lauweryns has shown that there are rarely lymphatic capillaries at the level of the "air-blood barrier" or the "interalveolar septum." The "air-blood barrier" is made up of the alveolar epithelial cell lining, the alveolar interstitium, and the blood capillary endothelial cells. The interalveolar septum is defined as the "septum between two neighboring alveolar lumina." Lymphatic capillaries are present between the alveolar walls and surrounding connective tissue. These are actually very close to the interlobular septa and have been described as being in the interlobular septa.

The valves in the pulmonary lymphatics, as stated previously, are different from other valves in other lymphatic systems of the body. The valves point in the direction of lymph flow and are suspended obliquely in the lumen of vessels. They are attached so that they cover the entire interior of the lymphatic. Their structure is such that they cannot easily be turned inside out by sudden pressure.

The lymphatics which accompany the pulmonary veins and branches drain toward the hilum. The valves sit in a position where they point inward to the hilum. The abundant network of lymphatics in the pleura unites with the main trunks which flow into the tracheobronchial lymph nodes. In the event that the nodes or channels are occluded as in lymphomas, lymph will go around these segments to the mediastinal channels. Flow in the bronchial and arterial lymphatics is toward the interior of the lung. The lymphatics situated in the alveolar walls have valves which point toward the pleura. This is the only connection between the pleural (superficial) lymphatics and parenchymatous (deep) lymphatics.

Lymph flow is in two main directions from the lung. One direction is forward to the internal mammary chain of lymph nodes and vessels, and the other is backward to the posterior mediastinum. Some of the lymphatics in the lower intercostal spaces then drain down through the diaphragm to the cisterna chyli. Some of the mediastinal lymphatics flow directly into the thoracic duct, while the majority join the pulmonary lymphatics and drain into the veins at the base of the neck near the thoracic duct.

Much research has been done on the role of lymphatics in disease. It is known that lymph flow increases considerably during most inflammatory disorders of the lung. In the presence of pulmonary lymphatic obstruction, a more severe degree of pulmonary edema is provoked than would be the case if the lymphatics were normal. Other studies on pulmonary edema show that lymph flow increases greatly during the acute phase and is slower in the recovery phase. Some researchers believe that interalveolar edema occurs as a result of insufficiency of the pulmonary lymphatic flow.

Pneumoconiosis is characterized by a chronic lymphangitis, perilymphangitis, and eventual mechanical insufficiency of the pulmonary lymph circulation. In emphysema, as the alveolar spaces become enlarged, pressure is applied to the surrounding lymph channels and the peripheral nodes. Therefore, lymph has to be conveyed by collateral channels in the pleura or along a proximal artery toward the region of the hilum.

The primary cause of hyaline membrane disease in infants remains questionable. Work has been done on the role that pulmonary lymphatics play in this disease. There is an increase in their diameters, but after experiments, it has been found that this increase is really a normal occurrence in the newborn and a defense mechanism against the increased alveolar transudation.

The significance of this lymphatic system should be emphasized in conditions such as hemorrhagic shock, gram-negative sepsis, respiratory distress of the newborn, and myocardial infarction leading to cardiogenic shock.

One anatomic fact, which has been long overlooked by the busy clinician, is that all human hearts and lungs are connected in series. Therefore, events taking place within the heart are directly reflected in the microcirculation of the lung and vice versa. The cardiologist might treat the failing heart while not realizing the lung is also in failure.

III. Pulmonary Embolism

One common form of embolization to the lung is that of fat globules which entered the blood as a result of crush injury to soft tissue or long bone fractures. It is now well established that orthopedic surgery, mobilization of stored lipid, or coalescing microspheres of free fatty acids can produce the same entity. If ruptured fat cells release liquid fat droplets into the circulation, a veritable myriad of fat globules form in blood as a result of their surface tension characteristics. These may diffusely embolize to the small pulmonary capillaries, which is the case in gram-negative sepsis when no bone injury has occurred. The patients who develop fat emboli in gram-negative sepsis, do so as the result of tissue destruction following bacterial invasion or free fatty acid increase with stress. Acute pulmonary circulatory obstruction results in profound hypoxemia, dyspnea, cyanosis, and tachypnea. Additionally, some of these fat emboli escape through the pulmonary network and are returned to the systemic circulation where they may also produce occlusion of peripheral capillaries. These emboli have been observed in the skin, brain, and kidneys. In the brain, they produce obstruction in small vessels of the white matter and cause the patient to have delirium, restlessness, or transient neurologic manifestations such as convulsions and twitching. Petechiae in the skin are most commonly found in such cases and may exhibit a brownish color rather than the usual reddish appearance. Glomerular lesions may be focal and bear no relation to renal cellular alterations. Renal function may sometimes not be impaired, but the urine in such patients is often characterized by globules of fat or chylomicrons dispersed on the surface.

The consequence of large pulmonary emboli or thrombosis in pulmonary arteries is well known. These emboli and thrombi are composed of aggregated erythrocytes, leukocytes, platelets, and fibrin. Embolism of this type usually occurs in trauma, particularly in young individuals who were previously healthy. In younger patients, survival occurs in a higher percentage than in elderly individuals who are predisposed to age factors and vascular disease. Venous stasis, which may be caused by incipient venous disease, immobilization, or gravity, is a well-recognized factor in producing phlebothrombosis. When pulmonary emboli are released from such thrombotic sites, infarcts are predominantly located on the right side in the lower lobes. Statistically, a greater percentage of these emboli are produced in the venous system of the left leg. This is apparently due to the anatomic distribution of the iliac vein and its relationship to the artery as it enters the left common iliac vein. Lower extremity wounds have been shown to predispose the patient to fatal pulmonary embolism, also.

A third type of pulmonary embolization consists of a microembolic shower of aggregated blood elements. This condition is also clinically important since it has been determined that human pulmonary embolism of this type is usually fatal because of massive mechanical blockage. These microaggregations are often found in the presence of other debilitating diseases and they are not necessarily the documented cause of death. Whether or not reflex vasospasm is important, is questionable. The rapidly tapering pulmonary arteries and arterioles which run in series with the remainder of the pulmonary circulation are consequently the most likely resting place for microemboli, excluding the portal bed. Emboli from the venous side or the right heart may obstruct the pulmonary vascular tree causing a relatively low blood volume to reach the systemic arterial side and overdistention of the pulmonary arteries, right heart, and systemic veins. Such changes in blood distribution can induce widespread reflex vascular activity. Some evidence indicates that pulmonary vascular resistance in arteries, capillaries, and veins is longitudinal while other investigators have indicated focal pulmonary vascular obstruction is caused by sphincteric action at the precapillary site.

IV. Shock and Related Capillary Phenomenon

Since 1965, an intensive investigation has been underway to determine the cause of a now recognized clinical entity called "shock lung." Briefly, numerous investigations have shown that part of the problem encountered in producing pulmonary vascular damage leading to progressive pulmonary insufficiency is generated by disseminated intravascular microaggregates (Fig. 5). Platelets, leukocytes, and, eventually, erythrocytes can obstruct flow in the pulmonary vascular network when stasis occurs. In hypovolemic and gram-negative septic shock, platelet aggregation occurs rapidly. This type of platelet aggregation has also been demonstrated after the injection of adenosine diphosphate (ADP), local injury to the capillary endothelium, administration of high concentrations of oxygen, endotoxin production by bacteria, and inhalation of oxident gases (e.g., nitrogen dioxide in relatively low concentrations). Debris which develops in stored whole blood from the breakdown of cellular elements may also be recovered from the microvascular network of the lung. Platelet aggregates, red cell clumps, polymorphonuclear leukocyte aggregates, and masses of cytoplasmic particles from degraded cells have been documented. In conjunction with this type of cellular degradation, the capillary endothelial cells appear swollen or edematous in most of these conditions. Morphologically, tight junctions between capillary endothelial cells are (Fig. 6) apparently damaged and allow fluid to extravasate into the interstitium of the lung through open zona occludens. This produces a characteristic, diffuse, hazy, hyalinized, ground-glass appearance on radiographic examination, caused by transudative interstitial edema. The most important therapeutic tool for this condition is a high index of suspicion. Second, serial chest roentgenograms obtained in the injured patient as soon as possible and followed with additional films every 2 to 3 hours may be extremely valuable after resuscitation with intravenous fluid therapy. The leaky lung capillary syndrome is becoming a well-recognized clinical entity. One of the most common clinical errors in resuscitation of such patients is failure to recognize that neither auscultation of the lung nor measurement of central venous pressure will provide a reliable diagnosis for the interstitial wet lung problem. These patients die with progressive pulmonary insufficiency, their lungs are the consistency of liver, and many of them have no audible rales at any time during their downhill course. This is in distinct contrast to the more classic picture of pulmonary edema associated with mitral stenosis. In the latter case, widespread rales and copious amounts of frothy sputum are both good clinical indicators. This fluid shift from the intravascular to the interstitial compartment occurs so rapidly that alveolar consolidation takes place in about 72 hours and ultimately involves entire lobes of the lung.

Positive end expiratory pressure adjusted to give the patient a better arterial oxygen saturation will help to remove much of this interstitial edema through the highly efficient lymphatic system previously described. Pharmacologic corticosteroidlike agents, such as methylprednisolone sodium succinate which seems to be specifically indicated in this condition, have been shown to decrease the edema and provide cellular protection during this type of insult. Anticoagulation wth heparin in some studies has also proven to be efficacious. This seems particularly true in the case of gram-negative septic shock which produces an identical picture. In contrast to the other types of shock, endotoxin maintains the ability to lyse endothelial cells and all the circulating blood elements, including platelets and leukocytes. Once these cells are lysed, lysosomal inclusions containing large quantities of hydrolytic enzymes and vasoactive peptides are released into the circulation where they are free to destroy the remaining normal cellular architecture and aggrevate the cascading condition. Between the ages of 3 and 37, shock lung with progressive pulmonary insufficiency is the leading killer of young Americans. Death from this condition usually occurs within 2 to 15 days after injury which is frequently unrelated to the thorax.

Much has been written about a biologic variable described as disseminated intravascular coagulation. Obviously, the lung with its gigantic capillary network which may be reactive to microemboli is a target organ for these disseminated aggregates. It may well be that the many shock states produce damage to the pulmonary capillary network via a common mechanism of intravascularly mediated chemical bombardment. Increases in pulmonary vascular resistance have been well documented both clinically and experimentally in many of these situations. Serotonin, histamine, protaglandins, and other vasoactive agents have been implicated, but the exact mediator is undetermined. Exposure to high oxygen concentrations will ultimately produce many of the same cellular changes found in shock, sepsis, and other acute pulmonary insults. Since the presence of an oxygen-rich environment does not seem to deter cell degradation, it appears that the question of cellular anoxia is unsettled at the present time.

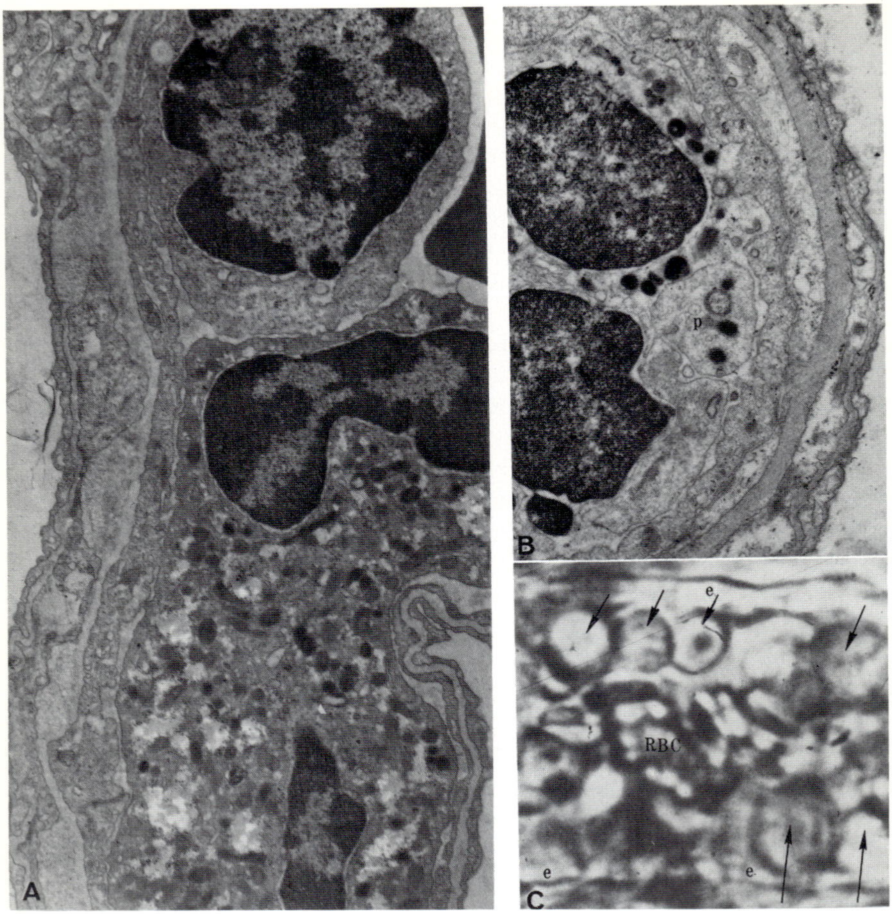

Fig. 5. (A) Human lung biopsy, following cardiopulmonary bypass, shows a septal capillary with two large leukocytes partially filling the lumen. These polymorphonuclear leukocytes have nonmembrane limited areas of decreased density in the cytoplasm (bottom), indicating an abnormal cell which does not show the usual changes associated with maturation or cell death. Glycogen particles are present in the cytoplasm, several lysosomes show a loss of their electron density (degranulation), and the cell has no pseudopod formation around its periphery. (19,800×.) (B) Human lung tissue, from a patient who died in hemorrhagic shock, illustrates a complex of leukocytes and platelets (p) which totally obstructed the lumen of this capillary. (15,600×.) (C) *In vivo* single frame from a 16-mm movie of dog lung in hemorrhagic shock. The white cells (arrows) are marginated against the endothelium (e) on both sides of this vessel. Erythrocytes (RBC) fill the central luminal space and are aggregated in a small rouleau formation. (360×.)

Fig. 5. (D) Platelets, having various morphologic appearances, undergo membrane lysis and release their vasocactive contents into the pulmonary capillaries. These plate-

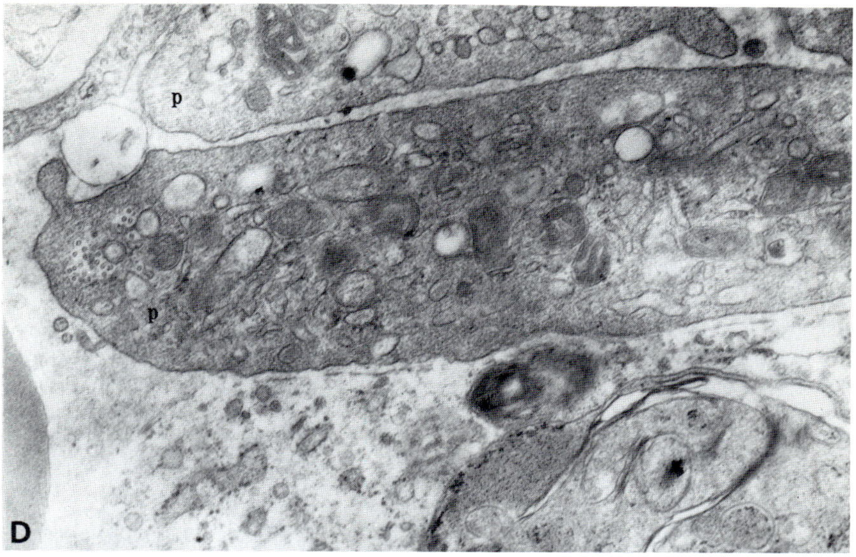

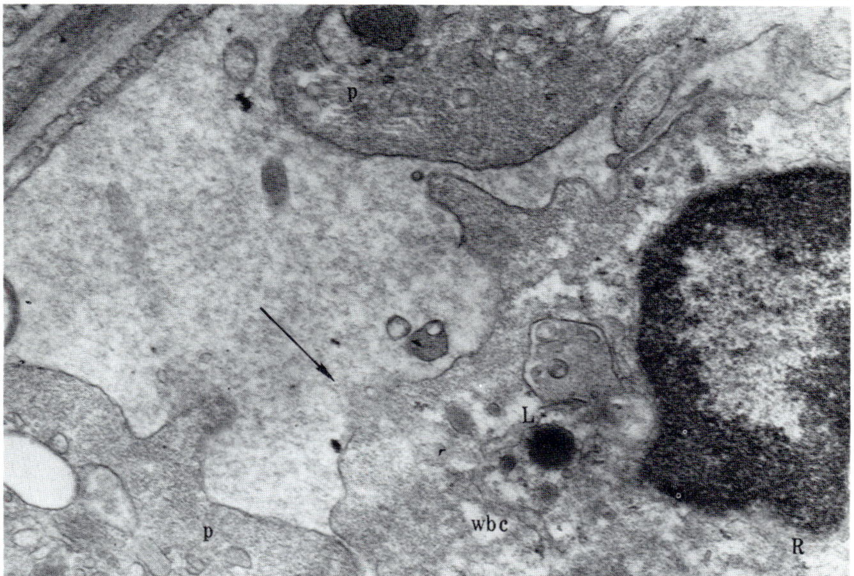

lets (p) show slight degranulation indicative of older thrombocytes. Membranes are intact, but the top platelet is adjacent to the endothelial cell, to which they sometimes adhere. (35,000×.) (E) Aggregates of white cells and platelets in animal lungs appear quickly in endotoxin-induced shock. This dog lung shows two platelets (p) which have aggregated with the leukocyte (wbc) at the lower right. This white cell shows only one lysosome (L) in this part of its cytoplasm and the plasma membrane (arrow) is disrupted. (35,700×.)

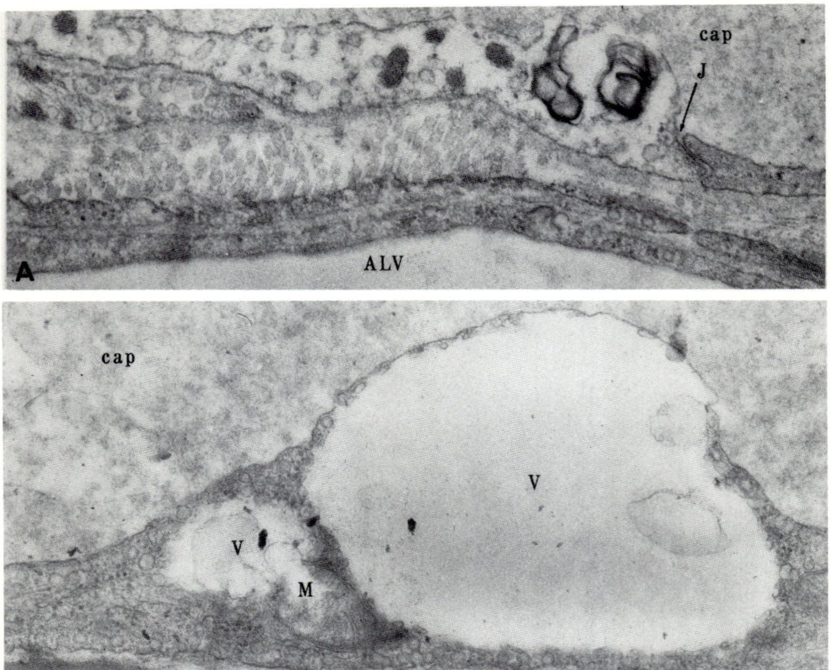

Fig. 6. (A) Endothelial cells in the septal capillaries (cap) of the alveoli (ALV) show focal cellular damage and swelling of their cytoplasm. The pinocytotic vesicles are decreased in number, myelin figures are also present in the rarefied cytoplasm, and a "tight junction" (J) is no longer normal in its appearance. This junctional disruption in the endothelial cells allows fluid to escape into the interstitial space. (29,250×.) (B)

V. Conditions That Occur More Often in the Right Lung

A certain group of pathologic conditions have been shown statistically to occur on the right side more often than on the left side of the chest. (1) Chylothorax, for one, is more frequent on the right and this predisposition is attributable to the fact that the thoracic duct in the chest lies to the right of the vertebral column in a greater part of its course. It also accounts for the high right lateralization of chylothorax development. (2) The "middle lobe syndrome" is believed to be produced by a lack of collateral ventilation through the pores of Cohn as opposed to obstruction of the bronchial system by enlarging lymph nodes. (3) Adults as well as children develop pneumonia and lung abscesses more often on the right side than on the left. (4) Likewise, sarcoidosis of the lung is preceded by hilar lymphadenopathy most usually found on the right side. This is also applicable to sarcoid enlargement of the tracheobronchial and paratracheal lymph nodes. (5) Carcinoma of the bronchogenic variety has been shown to develop in the right lung in 56 to 63% of all cases. Some investigators attribute this to the deposition of greater amounts of carcinogens in this location compared to the opposite side. (6) Pulmonary infarction is subsequently higher on the right side. (7) Unilateral pulmonary effusion is more frequently found in congestive heart failure, occupying the right pleural cavity. Virtually every case of interlobar effusion of the vanishing tumor of the lung (phantom lung tumor) has been observed on the right side. (8) Meig's syndrome produces the well-known hydrothorax which is detectable in the right hemithorax 70% of the time. In contrast, it occurs bilaterally 20% of the time and on the left in only 10% of the cases. The question arises as to the importance of anatomic, circulatory, and functional factors in these disease entities. Because the right lung is larger than the left, the volume of both gas and blood or lymph handled by it is greater than 50% (53 to 56%). Conversely, of the total lung volume, the left lung provides only 44 to 47%. The right mainstem bronchus runs in a more

---

Vacuolated areas (V) in the endothelial cell are filled with edema fluid and demonstrate the thin plasma membrane which prevents the cytoplasm from communicating with the capillary lumen (cap). A mitochondrion (M) is damaged and shows direct connection with a vacuolated appearing area of cytoplasmic rarefaction. Smooth muscle cells (SM) are present in this particular section at the lower border. (29,900×.) (C) Single mitochondria (M) show dilatation of the cristi system, distortion, and edema. This may be responsible for the later lesion seen in (B) above. Once these organelles are damaged and fluid fills the interstitium (I), plasma and cell elements quickly fill the space through open junctions (J) between interstitial supporting cells; capillary lumen (cap), endothelium (E). (29,900×.)

perpendicular course than the left. When the pulmonary circulation is carefully considered, it is found that approximately 55% of the blood volume from the right ventricle flows through the vasculature of the right lung where it is oxygenated. Another contributing factor may be the more negative intrapleural pressure on the right side as compared to the left. Authoritative investigators have shown that pulmonary function tests clearly indicate the vital capacity for the right lung ranges between 52 and 54%, the total volume 53 to 57%, and the minute volume 54 to 55%. From these total comparative pulmonary function tests, it is clear that the left lung plays a lesser role than the right. This interesting predisposition of the right hemithorax to disease deserves some clinical consideration on the basis of its statistical importance.

VI. Pulmonary Hemorrhage

Massive pulmony hemorrhage is frequently seen in the lungs of newborn infants during the first 2 weeks of life. No preferable location has been documented and the predisposing factors are unclear. Most cases present with an acute infection elsewhere and eventually develop pneumonia. Many of these infants have congenital heart disease, kernicterus, and intracranial hemorrhage. Small, subpleural, irregularly located hemorrhages may indicate shock, asphyxia, or breathing disorders associated with infections.

In the adult, hemorrhage is an entirely different matter and is usually a disruptive process resulting from local injuries such as the rupture of an aneurysm into the lung. Damaged pulmonary vessels may be caused by tuberculosis, carcinoma, polyarteritis, lymphatic disease, etc. Blast injuries producing negative pressure may also cause massive pulmonary hemorrhage. Usually this hemorrhage is accompanied by marked edema and congestion which produce a dense, airless, beefy red lung. Blunt trauma is capable of producing similar effects which have been shown to result from rupture of alveolar capillaries. All these injuries are very similar to the pictures seen after shock and trauma.

It has been observed that thin-walled, widened pulmonary arteries occur in patients who die without having undergone surgical procedures. In many cases, this atrophy of the pulmonary arterial media is an important factor in the origin of circulatory disturbances occurring in the lung. Thin pulmonary vascular walls are unable to resist sudden increases in flow and pressure, cannot withstand sudden massive contractions, do not compensate for rapid hemodynamic changes predisposed by surgical intervention, and may progressively undergo necrosis and allow communication with the perivascular space. In patients who have pulmonary stenosis and a surgical closure of a ventricular septal defect, the picture of the lungs at autopsy in nonsurviving patients is that of pulmonary edema, the escape of red blood cells into the perivascular space, and distention of the pulmonary arterioles, capillaries, and some venules. Extracorporeal circulation may also render the lung nonviable in some areas, depending on the extent of bleeding into the interstitium. Interstitial hemorrhage in the lung is analogous to hemorrhage into any other potential space in the body. The pulmonary interstitium is the lung's fascial space which runs from the hilum to the periphery. Once blood, fluid, or bacteria have gained access to this compartment, they are free to invade in either direction, with very little resistance, except for gravity influences. This type of pulmonary hemorrhage acts as an effective perivascular tamponade. This tamponade may serve as a protective mechanism to halt pulmonary hemorrhage from small vessels.

The entire sequence for interstitial hemorrhage may terminate in intraalveolar hemorrhage and the wet, congested, heavy lungs found at the autopsy table.

As red blood cells gain access to the perivascular space, they may produce characteristic perivascular and peribronchial hemorrhages which have been documented in both animal experiments and human lungs. With further cellular damage, anoxia, and hemodynamic changes, denudation of the basement membrane underlying the alveolar epithelial type I lining cells may take place. Subsequently, red cells which have gained access to the interstitial lung compartment are then allowed access to adjacent alveoli, and terminal congestion with intraalveolar hemorrhage, loss of plasma proteins, and lungs that weigh at autopsy are 800–1400 gm produced. The consequence of this hemorrhage, if the patient survives, is necrosis of lung tissue and a nonfunctional gas-exchanging membrane. The significance of this type of hemorrhage in small arterioles located at the precapillary level is very important.

Since the lymphatics have been documented as being located along arterioles, venules, and at the level of the larger bronchioles, some of the perivascular hemorrhage seen in microscopic sections at autopsy might be interpreted as leading into these lymphatic spaces. The hypothetical connection of these spaces with pulmonary veins under pathologic conditions, in which pulmonary venous pressure is increased, has never been conclusively documented. However, such a hypothesis is tempting since edema and hemorrhage into lymphatic vessels are recognizable in certain disease conditions. This is particularly true if these lymphatics are enlarged and can be easily identified on histologic sections. It is important to recognize, however, that the intraadventitial or perivascular spaces are not the same as the perivascular lymphatics. Some investigators have claimed that these perivascular spaces represent preexisting lymphatic vessels while others consider this condition to be a pathologic rather than a normal anatomic finding. It is logical that pronounced dilatation or bleeding into these spaces may lead to tearing of lymphatics, and, therefore, blood could gain access to lymphatic channels in this manner.

Hemorrhage into the interstitium of the lungs has largely been regarded as a consequence of abrupt physiologic changes rather than a pathologic process. Even though it may be experimentally produced in more than one way, the final outcome is essentially the same. Once blood or edema is interposed in the air-blood barrier between the alveoli and the vessels supplying a lung segment, the efficiency of gaseous exchange is significantly reduced. If fluid is interposed in this potential space, an effective alveolar capillary block is not only present at the level of the thin portion of the air-blood barrier, but may also dissect in a retrograde fashion toward the hilum and interfere with the exchange of gases in larger arterioles.

Tamponade produced by bleeding into the perivascular space may be extremely important in allowing the lung to halt or limit blood flow to damaged areas under certain pathologic conditions. It may also enhance the repair of these areas via revascularization and cell regeneration, following the vascular insult.

The importance of hemorrhage into the lung should not be minimized since it is one of the most common and most destructive lesions seen at autopsy. Hemorrhage is not always massive, but sometimes is continuous in very small quantities over extended periods of time. Slow, insidious hemorrhage is more usually associated with chronic inflammatory diseases of the lung rather than acute processes such as the insult documented in hemorrhagic shock. The destruction of blood vessels proceeds on a relatively large scale under the former conditions, but the total process of inflammation may be slow, thereby permitting ample time for the intima of these vessels to regenerate and afford closure of most of the damaged areas. With decreasing blood flow through a given area during a disease process, hemorrhage may also be minimized. The upper and middle lobes, which are not well perfused during hypovolemic shock, may also develop patterns of hemorrhage following the reinfusion of blood. Numerous investigators have suggested that this hemorrhagic interstitial leakage of blood, or red cell diapedesis, is caused by some injurious agent contained within the blood itself. This hypothesis is yet to be substantiated and the causative agent isolated.

The sequential development of perivascular and interstitial hemorrhages within the pulmonary parenchyma in hemorrhagic shock, experimental anaphylactic shock in rats, cardiopulmonary bypass procedures, homologous blood transfusions, etc., has been documented. This characteristic type of hemorrhage has also been shown to occur in patents after surgical repair of a tetralogy of Fallot and other specific surgical procedures. Documentation of cellular changes leading to the release of blood cells into the interstitium has explained why copious diapedesis is one of the characteristic changes found in autopsy lungs from patients who died in hemorrhagic shock after general surgery, or other nonthoracic trauma. The development of this lesion may subsequently lead to the escape of red cells into the alveoli and produce the terminal picture of intraalveolar hemorrhage. Perivascular tamponade also serves as a protective mechanism for the lung to halt bleeding from damaged vessels which may subsequently be repaired by revascularization and recanalization. It also allows collateral circulation to reach undamaged alveolar vessels and sustain gas exchange. This process, however, depends on the patient surviving the initial pulmonary vascular insult which produced the hemorrhages. Subtle hemorrhage into a limiting space is more readily tolerated by the lung than massive intraalveolar hemorrhage which may produce immediate death.

The perivascular lesion is shown in Fig. 7A–E.

Aspirated blood will eventually settle in the lower lobes and appear as a dark red focus accompanying intrabronchial congestion. If the volume of hemorrhage is sufficient, the patient may literally drown in his own blood. Aspiration is a life-threatening situation to the lung and is well known to produce pneumonitis. The source of such aspirated blood may be the stomach, oropharynx, nasopharynx, or even the lung itself. Tuberculous cavities, carcinoma, or destructive lesions may produce profuse hemorrhage. Many hemorrhagic types of infectious disease may produce patchy hemorrhages. Pulmonary infarcts are easily distinguished from hemorrhage owing to their well-defined margins and their position in the lung, which is not subpleural as are the hemorrhages. Many lobules may be spared, with diffuse hemorrhage allowing good aeration and ventilation in the presence of numerous blood-filled respiratory units. It is best to remember that capillary bleeding can quickly become massive if adequate hemostasis is not available. Hemoptysis is indicative of an important underlying disease and should never be ignored by the clinician.

VII. Idiopathic Pulmonary Hemosiderosis

Widespread pulmonary capillary hemorrhage of variable intensity and unknown etiology characterizes a condition known as idiopathic pulmonary hemosiderosis. Most commonly, this disease is seen in young children, but

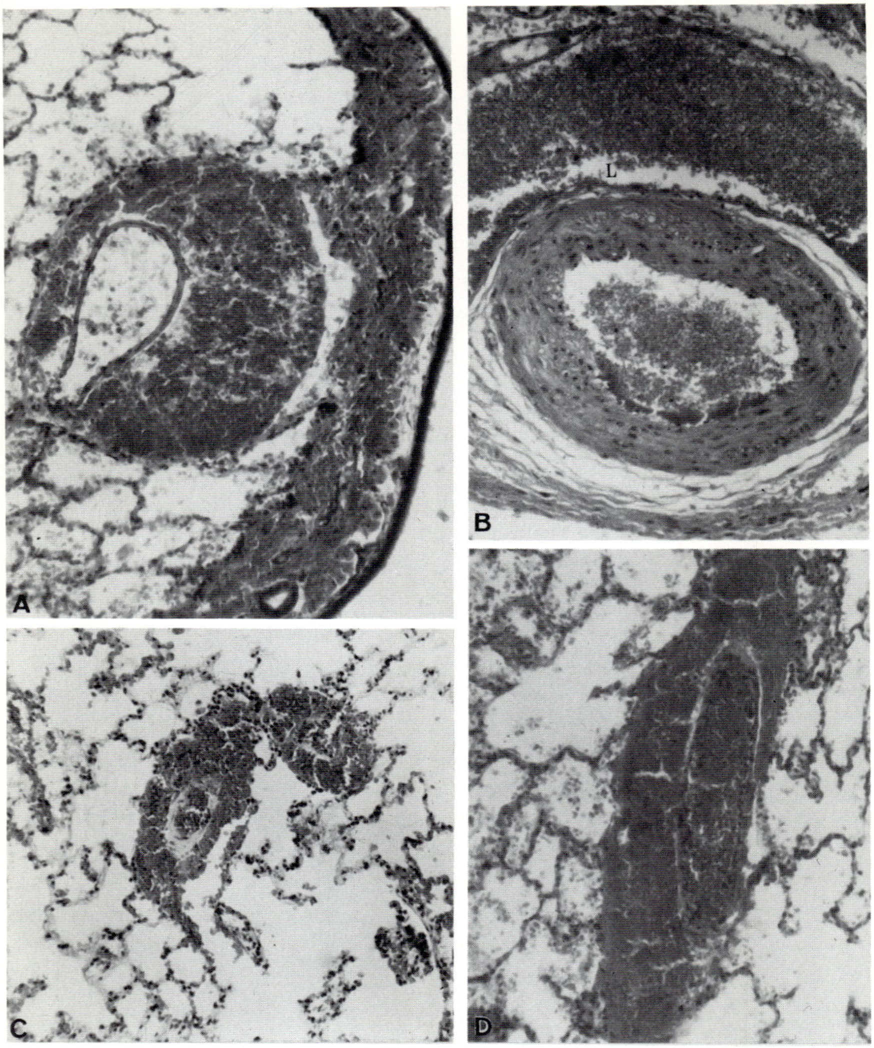

Fig. 7. (A) Dog lung. Hemorrhagic shock—perivascular and peribronchial hemorrhage is present in about 90% of the dogs studied after shock and retransfusion. Transfusion has been implicated as also producing this same kind of hemorrhagic lesion. (H & E, 114×.) (B) Human lung. Shock—perivascular hemorrhage is not present in this section, but lymphatic vessels (L) are filled with blood. They lie adjacent to the pulmonary arterioles. No direct connections between vessels of the blood and lymph networks have been demonstrated. (H & E, 96×.) (C) Rat lung. Anaphylactic shock—Perivascular hemorrhage is found in these animals studied in a Goodpasture's syndrome model using an anti-lung antibody. (H & E, 72×.) (D) Human lung. Hemorrhagic shock—postoperative bleeding was responsible for this patient's death. Perivascular hemorrhages are frequently found in such patients after surgery, trauma, and shock. (H & E, 108×.)

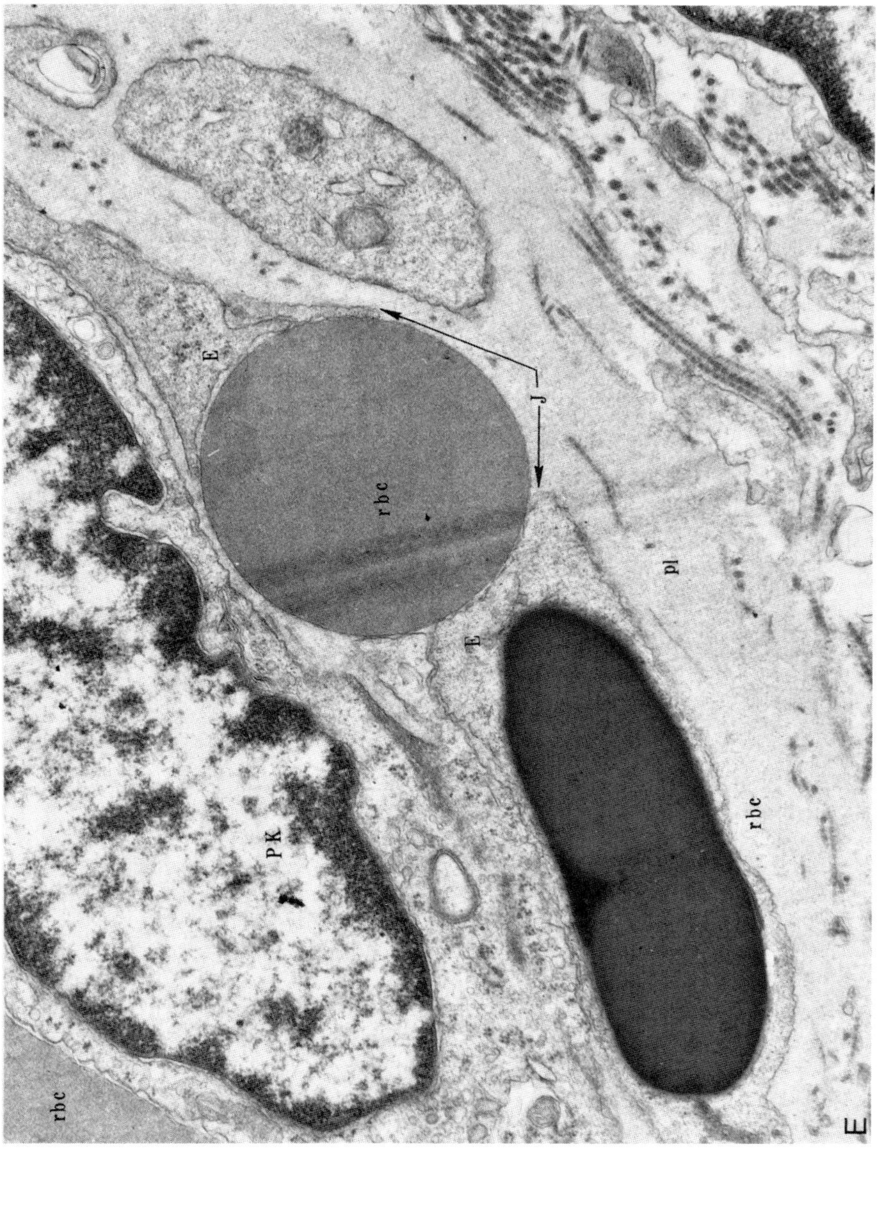

Fig. 7. (E) Human lung biopsy. Postcardiopulmonary bypass pump–an erythrocyte (rbc) sits in an open junction (J) between two endothelial cells (E). Plasma (pl) fills the interstitial space and one erythrocyte has escaped into the connective tissue space. The nucleus for the endothelial cell or perikaryon (PK) located at the upper left. (31,200×.)

does occur in adult life. The male is significantly more predisposed to developing this problem than the female. The onset is rather insidious with intermittent hemoptysis soon followed by a hypochromic anemia. Many patients have continued such a course for several years. Some exhibit massive hemorrhage with extreme dyspnea, fever, and cyanosis. The liver and spleen are frequently enlarged and sometimes clubbing of the fingers is present.

VIII. Electrolytes and the Pulmonary Capillary

Normally, sodium is retained within the pulmonary capillary network and the endothelium is relatively impermeable to the sodium ion. Sodium is, however, precipitously lost when the patient suffers acute pulmonary insufficiency following operation, trauma, or acute pulmonary insult. This loss is probably associated with the shifting of fluids from one compartment to another, which has been previously described. The extent of pulmonary capillary damage may also be important in determining sodium loss from the lung.

In shock and trauma, the lactic acidosis classically described is associated with increases in serum, potassium, and magnesium levels. Since these two ions are contained in the intracellular compartment, it is reasonable to assume that they are being lost due to changes in membrane permeability. Again, the vascular network, its cells, and the cells within its portals are the end organ which produces an array of uniform changes which are sequentially ordered and fast becoming predictable. Even in surgical procedures, such as cardiopulmonary bypass, the capillary circulation within the lung is severely affected, to the point of post-pump pulmonary insufficiency developing in numerous patients. Such diseases as emphysema have been attributed to vascular defects rather than destruction of the alveolus, and numerous investigators have implicated the pulmonary capillary as the site for original pulmonary injury resulting in loss of alveolar architecture. Recent studies have demonstrated that lysosomal contents within the polymorphonuclear leukocytes, when aerosolized at a neutral pH, can produce emphysematous changes in experimental animals. Allergic manifestations are also vascularly mediated and numerous vasoactive agents such as histamine, serotonin, prostaglandins, bradykinin, and heparin have all been found in the lung. These are either manufactured at specific sites by specialized cellular machinery or transmitted to the lung via the pulmonary vascular channels.

It has also been suggested that respiratory distress of the newborn, or hyaline membrane disease, is a disease of pulmonary hypoperfusion. Conversely, clinicians dispute this fact by claiming it is a hyperperfusion syndrome. Presently, it is unclear as to which is factual. But whether a vascular problem or not, respiratory distress of the newborn accounts for a mortality rate of approximately 25,000 infants per year. One certainty exists, that we need further investigation into both airway and lung development in these infants. For without a sufficient vascular supply, the lung will surely manifest cellular immaturity and fail to support extrauterine life.

IX. Summary

Though relatively unrecognized, the pulmonary microvascular dynamics are exceedingly important in the maintenance of life for healthy or diseased humans. Current arguments as to whether flow is of a turbulent nature in the lung's capillaries or is theoretically capable of working on a "sheet flow" basis are of importance. One promising feature of the advancement of medical knowledge is that clinicians are increasingly aware that the lung is an organ which does more than "just exchange gas." It is specifically an air–liquid interface with a large surface area exposed to environmental conditions. With increasing emphasis on air pollution control, the pulmonary capillary is a prime target for future investigation. At some time within its circulatory cycle, every red cell in the human body is halted from escaping into the atmosphere by only a thin wall which separates capillary blood from the alveolar gas. This wall, composed of two cells and an interstitial ground substance, never exceeds 0.15 to 0.3 μm in thickness. Lined by a continuous liquid film on the gas side, the estimated 500 million alveoli have a total surface area of approximately 650 ft^2. Most of the surface area is occupied by the pulmonary microvascular network. The first principle of basic respiratory physiology is that pulmonary alveolar ventilation is necessary for life. But ventilation without perfusion is like pseudocyesis, the result of delusion. No useful productive end is achieved.

Selected References

Abramson, D. I., ed. (1962). "Blood Vessels and Lymphatics." Academic Press, New York.

Cross, C. E. (1970). Pulmonary lymphatics. *Arch. Intern. Med.* **115,** 248.

Epling, G. P., and Wilson, J. W. (1971). Uniformity of sequence in pulmonary alveolar necrosis. *Amer. J. Vet. Res.* **32,** 471.

Ferencz, C. (1960). The pulmonary vascular bed in tetralogy of Fallot. II. Changes following a systemic-pulmonary arterial anastomosis. *Bull. Johns Hopkins Hosp.* **106,** 100.

Hagadorn, J. E., Vazquez, J. J., and Kinney, T. R. (1969). Immunologic studies of an experimental model resembling Goodpasture's syndrome. *Amer. J. Pathol.* **57,** 17.

Lauweryns, J. M. (1969). The ultrastructure of pulmonary lymphatic capillaries of newborn rabbits and of human infants. *Lymphology* **2,** 108.

Lauweryns, J. M., and Baert, A. (1968). The pulmonary lymphatics in neonatal hyaline membrane disease. *Pediatrics* **41,** 917.

Lauweryns, J. M., Baert, A., and Boussauw, L. (1970). The pulmonary lymphatics: Macroscopical and microscopical studies. *Amer. Rev. Resp. Dis.* **101,** 448.

Pennell, T. C. (1966). Anatomical study of the peripheral pulmonary lymphatics. *J. Thorac. Cardiov. Surg.* **52,** 629.

Ratliff, N. B., Wilson, J. W., Hackel, D. B., and Martin, A. M. (1970). The lung in hemorrhagic shock. II. Observations on alveolar and vascular ultrastructure. *Amer. J. Pathol.* **58,** 353.

Tobin, C. C. (1959). Pulmonary lymphatics: With reference to emphysema. *Amer. Rev. Resp. Dis.* **80,** 50.

Trapnell, D. H. (1963). The peripheral lymphatics of the lung. *Brit. J. Radiol.* **36,** 660.

Trapnell, D. H. (1970). Proceedings of the Thoracic Society. *Thorax* **25,** 254.

Vieth, F. J., Hagstrom, J. W., Panossian, A., Nehlsen, S. L., and Wilson, J. W. (1968a). Pulmonary microcirculatory response to shock, transfusion, and pump-oxygenator procedures: A unified mechanism underlying pulmonary damage. *Surgery* **64,** 95.

Veith, F. J., Panossian, A., Nehlsen, S. L., Wilson, J. W., and Hagstrom, J. W. (1968b). A pattern of pulmonary vascular reactivity and its importance in the pathogenesis of post-operative and post-traumatic pulmonary insufficiency. *J. Trauma* **8,** 788.

Wilson, J. W. (1970a). The "shock lung" in dogs and cats: Hemodynamic alterations. *Biochim. Biol. Sper.* **9,** 157.

Wilson, J. W. (1970b). Interstitial and intra-alveolar hemorrhage: The mechanism of a common response to various pulmonary insults. *Anat. Rec.* **166,** 398.

Wilson, J. W. (1971). Pulmonary morphologic changes due to extracorporeal circulation: A model for 'the shock lung' at cellular level in humans. *Excerpta Med., Shock Symp., Augusta, Mich.,* 1970 I. C. S., pp. 168–181.

Wilson, J. W. (1972). Treatment or prevention of pulmonary cellular damage with pharmacologic doses of corticosteroid. *Surg., Gynecol. Obstet.* **134,** 675.

Wilson, J. W. (1972). Leukocyte sequestration and morphologic augmentation in the pulmonary network following hemorrhagic shock and related forms of stress. *Advan. Microcirc.* **4,** 197–233.

Wilson, J. W. (1972). Intravascular phenomena in shock: The lung, a target for microaggregates and cellular debris. *In* "International Conf. on Intravascular Coagulation and Fibrinolysis (Physiopathology, Diagnosis and Therapy)," p. 4. Centre Hospitalier Universitaire, Sherbrooke, Quebec.

Wilson, J. W., Ratliff, N. B., and Hackel, D. B. (1970). The lung in hemorrhagic shock. I. *In vivo* observations of pulmonary microcirculation in cats. *Amer. J. Pathol.* **58,** 337.

Wilson, J. W., Young, W. G., Jr., and Miller, B. J. (1971). Polymorphonuclear leukocyte alterations in lungs from patients on cardiopulmonary bypass. *Fed. Proc., Fed. Amer. Soc. Exp. Biol.* **30,** 720.

11 SYSTEMIC INDICATORS OF THE LOW FLOW STATE

Biochemistry and Metabolism during Tissue Hypoperfusion

FRANCIS D. MOORE, M.D.

I. Introduction — Low Flow State

Prolonged deficiency of blood flow results from the interplay of four closely related vectors, a parallelogram of forces, acting to reduce the microcirculatory perfusion of body tissues. These forces are

1. Tissue injury
2. Reduction in effective circulating blood volume
3. Infection
4. Pump failure

A low flow state may be initiated by any one of the four, but in severe cases all four elements ultimately become involved no matter what the initial genesis.

Prolonged deficiency of microcirculatory blood flow is the mechanism by which tissues are damaged, organs fail, and death results. In the acute instance, this deficiency of blood flow is lethal when it occurs in the brain or heart. In sudden massive loss of blood, this is the mechanism of death: inadequate inflow pressure at the coronary ostia and circle of Willis with inadequate perfusion of heart and brain. As these two critical tissues die, the patient is dead in the medical and social sense of irreversible loss of life. At that moment many other tissues and organs are still alive. These other organs—kidney, liver, lung, spleen, for example—do not tolerate low flow states any better, but are in themselves not necessary for the minute-to-minute function of the rest of the body. Their beginning failure, therefore, does not alter the living process of the total patient, and by cold perfusion they can easily be resuscitated. The viability of these other organs and tissues has now been assessed in many instances, and they have been used successfully for transplantation even though death has overtaken their original owner, via the brain and/or heart. As between these two critical tissues, the brain is dominant—with brain death, cardiac performance may be continued for many hours or days if artificial respiratory support is given.

By contrast, in the more chronic state of low flow, the deficiency of blood flow stretches out over hours or days, each tissue suffering in proportion to the reduction in its perfusion:metabolism ratio. The *perfusion:metabolism ratio* is defined as the ratio of the total perfusion of a tissue or organ (providing oxygen and substrates) to its metabolic requirement (as determined by temperature and work). In its simplest terms this is the relationship of blood flow (expressed as ml/100 gm/min) to oxygen demand (expressed as ml/100 gm/min). If the metabolic requirement is sharply reduced, as in hypothermia, then hypoperfusion is well borne. If perfusion is normal but metabolism increased, as in muscular work by an individual with fixed vessel disease, a severely reduced perfusion:metabolism ratio results in the exercised muscle. This produces a local anaerobic state and oxygen debt, with local lactic acidosis and muscular spasms or cramps. If this process occurs acutely in the heart, the disorder is expressed first by acute cardiac arrhythmias, going on then to frank ischemia and infarction.

Fixed vessel disease also manifests itself in systemic hypoperfusion through the loss of autoregulation in the microcirculatory bed. Sharply lowered inflow pressures at the coronary ostia and circle of Willis, for example, can be borne transiently by young persons because of vascular flexibility. When atherosclerotic plaques encroach on the lumen of small arteries, the same reduced inflow pressures are followed by local tissue anaerobiosis and necrosis, as manifested by myocardial infarction or cerebrovascular occlusion.

These introductory comments on the low flow parallelogram, the perfusion:metabolism ratio, and the impact of degenerative vascular disease on the microcirculation will serve to explain our avoidance of the term "shock." This word, much overworked in the literature on trauma, surgery, and heart disease, has come to cover a meaningless hodgepodge of hypotension, psychological trauma, spinal cord injury, and highly artificial laboratory situations observed in rodents, frogs, or other lower forms whose vascular arrangements bear little relationship to the erect-walking biped whose blood vessels are usually far more pathologic than anything seen in the laboratory.* Since it is the prolonged deficiency of blood flow that is ultimately damaging to tissues, and the perfusion:metabolism ratio that determines the extent of that damage, we prefer to use the somewhat more clumsy term "low flow state" to indicate tissue hypoperfusion. The term can then be qualified to suit the clinical reality of the situation and to express the perfusion:metabolism ratio in numbers if possible.

In low flow states, tissue damage results from changes in the microcirculation. The body as a whole—the patient—suffers according to which tissues have the most profoundly reduced perfusion:metabolism ratio. In this chapter we will mention a variety of peripheral indicators, measured in the blood or urine, that reflect hypoperfusion. We will concentrate mainly on elevations in the blood lactate, metabolic acidosis, and functional changes in specific viscera as their perfusion:metabolism ratios are reduced.

II. Lactic Acidosis

Originally observed by Henderson (1928) in his studies on exercising normal volunteers, an understanding of blood lactate levels as indicators of a depressed perfusion:metabolism ratio is vital to the quantification of systemic changes in low flow states. Our current concepts of this subject are traceable largely to the work of Huckabee (1958a). Building on the older knowledge, he has developed several concepts and measurements of remarkable usefulness in the study of general and local hypoperfusion.

The production of lactic acid in body cells occurs when conditions are unfavorable for the direct entry of pyruvate into the Krebs cycle and favor-

*Writings on "shock" have led to a subculture of promotional pharmacology; one writer favoring some one drug or toxin, another pushing for a new vasoactive agent. In the laboratory it is possible to establish an animal model which will prove almost anything the investigator wishes it to establish.

able for the accumulation of lactate, produced initially as lactic acid. Several conditions favorable for this accumulation will be mentioned below, but the principal one of interest here is local tissue anaerobiosis due to hypoperfusion of the microcirculation. Adverse effects of this metabolic accumulation of intracellular acid are initially minor and consist solely in the donation of protons to the intracellular fluid with a resultant lowering of cell pH.

The lactate ion itself is a normal degradation product of 6-carbon sugars, and is quite harmless. Its accumulation in the peripheral blood is but an indicator of the extent of the cellular acidosis. The cell membrane is almost perfectly permeable to hydrogen ion, and as cellular pH falls, acidosis is also produced in the extracellular fluid bathing the tissue cell and ultimately in the entire extracellular fluid and blood.

When acid is added externally to the extracellular fluid as by the administration of a proton donor, such as ammonium chloride, the buffering effect of the blood and extracellular fluid buffers are first observed. There is a slight fall in blood pH. Minutes later the cellular buffers of the body are taken up as the protons pass into the cells, and the total body-buffering capacity becomes manifest. One may think of this external acid load, therefore, as being expressed by a titration curve with two components: one, the extracellular and blood buffers which are taken up first, and then the almost equal and large capacity of the cellular buffers.

When lactic acid is produced within the cells by hypoperfusion, the tissue buffers are taken up first. The total body titration curve is therefore shifted backward, and the effect of extracellular and blood buffering (manifested ultimately by the observed clinical change in blood pH and plasma bicarbonate) represents the end stage of a total body acid load. An acute lowering of blood pH associated with lactate accumulation due to a low flow state, such as that occurring after severe injury, for example, is, therefore, the harbinger of a far more massive load of hydrogen ion than would be the case where the observed extracellular acidosis to result from a simple external acid load alone.

Elevations of blood lactate are readily produced either by large loads of sugar or in the diabetic whose glucose levels are high and there is a relative shortage of blood insulin. In both of these situations pyruvate is proportionally increased, and the ratio of lactate to pyruvate, therefore, remains normal in the initial stages.

Huckabee (1965) demonstrated that in anoxia due to hypoperfusion the elevation of lactate is far greater than one would predict from the proportional increase in pyruvate. There was a specific shunting of 3-carbon fragments from pyruvate to the lactate stage, over and beyond that predicted from the level of pyruvate alone. The result was an elevated lactate at a markedly increased lactate:pyruvate ratio and a marked alteration in the activity of lactic dehydrogenase, favoring the production of lactic acid. The extent of the lactate elevation, when corrected for that predicted from a given level of pyruvate, is referred to as the "excess lactate," and the lactate:pyruvate ratio becomes greatly increased. The normal blood value for lactate is best expressed in millimoles per liter. The normal blood lactate is 1 mmole/liter or less, and the excess lactate value is essentially zero. The normal lactate:pyruvate ratio is 3.0 or less. With diffuse hypoperfusion and a lowering of the perfusion:metabolism ratio in body tissues, especially skeletal muscle, the excess lactate readily rises to values over 10 mmoles/liter, and the lactate:pyruvate ratio to levels of 15–30. In the paragraphs that follow, a few of the situations that cause elevation of lactate will be described.

A. Alkalosis

Mild degrees of alkalosis are associated with an increase in blood lactate (Anrep and Cannan, 1923), which can be associated with mild elevations of the lactate:pyruvate ratio and, therefore, with mild accumulations of excess lactate. In alkalosis, the total lactate may reach 2.0–3.5 mmoles/liter, and the excess lactate accounts for 0.5–1.5 mmoles of this elevation.

There are two mechanisms by which alkalosis might favor the production of lactate. One, notable in pure respiratory alkalosis (hypocarbia), could result from lowered tensions of carbon dioxide and the inhibition thereby of some step in the enzymatic reactions between lactate, pyruvate, oxalacetate, and acetoacetate. It was considered for some time that this "shortage of carbon dioxide" was the prime mechanism of elevated blood lactate in hypocarbia.

Haldi (1933) had demonstrated that infusions of sodium bicarbonate produced precisely the same effect. In this case the pCO_2 is normal or slightly elevated, and one must look elsewhere than lowered carbon dioxide tension for the cause. In our opinion the most probable cause is an acute left-shift of the oxyhemoglobin dissociation curve with a resultant defect in tissue oxygenation.

The position of the oxyhemoglobin dissociation curve may be quantified by the oxygen tension at which hemoglobin is half-saturated. This is known as the P_{50} value. The normal P_{50} for human blood is 27 ± 1.5 mm Hg. In accute alkalosis this value may shift as low as 20 mm Hg, and at this level 35–40% of the oxygen available to peripheral tissues will not be extracted at the oxygen tension observed in those tissues. With a left-shifted oxyhemoglobin curve, blood does not unload its quantum of oxygen as it passes through a tissue loop. An alkalosis-induced tissue hypoxia therefore results. This could be the cause of the mild lactate elevation seen in acute alkalosis.

Alkalosis is one of several stimuli to increased erythrocytic production of 2,3-diphosphoglycerate (2,3-DPG); in chronic alkalosis, therefore, the body compensates with increased synthesis of 2,3-DPG which shifts the curve to the right, toward normal.

The posttraumatic patient who is not in a low flow state is characteristically alkalotic (Lyons and Moore, 1966) owing to the interplay of transient hyperaldosteronism activated by volume reduction, the loss of gastric juice through nasogastric suction, the loads of sodium citrate (in transfused blood) oxidized to sodium bicarbonate, and mild hyperventilation. The posttraumatic alkalosis of the postoperative patient or the individual after severe injury is therefore associated with mild elevations of blood lactate. In this situation we have an interesting variation on the perfusion: metabolism ratio. The total perfusion and metabolic requirement may be normal, yet the delivery of oxygen is reduced, producing the same defect as a reduced ratio, without alteration in total blood flow.

B. Ventilatory Anoxemia

Ventilatory anoxemia is but a mild stimulus to the elevation of blood lactate. Breathing of a low oxygen mixture, or air at a low barometric pressure, will gradually produce slowing of the heart, unconsciousness, and then death, and yet this event may be associated with blood lactate elevations no higher than 4–5 mmoles/liter. There are a number of possible explanations for this inability of acutely anoxic tissues to produce lactate. The most probable explanation is that the acute oxygen lack itself inhibits the glycolytic cycle above the lactate step so that pyruvate production is inhibited, resulting in a far smaller elevation of lactate. Here again, the perfusion:metabolism ratio is apparently normal, but oxygen delivery is defective owing to arterial anoxemia.

C. Acute Muscular Exercise

Intense physical exertion of a single muscle, as in flexing the hand or forearm repeatedly, results finally in muscle fatigue or a muscle cramp or spasm. Measurement of lactate in the vein draining that muscle will demonstrate that it is markedly increased. This reflects a lowering of the perfusion: metabolism ratio due to greatly increased metabolism with normal or slightly increased perfusion.

A short-distance runner or sprinter will produce markedly elevated systemic blood lactate levels immediately after the race—levels as high as 15–20 mmoles/liter of lactate being observed. The runner will then sit down and overbreathe, finally oxidizing his lactate or excreting it in the urine. It is for this reason that the total body lactate was conceived of as an index of the total oxygen debt. This concept is easily confirmed quantitatively (Huckabee, 1958b) so long as one appreciates that the integral of the lactate curve represents the change in oxygen debt over time. Loss of lactate by oxidation or excretion is proceeding simultaneously. It is therefore difficult to express the oxygen debt at a single point in time, relative to a single value of lactate.

Only a small fraction of the potential energy yield of carbohydrate oxidation has been realized when the 6-carbon sugar reaches the lactate step. Regeneration of high-energy phosphates has been minimal. Most of the energy yield and adenosine triphosphate (ATP) regeneration occurs beyond the lactate step. The elevation of blood lactate in acute situations not only reflects oxygen debt, but is an expression also of unburned fuel from which the major caloric yield is yet to be gained.

This factor of muscular exercise with a lowered perfusion:metabolism ratio is of special interest in the heart. Where there are specific small areas of hypoperfusion of the myocardium due to fixed vessel disease, that portion of the heart muscle becomes a lactate donor, and the extent of its lactate production is an index of the extent of tissues involved with a lowered perfusion:metabolism ratio (Gorlin, 1966).

By the same token, sudden increase in cardiac work, when blood supply to the myocardium is inflexibly fixed by vascular disease, results in a fall in cardiac muscle pH that leads to arrhythmias and is potentially lethal by the mechanism of ventricular fibrillation.

D. Hypoperfusion and the Low Flow State

Hypoperfusion of body tissues, particularly of peripheral skeletal muscle, produces rapid and very marked elevations of blood lactate. In severe low flow states, as is seen in gram-negative bacillary infections, heart failure, trauma, or blood loss, all the conditions are perfect for lactate production. There is initially no anoxemia, and oxygen delivery is normal for each quantum of blood that actually reaches the microcirculation. Arterial oxygen tensions are normal, but venous oxygen tensions are markedly reduced as tissue oxygen extraction reaches the maximum value attainable for each tissue. There is no difficulty in the glycolytic cycle from glucose to the pyruvate step.

During tissue hypoperfusion large areas of skeletal muscle are shunted out of the circulation and exist anaerobically for prolonged periods of time. During the anaerobic phase they slowly "leak" lactic acid into the venous drainage. When perfusion is returned, large amounts of lactate produced locally in muscle are washed out of the muscle and into the circulation. This "washout acidosis" is seen with sudden returns of perfusion after a low flow state has been treated. If no treatment is given, the lactate ion leaks into the circulation from the hypoperfused microcirculatory beds, particularly in skeletal muscle, and the accumulation, while more gradual than that seen in the washout effect mentioned above, reaches very high levels.

Measurements of the pH of muscle surfaces done with a directly placed electrode demonstrate these alterations quite dramatically (Lemieux *et al.,* 1969; Couch *et al.,* 1971). With exercise of the muscle, or transient hypoperfusion, the drop in muscle surface pH is almost instantaneous as lactic acid is produced within the muscle cells. If the period of hypoperfusion is short or the area of tissue is small, there may not be any alteration in systemic blood lactate or pH. The small amount of lactate produced is quickly oxidized in other tissues, principally the liver, and the pH effect is completely buffered by the fluids and tissues of the rest of the body. This is the characteristic change seen in small venous hemorrhages in man, where alterations in muscle surface pH are readily demonstrated, but blood pH does not change at all (J. R. Dmochowski, personal communication, 1971). If the period of ischemia is longer, or the reduction in perfusion:metabolism ratio is imposed over a larger tissue mass, then there will be a gradual increase in blood lactate. In man, in prolonged periods of hypoperfusion, blood lactate levels in the range of 16–25 mmoles/liter may be observed. These high levels are frequently associated with a lethal outcome.

Where hypoperfusion affects all tissues instantaneously and equally, it appears that almost all the tissues of the body are lactate producers. This was nicely shown in a series of experiments by Schroeder *et al.* (1968) in the dog in which systemic circulatory perfusion was reduced by acute reversible cardiac tamponade. By measuring AV lactate differences over a variety of tissues, it was demonstrated that brain, kidney, tissue, and liver were all lactate producers during the low flow state. When flow was restored, liver became a lactate burner with a negative lactate clearance across its circulation. Large amounts of lactate were excreted in the urine, and muscle very slowly restored its normal balance.

It has been shown by Zierler (1966) that even in resting forearm muscle there is some lactate production, suggesting that in the normal resting skeletal muscle there are some areas of muscle that are not being perfused.

The body has adapted to holding bundles of muscle fibrils in reserve in a mildly anaerobic condition, pending their use in exercise. Slow, steady exercise restores this perfusion to the muscle, and if the exercise is mild, the restoration of perfusion completely obliterates the normal small lactate production of the resting muscle. Then, as mentioned above, when exercise increases stepwise to maximum exertion, abundant amounts of lactate are again produced.

In clinical hypoperfusion, as in any of the low flow states, the depression of the bicarbonate concentration is related in linear fashion to the amount of lactate present. The lactate accumulation accounts for about 85% of the bicarbonate reduction, suggesting that lactate has been the principal new anion produced, and that the new hydrogen ion presented to body buffers is virtually all from the lactic source. This finding is rationalized by the fact that pyruvate elevations are minimal, as one would expect when the lactate: pyruvate ratio is high, and excess lactate accounts for more than 75% of the total lactate. Other new organic acids, such as ketones, are not produced in any quantity unless there is inadequate insulin production or overproduction of free fatty acids. The latter is often the case where acute trauma and catecholamine discharge has occurred (see below), epinephrine and norepinephrine being potent inhibitors of insulin production. In the ordinary low flow state observed clinically the metabolic acidosis is therefore largely a lactic acidosis.

E. Lactate Infusion

The use of sodium racemic lactate in resuscitative fluids can lead to a factitious rise in plasma lactate concentration that is quite innocent of any damage to the patient. If one were to base his therapy on the observed lactate levels alone, this artificial elevation of plasma lactate might confuse the results.

Such solutions as Ringer's lactate contain lactate at concentrations of about 30 mmole/liter. Were one to carry out determinations that differentiate between the optical rotatory forms of lactate, it would be possible to approximate that component of lactate in the plasma due to the infusion of the racemic form from that produced endogenously, which is always of the levorotatory form.

If an individual is not clearing lactate normally due either to renal failure or hypoperfusion of tissues, or both, then the half time of infused lactate in the body is longer than that for a normal individual.

The elevation of blood lactate produced by Ringer's lactate infusion is quite harmless because the pH of the infusate is at or above the normal pH of body fluids, and the lactate, therefore, carries with it no extra hydrogen ion to take up the body buffers. One is dealing with a lactate load without an acid load. This makes it important again to emphasize that the increase in lactate concentration in low flow states is a significant barometer of the time course over which tissues have been critically hypoperfused, and is but an index of the burden of new hydrogen ions presented to extracellular and blood buffers.

F. Bacterial Growth

Certain bacteria produce lactic acid as a product of their metabolism of carbohydrate. In one or two patients with very large surface burns extensively colonized by gram-negative organisms, we have suspected that some fraction of the elevation of blood lactate observed was due to the absorption from the burned surface of lactic acid produced by bacterial growth. We know of no quantitative studies which would enable one to assess the importance of this factor.

III. Acidosis

Lactic acid produced in the microcirculation during periods of hypoperfusion takes up first the cellular and later the extracellular buffers (as described above) and contributes to a severe metabolic acidosis in patients who are in a low flow state. It is for this reason that acidosis is so characteristic of prolonged low flow physiology.

Although lactic acid is the predominant contributor to this acidosis, both of cellular and extracellular fluid, and although the reduction in bicarbonate concentration is almost wholly accounted for by lactate accumulation, other acids can enter the picture significantly.

Most prominent among these is carbonic acid when pulmonary shunting or hypoventilation, or both, contribute to an elevated carbon dioxide tension. This is usually a preterminal event in injured or postoperative patients who have had severely compromised tissue perfusion for many hours or days.

As can be imagined, the impact of even a small additional load of carbonic acid is quite devastating in a patient whose cellular buffers are already completely taken up by a large chronic load of lactic acid which has accumulated over the previous hours or days. It is for this reason that there is such a precipitous fall in pH in patients in late hypoperfusion, who then develop an elevated carbon dioxide tension.

The measurement of blood pH is an accurate biochemical indicator of the state of a patient whose microcirculation is underperfused systemically. In only rare instances (diabetes, pancreatectomy, and hyperinsulinism) is it necessary to measure the lactate concentration itself. Data on pH, pCO_2, pO_2, and buffer base obtained from arterial blood are essential to determine the intermixture of metabolic and respiratory acidotic vectors.

The pH values commonly observed in low flow states without respiratory embarrassment range in the vicinity of 7.30 ± 0.05. When the hypoperfusional state is severe and the plasma lactate elevation exceeds 10 mmoles/liter, the acidosis can reach a pH of 7.15, with a standard bicarbonate of 12–15 mmoles/liter.

When respiratory embarrassment with pCO_2 elevated to levels of 50–70 mm Hg is added to this, the blood pH quickly falls below 7.0. Levels of 6.85–6.95 are seen in the terminal phase.

The cessation of cardiac action, so characteristic of the terminal event in prolonged systemic hypoperfusion, occurs because of the combination of anoxia and acidosis. This is an environment in which myocardial irritability is severely depressed. The usual events after many hours or days of tachycardia are a slowing of the heart beat and a gradual disorganization of the ventricular complexes, followed by diastolic arrest. In this chemical environment, resuscitation is quite unavailing by the usual steps taken for myocardial stimulation.

In patients with chronic hypoperfusion (i.e., more than a few hours) and without acute changes in respiratory function, central venous blood gas measurements are valuable, and arterial puncture need not be performed. The normally elevated carbon dioxide tension of venous blood (45 mm Hg), lower pH (7.35), and pCO_2 (70–80 mm Hg) of venous blood must be taken into consideration in interpretation of central venous blood gases.

The acidosis of hypoperfusion causes a right shift of the oxyhemoglobin dissociation curve. The P_{50} is increased. Typical values are 30–35 mm Hg. This curve shifted to the right delivers a larger load of oxygen for each quantum of oxyhemoglobin perfused in tissues, and is a compensation that tends to improve the oxygen supply of poorly perfused microcirculatory beds. In severe low flow states this mild compensation in improved oxygen delivery has little impact on the overall anoxia of the tissues due to hypoperfusion. Any favorable effect of an oxyhemoglobin dissociation curve shifted to the right must depend on the actual presence of oxygenated blood in the microcirculation. When there are underperfused areas and diffuse shunting, leaving many regions of the microcirculation nonperfused, this oxyhemoglobin curve shifted to the right has little impact on tissue oxygenation. This entire set of events (acidosis and hemoglobin curve shifted to the right) is in contrast to the normal posttraumatic pathophysiology in the absence of low flow. As mentioned above, in normally perfused and well-resuscitated posttraumatic patients (after the injury episode is over), a mixed metabolic respiratory alkalosis with a curve shifted to the left and a mild elevation of lactate are regularly observed.

IV. The Function of Viscera

Space does not permit an enumeration of the many changes in visceral function that result from microcirculatory underperfusion of specific organs. In all cases, the visceral disorder results from a lowering of the perfusion: metabolism ratio, whether this be a reduction in bulk perfusion itself, as in low flow states, or a reduction in the transport function as is found in disorders of oxyhemoglobin dissociation. Mention will be made in this section of those viscera whose function is a valuable index of the overall state of the microcirculation.

A. Kidneys

In low flow states the volume of bladder urine is a linear function of the glomerular filtration rate. Its quantitative measurement, hour by hour, is therefore a valuable index of the perfusion of the kidney.

The quality of the urine, e.g., its concentration and sodium content, reflects tubular function. When tubular function is good and the kidneys are underperfused, sodium reabsorption will be maximal and the urine osmolality will be elevated to maximum values, most of the solute being urea. Typical values for underperfused kidneys with normal tubular function are a sodium concentration of less than 10 mEq/liter, and an osmolality of over 800 mosmoles/liter.

When parenchymatous renal failure supervenes and renal tubular function is severely compromised or destroyed, the low volume urine represents a continuing solute diuresis through a few remaining viable nephrons. The sodium concentration and osmolality of urine, therefore, approach that of plasma ultrafiltrate. Sodium concentrations above 50 mEq/liter are characteristic, and the urine osmolality falls to values approaching 300 mosmoles/liter.

In between these two extremes are the urinary findings in patients with fixed vessel disease and some degree of nephrosclerosis whose kidneys are challenged but not yet destroyed. In these cases the urine will have a fixed osmolality around 750 mosmoles/liter, exactly as is found with the administration of a solute diuretic; sodium concentrations usually vary between 10–40 mEq/liter.

It is thus evident that by following the quantity and quality of the urine over the course of time, not only is the circulatory state of the whole patient evaluated, but likewise the fate and future of the kidneys themselves may be predicted.

B. Heart

In young persons with flexible coronary arteries and arterioles, local autoregulatory mechanisms are so efficient that virtually normal cardiac irritability is maintained even after hours or days of hypoperfusion. A few minor electrocardiographic anomalies may be observed, particularly those of subendocardial ischemia. These anomalies result from a low inflow pressure at the coronary ostia and outright failure of perfusion of the myocardium.

By contrast, in older people with fixed vascular disease of the coronary arteries and some caliber encroachment by atherosclerotic plaques, a fall in inflow pressure at the coronary ostia is critically reflected by an immediate and drastic alteration in myocardial perfusion and oxygenation. Electrocardiographic anomalies are quickly evident. These may mimic the changes of myocardial infarction, and such patients may go on to a frank infarct if the low flow state is prolonged. With these electrocardiographic changes, severe arrhythmias and pump failure may occur, as well as the elaboration of lactate from the ischemic myocardium.

It is for these reasons that older patients are more "fragile"; they cannot tolerate hypoperfusion. In blood replacement for older persons it is well to recall that the need is even more demanding and urgent than it is in young persons. Any restraint on blood transfusion should be placed, not on speed or accuracy, but rather on the possible hazards of overreplacement.

The tachycardia characteristic of low flow reduces the diastolic filling time and, therefore, the stroke volume. In a normal individual, cardiac output increases as the pulse rate increases up to a critical level of about 140 beats per minute. Above this, diastolic filling time is so shortened that cardiac output goes no higher, and at rates over 200 the cardiac output falls drastically as evidenced, for example, by the cerebral ischemia suffered by elderly persons with paroxysmal ventricular tachycardia.

In persons with fixed vascular disease or with valvular disease of the heart, this "critical point" of heart rate above which cardiac output starts to fall lies in the vicinity of 100–120 beats per minute. For these reasons one should try to avoid excessive tachycardia in the severely hypoperfused patient, and the best way to do this in most instances is by quantitative volume replacement or by the control of infection.

The ability of the right heart to accept and propel its venous return is reflected by the right ventricular end-diastolic pressure which, in turn, is reflected by the right atrial and central venous pressure. For this reason the measurement of these pressures is a valuable index of the relationship between venous return and cardiac output. In most individuals in low flow states, an elevation of the central venous pressure signifies myocardial failure usually due to the impact of the low flow state itself, often complicated by atherosclerotic coronary arteries.

In other instances with trauma to the chest, this elevation of venous pressure may signify pericardial tamponade, mediastinal emphysema, pneumothorax, or other local traumatic events around the heart and great vessels. It is evident that the surgeon caring for such patients must use discrimination and avoid such obvious therapeutic errors as treating acute pericardial tamponade with digitalis.

C. Brain

Cerebral function, like cardiac function, is surprisingly well maintained in low flow states in young people. The typical young person after a severe accident, or the military casualty in shock, may be so severely hypoperfused as to be markedly acidotic and with beginning pump failure, as indicated by a rising central venous pressure. Despite this, he may be quite conscious and lucid.

In sharp contrast, the brain of any older individual or any person with fixed vascular disease of the carotid tree shows the same striking sensitivity to inflow pressure changes as does the myocardium under similar circumstances. It is not uncommon to observe older patients in which the state of consciousness (as evidenced by conversation or recognition of the attendants) is in quantitative relationship to blood pressure, coma resulting whenever the pressure falls below a critical value, typically in the region of 85–95 mm Hg.

The cerebral microcirculation is probably the single most critical area for the acute survival of the patient. The maintenance of normal cerebral function is remarkably important for all the viscera. There is no better index of this than the responses of the patient: reflexes, ocular activity, sensation, recognition, and the sum total of mental processes. If the patient is in coma for other reasons, either of a metabolic or locally traumatic nature, then the electroencephalogram can be added as a further index of the state of the cerebral microcirculation.

In older patients with fixed vascular disease who have prolonged periods of cerebral hypoperfusion, areas of cerebral infarction are a frequent result, manifested as cerebrovascular accidents with focal regions of paralysis or hemiparesis. In patients over 70 years of age who have prolonged periods of hypoperfusion, cerebrovascular accidents are a more frequent complication than are acute myocardial infarctions.

The cerebral circulation is also very sensitive to changes in the oxyhemoglobin dissociation curve and in acid–base balance. In alkalosis and hypocarbia, the curve shifted to the left tends to diminish cerebral blood flow and cerebral oxygenation. One will occasionally see individuals in whom coma can be rectified by the correction of these variables alone.

D. Lungs

The pulmonary microcirculation is normally a low pressure circuit. Data would suggest that general hypoperfusion, as in low flow states, has little immediate effect on pulmonary circulation or oxygenation. One can demonstrate a remarkable sensitivity of the pulmonary arterial tree and, therefore, the total pulmonary vascular resistance to norepinephrine (Hanson *et al.,* 1970). This hypersensitivity is observed after reduction in volume. Pulmonary hypertension of a mild variety is readily produced, and one might imagine that this would be associated with an increased tendency to pulmonary shunting, i.e., the opening up of new AV communications. Such has not been demonstrated.

Most cases of posttraumatic pulmonary insufficiency arise because of insults to the lungs (Moore *et al.,* 1969). These arise via the airway (explosive compression or decompression, inhalation of irritating substances such as smoke or gas, aspiration of gastric contents), via the bloodstream (multiple small emboli from poorly filtered blood transfusions, platelet emboli from peripheral areas of tissue ischemia, pulmonary thromboemboli), or by direct trauma to the chest wall (multiple rib fractures, hemothorax, pneumothorax). Many animal experiments alleged to demonstrate "shock lung" do not adequately control these other variables. There is little evidence from the laboratory or from man to state categorically that hypoperfusion in itself produces a disorder of pulmonary ventilation:perfusion relationships.

It is also noteworthy that maintenance of the patient in a single posture, such as the dorsal decubitus, during periods of hypovolemia, tends to redistribute the small amount of blood in the lungs toward the dorsal bronchopulmonary segments. This redistribution in itself leads to shunting and anoxia refractory to inhaled oxygen tensions. These are the characteristic early changes of posttraumatic pulmonary insufficiency. It is our interpretation of the available evidence that these changes are due to factors other than hypoperfusion per se. Quite clearly, reduced blood volume, hypoperfusion, posture, and the entire ambiance of the severely traumatized patient, all contribute to the gradual development of posttraumatic pulmonary insufficiency which may, in the end, be the cause of death.

V. Endocrine Effects

Many of the endocrine sequellae of low flow are produced by tissue injury itself, quite aside from alterations in the microcirculation. The posttraumatic endocrinology is activated by injury, even though tissue perfusion remains essentially normal and resuscitation is prompt.

In the case of the catecholamines, the incremental response is so much greater and so much more prolonged in low flow states than in ordinary trauma that their activity must be considered as one of the characteristic endocrine earmarks of generalized tissue hypoperfusion.

The adrenal medulla is the sole source in the body of epinephrine. Norepinephrine is produced throughout the body at neural synapses and neuromuscular junctions. Both these areas are stimulated to a maximum production of catecholamines by even modest reductions in tissue perfusion. The entire sensing arc and effector system for this increase in catecholamine secretion is not yet fully understood.

Increases in catecholamine concentration in the blood have several important effects relative to the low flow state itself. Most clearly understood is the diffuse increase in vasomotion and increased vascular resistance at the arteriole produced by diffuse arteriolar vasoconstriction. These effects are a result of stimulation of the alpha receptors, largely by norepinephrine. This effect appears to maintain inflow pressure at the coronary ostia and at the circle of Willis, and, therefore, appears superficially to be a teleogically advantageous evolutionary adaptation to reduced blood volume and tissue hypoperfusion. For the body to manifest this response, a basal level of glucocorticoids must be present from the adrenal cortex.

If this type of arteriolar vasoconstriction is long continued, it will, of itself, produce severe ischemia in microcirculatory beds distal to the arteriolar vasoconstrictive sites. The lethal effect of prolonged norepinephrine infusion results from this particularly prolonged alpha receptor stimulation, with tissue ischemia and necrosis.

Epinephrine is also a vasoconstrictor. Both epinephrine and norepinephrine have vasodilating effects on certain areas of the myocardial circulation, and both of them, particularly epinephrine, have a positive inotropic effect on the heart.

The catecholamines have important metabolic as well as hemodynamic effects. The most prominent is the inhibition of insulin release from the pancreas, decreasing the amount of insulin available to peripheral tissues. This state favors the release of amino acids from muscle and the hydrolysis of adipose tissue, neutral fat yielding glycerol and free fatty acids to the plasma. The sum total of these metabolic changes might be described as the primal endocrine-metabolic response to injury. Although readily activated by injury and without diffuse hypoperfusion, this activation is immensely exaggerated in prolonged low flow states. Diffuse hypoperfusion of microcirculatory beds is therefore associated with a most exaggerated mobilization of intracellular substances to the extracellular fluid and mobilization of free fatty acids. The biochemical and metabolic reflections include a massive increase in the urinary excretion of nitrogen and potassium and very high blood levels of free fatty acids.

Prolonged administration of catecholamines can result in such a large mobilization of free fatty acids that the reesterification of these free fatty acids in other tissues results in the diffuse deposition of neutral fat. This "fat mobilization syndrome" is sometimes seen after prolonged hypoperfusion, the fat being most notable in the myocardium, the liver, and peripheral skeletal muscle.

VI. Summary

Microscopic alterations in the small vessels that supply metabolic exchange to tissues and organs, and alterations in cellular fine structure, which result from hypoperfusion, are most prominent in the literature on microcirculation in "shock."

In this chapter we have attempted to describe a few of the systemic indicators seen in the whole organism which reflect this microcirculatory hypoperfusion. These changes are all related to reduction in the perfusion: metabolism ratio, that reduction occurring either as bulk decrease in blood flow or in disorders of oxygen transport or delivery.

Most prominent among those changes in the systemic circulation are increases in the blood lactate concentration associated with metabolic acidosis. This acid is released initially within body cells themselves; cellular buffers are taken up before the extracellular buffers. The final result observed by the physician measuring blood pH represents, therefore, an end stage of total body buffering. While the lactate ion itself is quite harmless, its absolute concentration provides an approximate index of the total time course, or integral, of cellular hypoxia due to hypoperfusion.

Other states that increase blood lactate and other causes of acidosis are briefly reviewed.

Finally, alterations in specific visceral function and in the activity of the endocrine glands likewise provide systemic indicators of tissue hypoperfusion. Of these changes, prolonged increases in the catecholamine level in blood are most significant, not only because of their hemodynamic effects, but because they produce diffuse metabolic changes characterized by release of amino acids from hydrolyzed muscle protein, the mobilization of free fatty acids from adipose tissue, and the entire sequence of endocrine and metabolic changes so characteristic of the posttraumatic state.

References

Anrep, G. V., and Cannan, R. K. (1923). The concentration of lactic acid in the blood in experimental alkalaemia and acidaemia. *J. Physiol.* (*London*) **58,** 244–258.

Couch, N. P., Dmochowski, J. R., VanDeWater, J. M., Harken, D. E., and Moore, F. D. (1971). Muscle surface pH as an index of peripheral perfusion in man. *Ann. Surg.* **173,** 173–183.

Gorlin, R. (1966). *In* "Proceedings of a Conference on Energy Metabolism and Body Fluid Utilization with Particular Reference to Starvation and Injury." Morgan, A., (ed), pp. 229–238. Harvard Printing Office, Cambridge.

Haldi, J. (1933). Lactic acid in blood and tissues following intravenous injection of sodium bicarbonate. *Amer. J. Physiol.* **106,** 134–144.

Hanson, E. L., Miller, J. T., Sheldon, G. F., Bartlett, R. H., Dmochowski, J. R., O'Connell, R., and Kagey, K. L. (1970). Pulmonary circulation: Effects of norepinephrine and hemorrhage in the human being. *Surg. Forum* **21,** 208–210.

Henderson, L. G. (1928). "Blood." Yale Univ. Press, New Haven, Connecticut.

Huckabee, W. E. (1958a). Relationships of pyruvate and lactate during anaerobic metabolism. I. Effects of infusion of pyruvate or glucose and of hyperventilation. *J. Clin. Invest.* **37,** 244–254.

Huckabee, W. E. (1958b). Relationship of pyruvate and lactate during anaerobic metabolism. II. Exercise and formation of O_2-Debt. *J. Clin. Invest.* **37,** 255–263.

Huckabee, W. E. (1965). Metabolic consequences of chronic hypoxia. *Ann. N. Y. Acad. Sci.* **121,** 723–730.

Lemieux, M. D., Smith, R. N., and Couch, N. P. (1969). Electrometric surface pH of skeletal muscle in hypovolemia. *Amer. J. Surg.* **117,** 627–631.

Lyons, J. H., Jr., and Moore, F. D. (1966) Posttraumatic alkalosis: Incidence and pathophysiology of alkalosis in surgery. *Surgery* **60,** 93–106.

Moore, F. D., Lyons, J. H., Jr., Pierce, E. C., Jr., Morgan, A. P., Jr., Drinker, P. A., MacArthur, J. D., and Dammin, G. J. (1969). "Post-Traumatic Pulmonary Insufficiency." Saunders, Philadelphia, Pennsylvania.

Schroeder, R., Eltringham, W. K., Gumpert, J. R., Jenny, M. E., Pluth, J. R., and Zollinger, R. M., Jr. (1968). Über die Bedeutung der Leber für die Hyperlactatämine in Schock. *Verh. Deut. Ges. Inn. Med.* **74,** 886–890.

Zierler, K. (1966). *In* "Proceedings of a Conference on Energy Metabolism and Body Fluid Utilization with Particular Reference to Starvation and Injury." Morgan, A., (ed), Harvard Printing Office, Cambridge.

12 THE MICROCIRCULATION IN HYPERTENSION

ROGER B. HICKLER, M.D.

I. Introduction

It is impossible to consider the pathophysiologic events leading to hypertension without focusing on the small vessels. The generation of an elevated arterial pressure indicates an alteration in vascular flow-resistance relationships. The arteriolar (precapillary) component of the microcirculation is the primary determinant of vascular resistance. The venular (postcapillary) component of the microcirculation is the major site involved in changes in blood volume, a primary determinant of cardiac filling pressure and output, and, therefore, of flow. It is not surprising that much of the current investigation on the origins of hypertension is focused on the hydraulic and humoral events taking place in the small vessels of the circulation.

Figure 1 describes the hemodynamic phenomena implicated in the generation of arterial pressure. Traditionally, attention has been focused on the resistance to flow, as determined by the critical factor of the radius of the arterioles. According to Poiseuille's formulation, the arteriolar radius is the most important determinant since the effect of the radius is proportional to its *fourth power*. To quote one authority: "Vascular radius is a function of three general factors: (1) the distending pressure: the difference between the pressure inside and that surrounding the vessel; (2) the

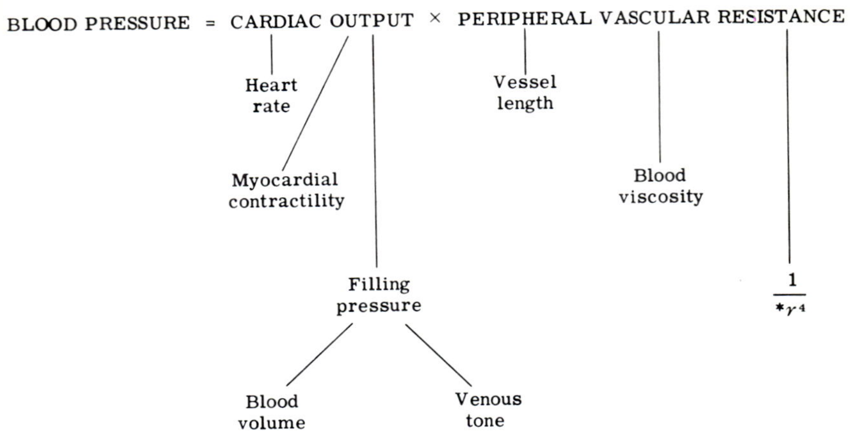

Fig. 1. The factors determining cardiac output and peripheral vascular resistance in the regulation of arterial blood pressure are shown. The asterisk indicates arteriolar radius.

geometry of the vessel: the wall thickness and the radius; (3) the elastic and the viscous properties of the vessel wall. The combined effects of factors 2 and 3 determine the extent to which a vessel will become stretched for a given distending pressure, and together, therefore, they specify what is usually called 'vascular tone'" (Peterson, 1966). It is evident that an increased resistance to stretch ("stiffening") will lead to an increase in arterial pressure. Initially, this may be evident only during periods of a high distending volume (increased cardiac output). As the vascular changes progress, hypertension becomes evident during a normal and, finally, even a low cardiac output. Aside from those rare instances of modest pressure elevation sometimes seen in conditions, such as macroglobulinemia and polycythemia, the factor of changes in blood viscosity is unimportant. Therefore, an explanation of the etiology of chronic sustained diastolic hypertension must unravel the events leading first to a loss of distensibility and then to a generalized narrowing of the arteriolar lumen.

II. Etiological Factors in Increased Arteriolar Resistance

A survey of the present status of our understanding of the initiating event leading to a high vascular resistance in sustained diastolic hypertension of various etiologies indicates that no common denominator can be identified.

A review of the important responses and endogenous factors known to increase vascular resistance at the level of the microcirculation is in order.

A. Sympathetic Nervous System—Catecholamines

Most readily understood are those instances of so-called "neurogenic" hypertension in which an increased sympathetic nerve activity on arteriolar smooth muscle is implicated. The hypertension is usually transient, relating to an increased neuroadrenergic outflow from medullary vasomotor centers. The clinical background is varied, including such conditions as acute central nervous system (CNS) hypoxia (e.g., pulmonary edema), sudden increase in CNS pressure (e.g., cerebral hemorrhage), and bilateral buffer nerve section. Further, few would contest that the α-adrenergic effect on the microcirculation of a high circulating level of norepinephrine, as released by a pheochromocytoma, accounts for the hypertension seen in this rare disorder. Less well known is the hypertension associated with the Guillain-Barré syndrome, which is currently thought to be related to a high level of circulating catecholamines, released in response to a pathologic alteration of the sympathetic nervous system (Mitchell and Meilman, 1967). However, as applied to essential hypertension and other forms of secondary hypertension, a *primary* neuroadrenergic-catecholamine mechanism has received very little substantiation. It has been known for a decade that the urinary excretion of catecholamines and their metabolites does not differ significantly from normal in patients with essential hypertension. Indeed, the available evidence indicates a *depression* of sympathetic nervous system reflex activity in essential hypertension (Hickler *et al.,* 1959; Fotino and Raiciulescu, 1964; Bristow *et al.,* 1969).

These generalities do not preclude the concept derived from more recent observations that a more subtle derangement in catecholamine metabolism may be part of the hypertensive equation. Thus, with an enzymatic double-isotope derivative technique it was shown that the mean plasma catecholamine concentration in 18 patients with essential hypertension was significantly higher than that for 32 normotensive controls (Engelman *et al.,* 1970). A study on the ultrastructure of sympathetic vasomotor nerves in sheep with experimental renal hypertension showed an increase in intra-axonal vesicles and in the size and density of their granular cores compared with control nerves (Burnstock *et al.,* 1970). Rats with spontaneous genetic hypertension and experimental renal hypertension have both neurogenically maintained and nonneurogenically maintained components to their hypertension (Smirk, 1970). The binding or retention of norepinephrine by the storage vesicle of the sympathetic nerves is considerably reduced in DOCA-salt hypertensive rats (DeChamplain *et al.*, 1969). While a *primary* role for the sympathetic nervous system in most forms of hypertension has not been established, it may quite regularly be playing a contributory role.

B. Renin–Angiotensin System

Another mechanism to which the resistance vessels of the microcirculation are sensitive is the renin–angiotensin system. The unique vasoconstrictor potency of angiotensin II as generated in the renin–renin substrate reaction is familiar to all. The level of activity of this system in hypertension in its various forms and stages has been well documented in a number of centers, including our studies from the Hypertension Unit of the Peter Bent Brigham Hospital. There is, now general agreement on these relationships which may be summarized as follows. In essential hypertension the level of activity is depressed in about 20% of the patients and is normal in all others. Therefore, no convincing case can be made at this time for a primary effect of angiotensin II on the microvasculature in the pathogenesis of essential hypertension. In primary aldosteronism the level of activity is uniformly depressed, reflecting the inhibitory effect on renin secretion of the chronically volume-expanded state of mineralocorticoid excess. This 20% of essential hypertensives and patients with primary aldosteronism have in common a lack of responsivity of the depressed level of renin secretory activity to stimulation by volume contraction (upright posture, sodium restriction, diuretics). However, the level of aldosterone secretion in the essential hypertensives with low plasma renin activity levels ranges from low to normal. Therefore, the mechanism for the renin depression in this subgroup remains to be explained. Only a very few can be related to the more exotic forms of nonaldosterone mineralocorticoid excess, such as excessive licorice ingestion (glycyrrhetinic acid), or the excessive adrenocortical production of 11-deoxycorticosterone (as in 11β-hydroxylase and 17α-hydroxylase deficiency) or of 18-hydroxydeoxycorticosterone (Melby *et al.*, 1971). The hypervolemia (Jose *et al.*, 1970) and superior blood pressure response to spironolactone therapy (Spark and Melby, 1971) reported for patients with hypertension with suppressed plasma renin activity do suggest the possibility of the excessive production of an unidentified mineralocorticoid.

There are two situations in which a high level of renin secretion and angiotensin generation may be directly implicated in the hypertensive state. The first is malignant or accelerated hypertension. In this condition there is a significant incidence of very high levels of peripheral renin activity. This increased activity pertains whether the underlying condition is essential hypertension or one of the secondary forms of hypertension. There is almost invariably an associated high level of aldosterone secretion, generally thought to be a consequence of the high level of generation of angiotensin II. In this setting, the malignant phase of the hypertensive disease is most likely a direct consequence of the peripheral vascular effects of elevated circulating levels of angiotensin and aldosterone. That this phenomenon may be as much a consequence as a cause in the vicious circle of progressive hypertensive vascular disease is indicated by the tendency for the hormonal changes to normalize following pharmacologic control of the hypertension (McAllister *et al.*, 1971).

The second is renovascular hypertension. Although the peripheral vascular effects of an elevated rate of renin secretion remains the best hypothesis to date to account for this secondary form of hypertension, there remains controversy and uncertainty with this formulation. In favor of the concept is the finding of a high level of renin activity in the renal venous blood from the involved kidney of most patients whose hypertension responds to revascularization procedures or nephrectomy. That this finding may be equated to a high level of renin secretion is supported by the human studies of Hollenberg *et al.* (1969). Against this concept is the finding that the incidence of a normal peripheral plasma renin activity in proven cases is in the range of 30%. Further, in the laboratory animal, hypertension persists although the elevated levels of circulating renin tend to normalize after the acute phase of experimental narrowing of a renal artery. Immunological studies involving the active generation and passive transfer of antibodies to renin and angiotensin in experimental renovascular hypertension are conflicting. Some support and some refute a role for the renin–angiotensin system in this form of hypertension. It is not unlikely that once the hypertensive state is established, other mechanisms reinforce the vascular changes such that in the chronic state a very small elevation in the rate of renin secretion is all that is required to perpetuate the hypertension. Conceptual support for this comes from the many studies indicating a potentiating effect of small amounts of angiotensin on the sympathetic nervous system. Khairallah *et al.* (1971) have shown that angiotensin II inhibits the uptake and, hence, the inactivation of norepinephrine, which would augment the effect of norepinephrine released by sympathetic nerves into the adventitial–medial border of the small vessels.

No discussion of the role of the renin–renin substrate system in hypertension would be complete in this age without citing current concepts concerning the evolution of hypertension in females on oral contraceptives, the incidence of which is in the range of 1% (Smith, 1972). It is well known that the high estrogen effect of "the pill" causes a sharp increase in renin substrate concentration in the circulation. This leads to a significant increase in plasma renin activity and in plasma angiotensin II concentration. There is an associated increase in aldosterone excretion. These changes are partially compensated by a negative feedback mechanism, leading to a depression of the actual concentration of renin in the circulation. These relationships have been well documented (Weinberger *et al.,* 1969; Saruta *et al.,* 1970; Cain *et al.,* 1971). Saruta *et al.* (1970) found that the depression of plasma renin concentration was less in the females who became hypertensive than in those who did not, which suggests a breakdown in a negative feedback mechanism at the level of the renal juxtaglomerular cell as a possible explanation for this phenomenon and the associated hypertension. Changes comparable to those cited above are associated with the estrogen effect of normal pregnancy. To what extent an aberration in these humoral–vascular adjustments of pregnancy may account for the hypertension of toxemia remains to be determined. In this regard it is impressive that there is a greatly increased incidence of hypertension from "the pill" in women who have a previous history of hypertension in pregnancy (Saruta *et al.,* 1970).

C. Adrenocortical Steroids and Electrolytes

The regular association of hypertension with hypersecretion of adrenocortical steroids, principally cortisol as manifested in Cushing's syndrome, and aldosterone as manifested in Conn's syndrome, invites an examination of the influence of these and related steroids on the microvasculature. A direct relationship is indicated by the numerous clinical reports of the development of hypertension in normotensive individuals following the excessive administration of either gluco- or mineralocorticoids.

In Cushing's syndrome, hypertension develops in 80% of the cases and should be attributed to the high level of glucocorticoid secretion; only rarely is there a concomitant elevation of mineralocorticoid secretion. Kalsner (1969) has shown that hydrocortisone potentiates the contraction of rabbit aortic strips in response to epinephrine and norepinephrine, apparently by inhibiting catechol-*O*-methyltransferase activity in the vascular tissue. Thus, the high circulating cortisol level in Cushing's syndrome may lead to hypertension by potentiating the effect of a normal level of sympathetic nerve activity and circulating catecholamines on the microcirculation. This condition could occur without any readily demonstrated abnormality in circulating and urinary excretion levels of catecholamines or their methoxylated derivatives. The moderate mineralocorticoidlike activity of cortisol could contribute to the development of hypertension, as well, as described below.

In Conn's syndrome, hypertension is a constant feature and should be attributed to the high level of mineralocordicoid secretion. Schmid *et al.* (1966) showed that pretreatment of normal subjects with the potent mineralocorticoid, 9α-fluorohydrocortisone, augmented the increase in vascular resistance response and decrease in blood flow response of the forearm to the intravenous infusion of norepinephrine. It is well known that the sodium and water content of the arterial wall is increased in human and in the various forms of experimental hypertension. Whether this is a fundamental causative factor or simply an effect, or both, of the hypertensive state is unresolved (Hollander *et al.,* 1968). However, it is established that vasoconstriction is associated with a movement of sodium into and vasodilation with a movement of sodium out of smooth muscle cells. Friedman and Friedman (1965) showed in the tail of the rat that the withdrawal of sodium from these cells decreased and its restoration increased the vascular resistance during a steady infusion of norepinephrine. Heistad *et al.* (1971) showed that the vasoconstrictor response to the injection of norepinephrine and angiotensin into the brachial artery of man is augmented by a high and reduced by a low plasma sodium concentration. It is well known that aldosterone fosters the intra- as well as extracellular accumulation of sodium. An acceptable hypothesis for the hypertension in primary aldosteronism, then, would be an enhancement of the vascular smooth muscle response to sympathetic tone related to an increase in intracellular sodium content. An additional component would be luminal narrowing of resistance vessels due to the "waterlogging" effect of the sodium accumulation, per se. Comparable mechanisms may be postulated for those rarer forms of nonaldosterone mineralocorticoid hypertension cited previously in the section on the renin–angiotensin system.

If it is true that hypertension of itself increases the sodium and water content of vessel walls and that this both congests them and enhances their response to a normal level of sympathetic tone and circulating vasoconstricting factors, then it would not be surprising that both a neurogenic and nonneurogenic component can be identified in hypertension, irrespective of etiology as identified by Smirk (1970).

It is known that minimal tissue levels of potassium, as well as sodium, are required for normal vascular responsiveness to norepinephrine (Burks *et al.,* 1971), and that vasoconstriction is associated with an efflux of potassium from, as well as an influx of sodium into, vascular smooth muscle (Johansson and Jonsson, 1968). More fundamental to the contractile mechanism than the effect of sodium or potassium ion on the response to neuroadrenergic activity may be calcium flux. Based on their studies, Seidel and Bohr (1971) have stated: "It seems possible that vasoactive agents may cause their effects by producing quantitative changes in the handling of Ca by the plasma membrane. Increased activator calcium, and the resultant vasoconstriction, could be produced by increasing calcium influx and/or decreasing efflux. Vasodilation, on the other hand, could be produced by decreasing influx and/or increasing efflux." Hudgins and Weiss (1967) demonstrated that norepinephrine inhibited calcium efflux from the rabbit aorta.

That other ions and physical factors are important in the contractile process and may be implicated in the hypertensive state is evident from an extensive literature on the subject.

III. Antihypertensive Function of the Normal Kidney

There is an extensive literature documenting the antihypertensive function of the normal kidney. That the normal kidney through a nonexcretory mechanism can inhibit the evolution of various forms of experimental hypertension is well known. Clinically, it has been shown that the majority of patients with hypertension associated with end stage renal disease of various etiologies do not have an increased level of circulating renin. In these patients, achievement of "dry weight" through restriction of dietary sodium and the use of diuretics generally results in a significant reduction in blood pressure. This "salt- and water-sensitive" hypertension of the uremic patient may relate simply to a loss of renal excretory function, leading to volume expansion, increased cardiac output, and, finally, an increase in peripheral vascular resistance through circulatory autoregulation. However, the chronic renal failure patient is frequently disproportionately sensitive to volume overloading in terms of hypertensive response. This has led to the concept that this unique susceptibility relates to the loss of some renal antihypertensive secretory factor in the course of the renal parenchymal destruction that protects the normal patient against the acute pressor effect of volume overloading.

A search for a specific renal mediator to account for these experimental and clinical phenomena has focused on lipid-soluble factors extractable from the renal medulla of mammalian kidney. Muirhead *et al.* (1972) have reported extensively on a neutral lipid in renal medulla, not yet chemically characterized, that in very low dosage protects against several forms of experimental hypertension. Lee and Hickler have identified a high concentration of prostaglandin in the renal medulla, subsequently identified as being largely in the form of prostaglandin-E_2 (Daniels, 1970). The *sustained* antihypertensive property of several of the prostaglandins in experimental models has been demonstrated (Alpert and Hickler, 1971; Muirhead *et al.*, 1969). Much attention has been focused on the osmiophilic droplets of the renomedullary interstitial cell, identified as the source of these lipids (Tobian and Azar, 1971). As well as possessing a sustained antihypertensive property, many of the prostaglandins have a potent vasodilator effect on resistance vessels. It remains to be demonstrated that they normally circulate in a concentration sufficient to influence directly the tone of the peripheral vasculature. An *in situ* effect on the renal vasculature and tubular transport mechanisms would account for the potent natriuretic and diuretic effects of the vasodilator prostaglandins. Such an effect on renal excretory function must be included in any consideration of their antihypertensive activity. At this time a deficiency of these renomedullary lipids must be included in the etiologic possibilities for essential hypertension and for the hypertension of chronic renal disease not associated with a high level of circulating renin activity.

IV. Hemodynamic Studies in Essential Hypertension

In spite of our understanding of a number of hypertensive mechanisms, as detailed in the preceding review, we still lack a clear concept of the primary disorder leading to essential hypertension. The best approach has been to study the disorder before it is fully expressed and before secondary phenomena obscure its fundamental manifestations. Hemodynamic measurements in borderline hypertension reveal a significant elevation in cardiac index, heart rate, and mean blood pressure; peripheral vascular resistance does not differ significantly from that of control subjects (Julius *et al.*, 1971a). Plasma volume tends to be decreased below normal in proportion to the degree of blood pressure elevation (Julius *et al.*, 1971b). The borderline hypertensive with a high cardiac output has been shown from the response to β-adrenergic blockade to have an increased sympathetic cardiac stimulation (Julius and Pascual, 1971). Once borderline or labile hypertension progresses to the stage of sustained diastolic hypertension, hemodynamic measurements reveal a normal cardiac index and an increase in heart rate and peripheral vascular resistance; plasma volume is depressed (Frohlich *et al.*, 1970). This progression from "high output" to "high resistance" hypertension may well prove to be a regular feature of the natural history of essential hypertension. Active vascular beds maintain an almost constant flow despite changes in perfusion pressure in the process of "autoregulation," relating to local myogenic vascular responses. This process is highly active in the cerebral and renal beds and is moderately

TABLE I

OUTLINE OF THE PRIMARY DISORDER IN VARIOUS CLINICAL FORMS OF HYPERTENSION AND THE EFFECT ON THE MICROCIRCULATION AND FINAL STATUS OF THE ADRENERGIC MECHANISM

Form of Hypertension	Primary Disorder	Effect On The Microvasculature	Status of The Adrenergic Mechanism
Neurogenic	↑ Sympathetic nervous system outflow	Vasconstriction	Enhanced
Pheochromocytoma	↑ Circulating catecholamines	Vasconstriction	Enhanced
Renovascular	↑ Renin — ↑ Angiotensin	Vasconstriction ↑ Norepinephrine uptake in sympathetic nervous system	Enhanced
Malignant	↑ Renin — ↑ Angiotensin ↑ Aldosterone	Vasconstriction ↓ Norepinephrine uptake ↑ Vascular muscle Na	Enhanced
Oral contraceptives ? toxemia	↑ Renin substrate — ↑ angiotensin	Vasoconstriction ↓ Norepinephrine uptake	Enhanced
Cushing's syndrome	↑ Cortisol	↓ Vascular catechol-*o*-methyltransferase activity	Enhanced
Primary aldosteronism	↑ Aldosterone	↑ Vascular muscle Na	Enhanced
Chronic nephritis	?↓ Antipressor renal function (↑ Renin — ↑ Angiotensin)	Vasoconstriction (↓ Norepinephrine uptake)	? Enhanced (unopposed) (Enhanced)
Essential	? High cardiac output ?↑β-adrenergic state ? Renal Na retention	? Myogenic vascular response w/ vasoconstriction and ↓ cardiac output	? Enhanced cardiac β-adrenergic

active in skeletal muscle and cardiac muscle beds (Green *et al.,* 1965). Such an intrinsically determined arteriolar vasoconstriction in response to an initially high cardiac output may well account for the changing hemodynamic pattern observed as the disorder evolves. If true, then a central point of interest must be the factor, or factors, leading to a state of heightened cardiac output. Under study in this regard are two possible mechanisms: (1) an intrinsically augmented level of sympathetic nervous (β-adrenergic) tone on the myocardium (Julius and Pascual, 1971); and (2) a chronically expanded plasma volume due to some intrinsic defect in the capacity of the kidney to excrete our customary dietary sodium loads. The ensuing relationships in this second formulation have been well described by Guyton *et al.* (1970) and raise the question of a fundamental defect in the "volume-sensing" mechanism. The generally higher than normal levels of plasma renin activity described in patients in the labile phase of hypertension (Frohlich *et al.,* 1970) is consistent with the latter concept. A heightened level of renal sympathetic stimulation or renin secretion could underly this important finding. The failure to find an increase in plasma volume in the labile phase of essential hypertension seems at odds with an expanded plasma volume to account for a high cardiac output. However, a "pressure diuresis," as manifested by the enhanced capacity of the hypertensive patient to excrete a saline load (Buckalew *et al.*, 1969), could obscure a state of volume expansion when hypertension develops and secondary vascular mechanisms enter into the equation.

Table I summarizes the current status of our knowledge with respect to the primary disorder in various clinical forms of hypertension and the effect on the microcirculation. It is of interest to note how regularly an increase in adrenergic effect seems to be playing at least a contributory role in the hypertensive state.

V. Summary

A summary of fundamental mechanisms leading to the various forms of clinical and experimental hypertension is presented. While a number of different primary events may start the process, certain common denominators can be found in the microcirculation that perpetuate the elevation of blood pressure. These factors would appear to include vascular stiffening from an increase in smooth muscle sodium content associated with an enhancement of the vascular response to sympathetic stimulation. Thus, a nonneurogenic and a neurogenic component may be generally identifiable in the hypertensive state, irrespective of the underlying etiology.

References

Alpert, J. S., and Hickler, R. B. (1971). Calcium and vascular smooth muscle contraction. *Circ. Res.* **28,** Suppl. 2, 88.

Bristow, J. D., Honour, A. J., Pickering, G. W., Sleight, P., and Smyth, H. S. (1969). Diminished baroreflex sensitivity in high blood pressure. *Circulation* **39**, 48.

Buckalew, V. M., Jr., Puschett, J. B., Kintzel, J. E., and Goldberg, M. (1969). Mechanism of exaggerated natriuresis in hypertensive man: Impaired sodium transport in the loop of Henle *J. Clin. Invest.* **48,** 1007.

Burks, T. F., Spalding, C. T., and Jones, V. D. (1971). Influence of sodium and potassium content on arterial responsiveness. *Circ. Res.* **29,** 525.

Burnstock, G., Gannon, B., and Iwama, T. (1970). Sympathetic innervation of vascular smooth muscle in normal and hypertensive animals. *Circ. Res.* **27,** Suppl. II, 55.

Cain, M. D., Walters, W. A., and Catt, K. J. (1971). Effects of oral contraceptive therapy on the renin-angiotensin system. *J. Clin. Endocrinol. Metab.* **33**, 671.

Daniels, E. G. (1970). Extraction of renomedullary prostaglandins. *In* "Kidney Hormones" (J. W. Fisher, ed.), pp. 507–524. Academic Press, New York.

DeChamplain, J., Krakoff, L., and Axelrod, J. (1969). Patterns of catecholamine excretion in urine in hypertension. *Circ. Res.* **24,** Suppl. I, 75.

Engelman, K., Portnoy, B., and Sjoerdsma, A. (1970). Plasma catecholamine concentration in patients with hypertension. *Circ. Res.* **27,** Suppl. I, 141.

Fotino, S., and Raiciulescu, N. (1964). Hypertension with aldosterone excess and low plasma-renin: Preoperative distinction between patients with and without adrenocortical tumour. *Lancet* **1,** 1182.

Friedman, S. M., and Friedman, C. L. (1965). Aldosterone and vasopressin as regulators of salt metabolism and of blood pressure. *In* "International Club on Arterial Hypertension" (P. Milliez and P. Tcherdakoff, eds.), pp. 240–258. L'Expansion Scientifique Française, Paris.

Frohlich, E. D., Kozul, V. J., Tarazi, R. C., and Dustan, H. P. (1970). Physiological comparison of labile and essential hypertension. *Circ. Res.* **27,** Suppl. I, 55.

Green, H. D., Schmid, H. E., Jr., and Rapelar, C. E. (1965). Autoregulation in vascular beds—possible role of autoregulation in the increased resistance to flow in hypertension. *In* "Hypertension Monographs" (Simon Rodbard *et al.* eds.), Vol. XIII, pp. 144–159. Amer. Heart Ass., Inc., New York.

Guyton, A. C., Coleman, T. G., Bower, J. D., and Granger, H. J. (1970). Circulatory control in hypertension. *Circ. Res.* **27,** Suppl. II, 135.

Heistad, D. D., Abboud, F. M., and Ballard, D. R. (1971). Relationship between plasma sodium concentration and vascular reactivity in man. *J. Clin. Invest.* **50,** 2022.

Hickler, R. B., Hanlin, J. T., III, and Wells, R. (1959). Plasma norepinephrine response to tilting in essential hypertension. *Circulation* **20,** 422.

Hollander, W., Kramsch, D. M., Farmelant, M., and Madoff, I. V. (1968). Arterial wall metabolism in experimental hypertension of coarctation of the aorta of short duration. *J. Clin. Invest.* **47,** 1221.

Hollenberg, N. K., Epstein, M., Bosch, R. I., Merrill, J. P., and Hickler, R. B. (1969). Renin secretion in the patient with hypertension. *Circ. Res.* **24,** Suppl. I, 113.

Hudgins, P. M., and Weiss, G. B. (1967). Differential effects of calcium removal upon vascular smooth muscle contraction induced by norepinephrine, histamine, and potassium. *J. Pharmacol. Exp. Ther.* **159,** 91.

Johansson, B., and Jonsson, O. (1968). Cell volume as a factor influencing electrical and mechanical activity of vascular smooth muscle. *Acta Physiol. Scand.* **72,** 456.

Jose, A., Crout, J. R., and Kaplan, N. M. (1970). Suppressed plasma renin activity in essential hypertension. *Ann. Intern. Med.* **72,** 9.

Julius, S., and Pascual, A. V. (1971). Different hemodynamic patterns in borderline hypertension. *Circulation* **45,** Suppl. II, 128.

Julius, S., Pascual, A. V., Sannerstedt, R., and Mitchell, P. L. (1971a). Relationship between cardiac output and peripheral vascular resistance in borderline hypertension. *Circulation* **43,** 382.

Julius, S., Pascual, A. V., Reilly, K., and London, R. (1971b). Abnormalities of plasma volume in borderline hypertension. *Arch. Intern. Med.* **127,** 116.

Kalsner, S. (1969). Mechanism of hydrocortisone potentiation of responses to epinephrine and norepinephrine in rabbit aorta. *Circ. Res.* **24,** 383.

Khairallah, P. A., Davila, D., Papanicolaou, N., Glende, N. M., and Meyer, P. (1971). Effects of angiotensin infusion on catecholamine uptake and reactivity in blood vessels. *Circ. Res.* **28,** Suppl. II, 96.

McAllister, R. G., Jr., Van Way, C. W., III, Dayani, K., Anderson, W. J., Temple, E., Michelakis, A. M., Coppinger, W. S., Jr., and Oates, J. A. (1971). Malignant hypertension: Effect of therapy on renin and aldosterone. *Cir. Res.* **28,** Suppl. II, 160.

Melby, J. C., Dale, S. L., and Wilson, T. E. (1971). 18-Hydroxy-deoxycorticosterone in human hypertension. *Circ. Res.* **28,** Suppl. II, 143.

Mitchell, P. L., and Meilman, E (1967). The mechanism of hypertension in the Guillain-Barré syndrome. *Amer. J. Med.* **42,** 986.

Muirhead, E. E., Daniels, E. G., Pike, J .E., and Hinman, J. W. (1969). Renomedullary antihypertensive lipids and the prostaglandins. *In* "Nobel Symposium 2—Prostaglandins" (S. Bergström and B. Samuelsson, eds.), pp. 183–196. Alqvist Wiksell, Stockholm.

Muirhead, E. E., Brooks, B., Pitcock, J. A., and Stephanson, P. (1972). Renomedullary antihypertensive function in accelerated (malignant) hypertension. Observations on renomedullary interstitial cells. *J. Clin. Invest.* **51,** 181.

Peterson, L. (1966). Physical factors which influence vascular caliber and blood flow. *Circ. Res.* **13,** Suppl. I, 3.

Saruta, T., Saade, G. A., and Kaplan, N. M. (1970). A possible mechanism for hypertension induced by oral contraceptives. *Arch. Intern. Med.* **126,** 621.

Schmid, P. G., Eckstein, J. W., and Abboud, F. M. (1966). Effect of 9-fluorohydrocortisone on forearm vascular responses to norepinephrine. *Circulation* **34,** 620.

Seidel, C. L., and Bohr, D. F. (1971). Calcium and vascular smooth muscle contraction. *Circ. Res.* **28,** Suppl. II, 88.

Smirk, F. H. (1970). The neurogenically maintained component in hypertension. *Circ. Res.* **27,** Suppl. II, 55.

Smith, R. W. (1972). Hypertension and oral contraception. *Amer. J. Obstet. Gynecol.* **113,** 482.

Spark, R. F., and Melby, J. C. (1971). Hypertension and low plasma renin activity: Presumptive evidence for mineralocorticoid excess. *Ann. Intern. Med.* 75, 831.

Tobian, L., and Azar, S. (1971). Functions of renal papilla. *Clin. Res.* **19,** 577.

Weinberger, M. H., Collins, R. D., Dowdy, A. J., Nokes, G. W., and Luetscher, J. A. (1969). Hypertension induced by oral contraceptives containing estrogen and gestagen. *Ann. Intern. Med.* **71,** 891.

13 HEMATOLOGIC DISORDERS: HEMATOLOGY AND THE MICROCIRCULATION

JOHN R. MURPHY, M.D.

I. Introduction

The concept of microcirculation in relation to hematology is in essence the dynamic or functional state of hematology. Microcirculation as the functional unit of the circulation is not a new concept, yet it is not generally thought of in regard to the pathology of disease. The physiologist deals with the function of organ systems. Consideration of the circulatory system and its control, until recently, has been primarily concerned with the heart and larger blood vessels. The pathologists have been concerned with changes that occur in tissues, primarily on a morphologic basis. The term microvasculature denotes structure, whereas microcirculation includes both structure and function, the latter being intimately related to the properties of blood. Although the microcirculation represents the functional component of the circulatory system, it is inappropriate to consider the microcirculation as a single unit, the microcirculation should be thought of as a variety of units, each unique to a different tissue or organ.

Microcirculatory manifestations of disease involve the interrelationships between the microvasculature and the blood. Abnormalities in the blood are associated with a spectrum of pathologic changes in different tissues, in part, due to the differences in the microvasculature in different tissues. The pathophysiology and clinical manifestations of primary hematologic disorders emphasize the uniqueness of the microvasculature in different tissues. In addition to the structural or anatomic differences in the microvasculature in different tissues, the control or regulation of the microcirculation differs in various tissues. In this chapter I will attempt to deal with the hematologic aspects of the microcirculation. Although the fluidity of blood is paramount to blood flow, this review will not be concerned with coagulation phenomena or those systems within blood which are related to the prevention and propagation of clotting.

II. Rheology—Viscosity

A. Components

The discipline of rheology is an important aspect in the understanding of hematologic phenomena in the microcirculation. However, a working knowledge of rheology does not require the detailed comprehension of mathematical formulations. The rheology of blood or its flow properties include the intrinsic properties of blood and the influence on these properties by the system in which flow is concerned. An example of the latter is the Fahraeus-Lindqvist (1931) effect, which is the apparent decrease in viscosity of blood when measured in capillary tubes of decreasing diameter up to the point that flow ceases. This phenomenon has an obvious relationship to the *in vivo* behavior of blood in regard to the range in diameter of blood vessels, as well as to the functional changes in vessel size which occur in the process of regulation or control of blood flow. The relationship of cell size to capillary diameter is another factor in regard to rheologic behavior of blood in the microvasculature. The normal erythrocyte undergoes profound changes in shape in many areas of the microvasculature. In considering the intrinsic rheologic or flow properties of blood, it is convenient in relation to both physiologic and pathologic states to categorize the flow properties as to (1) media or plasma, (2) particles or cells, and (3) interrelationships between cells and plasma and cell–cell interactions altered by plasma constituents. Most hematologic abnormalities in the microcirculation can be defined within the above dimensions.

The viscosity of blood is one of several rheologic properties and denotes the resistance to flow. Viscosity is the ratio of shear stress (force imposed per unit area of fluid plane) to shear rate (difference in the velocity of two planes divided by the distance between them—velocity gradient). Blood is a heterogeneous suspension and, in contrast to a homogeneous solution, differs from many other liquids. The viscosity of a homogeneous liquid, such as oil, is not related to the shear rate or velocity gradient and is termed a Newtonian fluid. The viscosity of blood changes in relation to shear rate and is termed non-Newtonian. A number of factors have been defined for blood, which contribute to its non-Newtonian behavior. These include fluid properties of cells and cell–cell interactions. In a sense, the viscosity of blood or its resistance to flow influences the energy required to maintain flow, or the work performed in maintaining circulation. The viscosity of plasma is greater than that of water, yet represents only a small fraction of the viscosity of blood at a normal hematocrit. The concentration of red cells in normal plasma has a profound influence on the viscosity of blood. Doubling the hematocrit of blood results in more than a twofold increase in viscosity. Thus, the relationship of viscosity to hematocrit is not linear but exponential. That portion of blood viscosity related to red cells reflects the fluid properties of the cell itself and cell–cell interactions. Both these factors contribute to the non-Newtonian behavior of blood. The cell–cell interactions are profoundly altered both by changes in hematocrit and by substances in the suspending media, such as fibrinogen and certain abnormal proteins which can cause rouleaux, agglutination, or aggregation of cells. Aggregation of cells results in an increased viscosity and, in part, accounts for the progressive increase in viscosity at decreasing shear rates. In contrast, with higher shear rates, the shearing forces of flow result in the dispersion of aggregates and a lower viscosity.

The important relationship of aggregation and shear rate to microcirculatory phenomena may be better understood with an appreciation of those factors which influence aggregation and shear rate. Aggregation and rouleaux of cells with the dysproteinemias or increased fibrinogen are both greater with a higher concentration of cells. The forces of fluid shear are primarily a function of vessel diameter and pressure gradient. The higher pressures and smaller size vessels in the arterial system are associated with greater shear rates with less aggregation. Thus, aggregation is more likely to occur in the venous system. Inasmuch as only a fraction of the microcirculation is being perfused at any one time, there are areas with minimal or no flow as well as areas with reversal of flow. In these areas of the microvasculature where flow is reduced, aggregation would be greater.

Another factor which contributes to the non-Newtonian viscosity of blood concerns the rheologic properties of the individual red cell. The red cell undergoes shape changes both in large vessels because of shearing forces, and in capillaries because of the restrictions of vessel size. The deformability of the red cell is related to its internal viscosity and to changes in the ratio of surface area to volume. The internal viscosity of the red cell is primarily dependent on the concentration and state of the hemoglobin. The significance of the relationship of membrane surface area and cell volume to deformability of the cell can be appreciated by comparing the deformability of a basketball, either half full or full of water. The basketball which is only half full would be more deformable than that which is full. Thus, the excess surface area of the red cell provides the cell with the potential to undergo considerable deformation.

B. Measurement

The rheologic properties of blood can be observed in a number of different ways. The early studies of blood viscosity were carried out in Ostwald or capillary type of viscometers which have certain limitations. The Ostwald viscometers measure viscosity at relatively high shear rates, which for the most part are greater than those which occur *in vivo*. In a non-Newtonian fluid such as blood, it is important to measure viscosity at both low shear rates and at variable shear rates. More recently, instrumentation has been developed which determines viscosity at very low shear rates, well within the physiological range (Gilinson *et al.,* 1963). It is appropriate to think of blood viscosity, as determined in these instruments, as the viscosity in a bulk flow system and as a homogenous suspension. This situation is in contrast to the flow of individual cells through the smallest components of the microvasculature. In a capillary, for example, where individual cells are separated by plasma, the elements of cell deformability and plasma viscosity may be more significant than the element of cell–cell interaction. Other systems for observing cell deformability have been developed which, in general, measure the flow of cell suspensions through microchannels of filters (Jandl *et al.,* 1961; Nicolau *et al.,* 1964; Murphy, 1967) and the movement of individual cells into micropipettes (Rand and Burton, 1964). Thus, there is no single measurement of the rheologic properties of blood which can be correlated with microcirculatory behavior.

III. Physiology

A. Microvasculature—Control of Flow

The concept of microcirculation includes the element of control of blood flow as part of its function. The microvasculature is more than just a system of tubes, but rather a group of systems with complex, interrelated controls. Zweifach (1961) has emphasized that the function of the microvasculature is not simply the delivery of substrates and removal of waste products, but of equal importance is the property of controlling the rate of blood flow to tissues. In the basal state, approximately one-fifth of the total microvasculature is being perfused at any one time. There is not space in this discussion to review recent studies in this area (Rodbard, 1971). Numerous substances have been identified which influence blood flow in the microcirculation, including pH, pO_2, polypeptides, potassium, phosphates, and osmolality (Scott and Radawski, 1971). Obviously, the control of blood flow determines the gradients for various substances to be delivered to or removed from tissues. The distance between vessels and tissue cells, or parts of a cell, also is an important factor influencing gradients. The distance which oxygen (O_2) must move from the hemoglobin molecule in the red cell to the mitochondria in a tissue cell influences the availability of O_2 in tissues. Shortening this distance by increasing the number of capillaries in a tissue would have a profound influence on substrate gradients. There is a need to identify the factors which control or determine the number or density of capillaries in different tissues, particularly in the repair processes involved in occlusive vascular disease.

B. Oxygen Transport

The phenomenon of O_2 transport occupies a key position in considering the relationships between hematology and the microcirculation. The function of the red cell is to transport O_2 and carbon dioxide (CO_2). The stimulation of erythopoiesis by anoxia, leading to an increase in the red cell mass, has been well defined. Recent studies have demonstrated the relationship of red cell metabolism to the affinity of hemoglobin (Hb) for O_2. The amount of O_2 bound to Hb at different levels of pO_2 represents the O_2 dissociation curve for Hb. The position of this curve or the comparative value describing changes in the affinity of Hb for O_2 is indicated as the P_{50}, i.e., the O_2 tension at which 50% of the Hb is saturated with O_2. An increase in the P_{50} value, or "shift to the right" in the position of the O_2 dissociation curve, reflects a decrease in the affinity of Hb for O_2. This change facilitates the delivery of O_2 to tissues at normal tissue pO_2 levels. Conversely, a "shift to the left," or a decrease in the P_{50} value, is associated with less dissociation of O_2 from Hb at a normal tissue pO_2, or an increase in the affinity of Hb for O_2. Any change in the affinity of Hb for O_2 has a significant effect on the availability of O_2 in tissues and little influence on the uptake of O_2 by the blood in the lungs. The important physiological factors which alter the affinity of Hb for O_2 include H^+ ions, CO_2, and the red cell 2,3-diphosphoglycerate (2,3-DPG). An increase in the concentration of 2,3-DPG, a glycolytic intermediate, in the red cell results in a decrease in the Hb affinity for O_2, which in turn increases the availability of O_2 for tissues. Similar changes in O_2 availability or the O_2 dissociation for Hb occur with increases in CO_2 or H^+ ions.

Changes in the Hb affinity for O_2 occur in many pathological states and are part of the compensatory processes involving microcirculatory function. For example, in many anemic states there is an increase in the red cell 2,3-DPG which facilitates the delivery of O_2 in the presence of a reduced O_2 carrying capacity of blood (Torrance *et al.,* 1970). Anemia is associated with a lower blood viscosity and less myocardial work at a constant cardiac output. In congestive failure, there is an increase in the red cell 2,3-DPG with a concomitant decrease in Hb affinity for O_2 which results in an increase in the quantity of O_2 available to tissues per rate of flow and concentration of Hb (Woodson *et al.*, 1970). This mechanism of compensation may well prevent the increase in erythropoiesis and polycythemia that would otherwise result from tissue anoxia. Polycythemia with the associated increase in viscosity would be detrimental to tissue perfusion in congestive failure. Changes in blood pH are another pathophysiologic state which influences the microcirculation and O_2 transport. An increase in H^+ ion concentration (a decrease in pH) causes both vasodilatation and a decrease in the affinity of Hb for O_2 which is reflected in the O_2 dissociation curve as a shift to the right with an increased P_{50}. This change in the P_{50} with a change in pH is immediate. However, over a period of several hours, there is a compensatory change in the concentration of 2,3-DPG in the cell resulting from the influence of a lower pH on red cell glycolysis. With a lower pH, 2,3-DPG decreases in the cell resulting in a greater affinity of Hb for O_2 with a lower P_{50}. This cellular compensatory mechanism for maintaining a relatively constant P_{50} becomes important clinically in the rapid correction of acidosis when it has been present for several hours. A rapid correction in pH would result in an increase in affinity of Hb for O_2 and a lower P_{50}. This could lead to tissue anoxia until there was time for the 2,3-DPG to accumulate at the higher pH and correct the P_{50} back to normal.

Recent studies of O_2 affinity for certain abnormal Hb's have improved our understanding of O_2 transport in both polycythemic and anemic states. Several abnormal Hb have been found to have high O_2 affinity or a low P_{50} and include Hb Chesapeake, J-Cape Town, Yakima, Kempsey, Ypsi, Hiroshima, Rainier, and Bethesda (Stamatoyannopoulos *et al.*, 1971). In those abnormal Hb's which are stable and not associated with a hemolytic anemia there is a compensatory increase in hematocrit resulting in polycythemia. Thus, the low P_{50} or high O_2 affinity for these Hb's leads to an increase in erythropoiesis and a greater concentration of Hb per unit volume of blood. Hb Seattle has a low O_2 affinity and is associated with anemia without reticulocytosis or increase hemolysis.

C. Altitude Adaptation

The adaptation of man to high altitude is another example of the relationship of O_2 transport to the hematologic aspects of microcirculatory phenomenon. When man moves to high altitudes, there is an increase in plasma and urinary erythropoietin, followed by an increase in the red cell mass and hematocrit. In addition, an increase in the red cell 2,3-DPG leads to an increased availability of O_2 for tissues (Lenfant and Sullivan, 1971). Some individuals who have been acclimatized to high altitudes develop a syndrome termed chronic mountain sickness characterized by dyspnea, fatigue, headache, and dizziness. These individuals have a further increase in hematocrit, a decrease in arterial O_2 saturation, and hypoventilation. The hypothesis that excessive polycythemia and secondary hypoventilation cause the decompensation has not been proved. Monge *et al.* (1965) observed three patients with chronic mountain sickness before and 24 hours after phlebotomy. This is in contrast to the statements of Penaloza and Sime (1971) who described temporary relief of symptoms with phlebotomy. The relationships of polycythemia, increased viscosity, and congestive failure need further definition in chronic mountain sickness as well as in other disease states, particularly chronic obstructive pulmonary disease.

Polycythemia is a classic feature of the dysventilation syndromes as classified in a discussion of cor pulmonale by Hecht (1966). In these conditions, congestive failure is frequently preceded by a further increase in hematocrit (Hecht, 1966). In the secondary type of polycythemia, the stimulus for the increased erythropoiesis is anoxia acting through the erythropoietin to increase red cell mass. However, what is not clear is what constitutes the optimal hematocrit in these anoxic states. This problem cannot be resolved with our present state of knowledge. Replogle and Merrill (1970) induced acute normovolemic polycythemia in dogs and observed a decreased cardiac output and perpheral O_2 consumption and an increased arteriovenous O_2 difference with an increase in the ratio of lactate to pyruvate. These studies indicated that tissue anoxia was associated with the increased viscosity of the blood and decreased tissue perfusion. Although cardiac output decreased with the increased O_2 carrying capacity, a more fundamental problem concerns the work load of the heart in the polycythemia states. To what extent does blood with an increased viscosity require more energy from the heart to maintain perpheral circulation?

IV. Hematologic Abnormalities

Prior to considering the relationship of hematologic abnormalities and the microcirculation, it is appropriate to briefly reexamine and classify the factors that influence the flow properties of blood. Although this is an arbitrary classification, it does have bearing on pathologic states. The flow properties can be separated into three areas: (1) the relative concentration of cells in the media, since the element of cell–cell interaction is obviously enhanced with a higher hematocrit such as in polycythemia states; (2) the viscosity of plasma, particularly in the dysproteinemias; and (3) the physical properties of the individual cells such as deformability in sickle cell anemia. Interrelationships between these categories will be evident in the following discussions. Hematologic abnormalities will be considered in these three general categories.

A. Polycythemia

Secondary polycythemia is primarily related to hypoxia resulting from chronic lung disease, congenital heart disease, and altitude. In these conditions, the polycythemia represents a compensatory process. What are the effects of the polycythemia on different tissues? The problem of myocardial work and congestive failure have been noted. Although not all patients with chronic mountain sickness develop congestive failure, the disease is characterized by dyspnea and easy fatigability. Evidence of central nervous system dysfunction is suggested by the common symptoms of headache, dizziness, paresthesia, and sombulence. Indeed, in polycythemia vera the same symptoms occur, particularly fatigue and dyspnea on exertion. This symptomatology strongly suggests that in polycythemia the increased viscosity results in tissue hypoxia and dysfunction.

Other microcirculatory phenomena can occur with polycythemia vera, including hemorrhage and thrombosis. Whether or not these two vascular manifestation are related to a similar process remains to be shown. The skin shows the characteristic "rubor," a reddish-blue color due to vasodilation. The sensitivity to cold in these patients is thought to be due to "slow" circulation and vasodilation. Funduscopic evaluations show marked engorgement and tortuosity. The engorgement and vasodilation, which is in part related to the increased blood volume, may well influence the apparent blood viscosity in these vessels simply by the increase in vessel diameter. Bleeding into the skin and mucous membranes is common. These patients not infrequently bleed from the GI tract and present with iron deficiency anemia, splenomegaly, and thrombocytosis. It is difficult to estimate the frequency of thrombosis in this disease. In one series of 250 cases, 50% of 49 untreated patients died within 18 months of the onset of symptoms with 40% of the total deaths in this series ascribed to thrombosis (Chievetz and Thiede, 1962). In contrast, the incidence of thrombosis in secondary polycythemia is low. Three factors which probably contribute to the phenomenon of thrombosis and bleeding are the abnormalities in platelets, the increased viscosity, and the increased blood volume. Platelet counts over one million with prolonged bleeding times are not uncommon in polycythemia vera. Although there are no specifically defined mechanisms, it may be logical to think of the bleeding as a result of the abnormal platelets and distention of the microvasculature with the increased viscosity and with a prolonged circulation time. Other specific organ dysfunctions are difficult to define. A small number of patients do present with or develop congestive failure which is improved with phlebotomy and reduction of blood viscosity. The observations of Lertzman *et al.* (1964) suggest that there are changes in cardiopulmonary function in polycythemia vera. They found decreased arterial O_2 saturations (less than 80 mm Hg) in 11 out of 26 patients without evident heart or lung disease and normal ventilatory function. These observations indicate that the arterial pO_2 value alone cannot be used to separate primary and secondary polycythemias.

B. Plasma Protein Abnormalities

The flow properties of blood are subject to major alterations with changes in the plasma proteins. Abnormalities in either plasma proteins or polycythemia are the major causes of the hyperviscosity state. Although many of the symptoms and physical findings associated with the hyperviscosity state are similar, irrespective of the cause, there are fundamental differences in the rheological properties depending on the cause of the hyperviscosity condition. In either condition, polycythemia or dysproteinemia, the viscosity of the blood is increased in a bulk flow system such as the cone-plate or couette viscometer. However, it has not been possible to correlate blood viscosity values in these different conditions with clinical manifestations. In the smallest vessels of the microcirculation where blood would not retain its homogenous character because of the similarities of red cell size and vessel diameter, the rheological behavior of the plasma itself becomes a significant factor. Some of the dysproteinemias have an additional effect on rheological behavior through changes in cell–cell interactions, resulting in aggregation of cells. Increased concentrations of the normal protein, fibrinogen, have a similar effect with rouleaux formation. Cold agglutinins and macroglobulinemia would have a similar influence on cell–cell interactions. Although both of these elements of abnormal rheologic properties can be identified, it is not possible at the present time to correlate specific abnormalities with clinical findings.

In most of the dysproteinemic states there is a significant degree of anemia which in some respects is beneficial to the patient in that the viscosity of blood would be less abnormal. Cline *et al.* (1963) has demonstrated that there are multiple causes for the anemia in macroglobulinemia, including (a) shortened red cell life span and (b) impairment of red cell production or an aregenerative anemia. It is interesting to note that there is rarely any red cell morphologic evidence for mechanical destruction such as that seen in microangiopathic hemolytic anemia.

There are two "normal" physiologic processes in which a change in a normal plasma protein alters the rheologic properties of blood in the microcirculation. The plasma fibrinogen increases during pregnancy and in the response to an inflammatory stimulus. Although there is little change in the viscosity of plasma with an elevated fibrinogen, there are marked changes in the viscosity of whole blood, particularly at low shear rates (Merrill *et al.*, 1963). In normal or uncomplicated pregnancy, the change in fibrinogen does not appear to result in a pathological process. However, in patients with Hb SC or SS disease there are major clinical problems during pregnancy which will be discussed with the hemoglobinopathies. The changes which occur in the microcirculation with tissue inflammation will not be discussed here although this process involves all the formed elements in the blood, many of the plasma proteins, particularly the proteins involved in clotting, and finally changes in the microvasculature, particularly the endothelium. Vasodilation, hemorrhage, and thrombosis are all part of the microcirculatory response to injury.

The clinical presentation of patients with dysproteinemia and increased plasma viscosity usually is related either to anemia or specific organ dysfunction. Symptoms related to CNS anoxia including mental confusion, vertigo, and nystagmus are common. Hemorrhage and a bleeding diathesis with purpura and epistaxis have been ascribed to the complexing of clotting factors and interference with platelet aggregation by the abnormal protein, usually a macroglobulin. It should be noted that precise documentation of organ dysfunction resulting from anoxia is lacking in many of these conditions. Support for a causal relationship of hyperviscosity to clinical abnormalities has been based primarily on changes in the clinical condition with treatment of the hyperviscosity state by plasmaphoresis (Fahey, 1963). However, the mechanism whereby increases in plasma viscosity result in tissue dysfunction is not entirely clear. Rosenblum and Asofsky (1968) have pointed out the importance of the hematocrit in the presence of the abnormal plasmaviscosity. The anemia which is present in most of these patients may prevent more serious problems. There are a number of questions which remain to be answered. What are the specific metabolic abnormalities in different tissues when plasma viscosity is increased? Are these abnormalities similar when blood viscosity is increased in polycythemia as compared to increases in plasma viscosity with macroglobulinemia? It is not difficult to understand congestive heart failure in these conditions because of the increased energy required to maintain flow. The similarity of symptoms related to the nervous system in both kinds of hyperviscosity is striking and possibly is related to the susceptibility of the central nervous system to hypoxia. Although there are similarities in the appearance of the eyegrounds with polycythemia and increased plasma viscosity, the incidence of visual disturbances with the dysproteinemias is very high. Do the abnormal proteins, particularly the macroglobulins, alter tissue function in some manner in addition to the changes in plasma viscosity? That there are differences in the microcirculation in the different tissues is clearly indicated by the spectrum of tissue dysfunction in the various hyperviscosity states. Abnormalities in function of the various endocrine glands have not been demonstrated. Liver and kidney function are minimally altered.

The ophthalmologic manifestations in hyperviscosity states often provide important clues to the diagnosis as well as an opportunity to observe physical changes in relatively large vessels with the aid of an ophthalmoscope. Visual disturbances are associated with venous distention or engorgement, tortuosity, sausage-shaped veins, and hyperemia of the disc (Carr and Henkind, 1963). Hemorrhages and exudates are also seen. Histologically, microaneurysms and capillary proliferation are seen in the retina. In the dysproteinemic hyperviscosity state, "plug flow" or the "boxcar" appearance can be seen in the retinal veins. This consists of the movement of large aggregates of cells (clumps) in a vein with changes in the diameter of the vein as the clumps of cells move along the vein.

The macroglobulinemia of Waldenstrom (1944) represents the classic disease process in which the hyperviscosity syndrome occurs. In this particular disease the abnormal protein is a IgM macroglobuiin. Macroglobulinemia can occur with neoplastic, collagen, and chronic infectious diseases, but usually with a lower concentration than in primary macroglobulinemia. Some of the IgM macroglobulins have properties of cryoglobulins in that they form precipitates or gel at temperatures below 37°C. Cryo properties are also observed with other proteins. IgG and IgA cryoglobulins can be associated with clinical manifestations, primarily in the skin and the extremities, including Raynaud's phenomenon, cold urticara and sensitivity, and tissue necrosis with gangrene due to vascular occlusion. In most cases of multiple myeloma, the increase in globulins, primarily the low molecular weight proteins, IgG and IgA, causes a mild increase in serum viscosity without the clinical manifestations of hyperviscosity. Extremely high concentrations of IgG or IgA protein can occur with sufficient increase in serum viscosity to cause the hyperviscosity syndrome. However, there have been some patients described with a hyperviscosity state without the very high concentrations of myeloma proteins. The IgG or IgA proteins which cause the hyperviscosity state at relatively low concentrations have been shown either to form molecular aggregates or to have an unusual molecular shape (Mackenzie *et al.*, 1970).

C. Platelets

The platelet occupies a rather unique position in regards to hematology and the microcirculation. Its function is best characterized by its role in maintaining the integrity of the microvascular system. Platelets are intimately involved in the very complex and interrelated microcirculatory processes of injury, inflammation, and hemostasis. Clinical manifestations of abnormalities in platelet function occur in widely differing disease states with either decreased, increased, or essentially normal numbers of platelets. This review will in no way attempt to cover the bleeding and clotting abnormalities with their intricate interrelationship to the microcirculation. The process of disseminated intravascular coagulation is covered elsewhere.

It is appropriate to point out some of the simple clinical phenomena that involve microcirculation and hemostasis. The mechanism of formation of the petechia in thrombocytopenia remains to be explained. How do these small hemorrhages occur primarily in the skin and mucosal surfaces with thrombocytopenia? The relationship of intravascular pressure to the formation of petechiae is well demonstrated by their predominance in the lower extremities in ambulatory patients and by their formation in response either to the tournique test or to a suction cup. The *de novo* appearance of petechiae in relatively nontraumatized areas of the skin in severe thrombocytopenia raises some interesting questions. In experimental injury to small vessels, platelets can be seen to adhere to the damaged endothelium, to aggregate, and finally form the "platelet plug" and subsequently a thrombosis. Is there a process of rupture or loss of integrity of the microvascular endothelium going on all the time which is continually repaired by platelets? Does the presence of platelets in the circulation in some way influence the integrity of the endothelium and thus prevent bleeding in the small vessels of the skin? Bleeding into joint spaces is extremely rare in both thrombocytopenia and with excessive anticoagulent therapy. In hemophilia, bleeding into joint spaces is common and is thought to result from trauma within the joint. Obviously, there must be certain differences in either the tissue or the microvasculature of joint tissue to account for these various clinical phenomena. The response of the platelet to endothelial injury has in recent years renewed interest in the complex area of thrombosis-coagulation-atherosclerosis (French, 1971). A key question in this area is what initiates the process of microthrombus formation or what constitutes the injury of the vascular endothelium?

D. Leukocytes

A full consideration of the role of leukocytes in the microcirculation is beyond the scope of this chapter. However, there are several unique features in regard to microcirculatory phenomena and leukocytes in normal physiologic states. Leukocytes, including both granulocytes and lymphocytes, function primarily outside of the vascular system. The microcirculation provides a transport system. Granulocyte function involves the response to inflammation, whereas lymphocytes are involved in immunologic processes. Numerous factors involved in the inflammatory process are concerned with the mobilization of granulocytes to inflamed tissue. Granulocytes have a relatively short half-life in the peripheral blood, 6–8 hours; and once they leave the vascular system through the endothelium, they do not return to the blood (Boggs, 1967). The pool of granulocytes which are circulating in the peripheral blood at any one time is in equilibrium with a similar size pool of granulocytes in what has been termed a marginal pool. The marginal pool represents granulocytes which are in the vascular system but are "attached" to vascular endothelium, primarily in the lungs. This pool of cells can be mobilized very rapidly (by epinephrine and exercise) and represents what was previously thought of as a splenic reservoir.

Granulocytes have little effect on blood viscosity as measured with a cone-plate viscometer. Viscosity studies on blood from a patient with chronic myelogenous leukemia revealed a 10–15% increase in viscosity with 300,000 WBC/mm^3 compared to the same blood without WBC's at a similar hematocrit of 60% (Murphy, unpublished). Specific microcirculatory abnormalities related to increased number of leukocytes have not been defined. Changes in organ functions in patients with leukemia, particularly in the brain, probably result from the perivascular infiltrates of abnormal cells.

The most unique aspect of the lymphocyte in regard to microcirculatory phenomena concerns its recirculation through the lymphatic system. This cell, particularly the small lymphocyte which may live for years, can leave the blood in the various lymphoid tissues, remain there for long periods of time, and then return to the blood vascular system either directly or through the lymphatic-thoracic duct system. The extensive movement of lymphocytes out of the blood stream and passing through endothelium into lymphoid tissue denotes a specialized function for the vascular endothelial cells in these tissues. The lymphocyte leaves the blood vascular system by passing through the cytoplasm of the endothelial cells in the postcapillary venules of lymphoid tissue (Marchesi and Gowans, 1964). This is in contrast to the movement of granulocytes which leave the microvascular system by passing between endothelial cells in small and medium-sized venules of other tissues (Marchesi and Florey, 1960). The phenomenon of the "traffic of lymphocytes" has recently been reviewed and related to the immune defense mechanisms by Ford and Gowans (1969).

E. Red Cells—Normal Processes

There are, within the microcirculation, many processes involving specific interrelationships between normal cells and the microvasculature that are concerned with the development and release of normal red cells from the bone marrow and the removal of senescent red cells from the circulation. The development and maintenance of normal bone marrow activity, erythropoiesis, is dependent on the microcirculatory environment of the marrow. Direct microscopy studies of marrow have suggested that two different microvasculature systems exist in functional marrow: one related to bone metabolism and the other related to hematopoietic activity (McClugage *et al.*, 1971). Recently reported studies (Knospe and Crosby, 1971) have suggested that irradiated marrow does not regenerate without replacement of vascular stem cells. The significance of these observations, particularly in regard to aplastic anemia, remains to be determined. Could repeated microinfarcts of the marrow microvasculature in Hb SS disease cause a relative insufficient production of red cells? There is virtually no understanding of the process whereby developing red cells are held in the marrow until after the nucleus is extruded. It is obvious that the nucleated red cell would be less deformable than a nonnucleated red cell. However, there is no evidence that such a difference actually controls the release of the cell from the marrow. It is presumed that there must be some particular physical–chemical interaction between the relatively mature red cell and the endothelium of the microvasculature in the marrow which controls the release of cells. The process of removal of senescent red cells is equally as poorly understood. Many investigators have proposed that these cells are destroyed in the spleen, a hypothesis for which there also is no evidence. LaCelle (1970) has proposed that severe deoxygenation of "old" red cells results in a more rigid cell as measured by sucking cells suspended in a tris buffer into micropipettes. Other studies have failed to show any change in bulk viscosity or filterability of fresh deoxygenated cells in serum. However, in tris buffer, progressive deterioration of red cells was evident by changes in both volume and osmotic fragility (Brereton and Murphy, 1971). Where and how the normal red cell is removed from the circulation and destroyed remain to be shown. That information in itself is critical for the understanding of various disease states. How is the removal of the aged normal red cell related to its physical properties and some unique function of the microvasculature in certain tissues?

1. *Physical Trauma to Red Cells*

The destruction of red cells by physical trauma has been beautifully defined in two completely different situations. The very eloquent studies reported by Davidson (1969) regarding march hemoglobinuria have demonstrated that in distance runners, trauma to the feet results in the intravascular destruction of red cells, probably in the microvasculature of the feet. Red cell destruction and hemoglobinuria were prevented by running on soft surfaces or using cushioned innersoles in their shoes. The syndrome of microangiopathic hemolytic anemia with fragmentation of red cells in the vascular system has been developed around the studies of Brain and Hourihane (1967). Visual demonstrations of red cells trapped, or "hung up" on strands of fibrin as if the cells were hung on a clothes line, with the subsequent buffeting by the blood flow around the cell clearly shows the mechanism of damage to cells in this syndrome. The relationship of this process to disseminated intravascular coagulation is discussed elsewhere. The identification of the morphologic change in the appearance of these damaged red cells have allowed the hematologist to group together anemias from a number of different disease states into the group of microangiopathic hemolytic anemias. The exact fate of the damaged cells seen in the peripheral blood film is not known. In most situations these are low grade hemolytic processes. In patients with cardiac prostheses, the hemolytic process can be quite severe with significant intravascular hemolysis.

Continuous intravascular hemolysis, irrespective of the cause, can lead to the development of iron deficiency through loss of iron with hemoglobinuria and hemosiderinuria.

2. *Intravascular Hemolysis*

Intravascular hemolysis can also occur in other conditions such as severe burns, transfusion reactions, paroxysmal nocturnal hemoglobinuria (PNH), autoimmune hemolytic anemia (AHA), chemical or drug toxicity, and severe infections. One of the unique features of PNH is the high incidence of venous thrombosis. This has been thought to be related to the initiation of the clotting process by phospholipids in the red cell membrane which are similar to those in platelets and can activate the early stages of clotting (Troup *et al.*, 1960). Why venous thrombosis and intravascular clotting are not seen more frequently in other conditions with intravascular hemolysis remains unexplained. There is also no explanation for the severe generalized pain which occurs with intravascular hemolysis as seen in transfusion reactions and acute autoimmune hemolytic anemias. Many of these patients have mid to low back pain associated with tenderness to light percussion of the kidneys. It is evident that our understanding of the effects of intravascular hemolysis on the microvasculature in different tissues is poorly understood.

In most disease states and probably in the normal aging process of cells, the destruction of red cells takes place outside of the vascular system and within the reticuloendothelial system (RES). The exact process for the removal of the aged or damaged cell has not been defined in most diseases. When the cell is lysed in the intravascular system, how is the stroma removed? Phagocytosis of the antibody-coated cell has been amply demonstrated (LoBuglio *et al.*, 1967).

3. *Hereditary Spherocytosis—Splenic Destruction*

Considerably more information is available concerning the process of cell destruction in one of the congenital hemolytic anemias, hereditary spherocytosis (HS). The abnormal red cell in HS is removed from the circulation by the spleen (sequestration) and subsequently destroyed there. A few of the cells which have been altered or damaged escape from the spleen and circulate for a relatively short period. These cells are very spheroidial (microspherocytes) and are thought to have been conditioned in the spleen (Weisman *et al.*, 1955).

The spleen is the only tissue which recognizes the HS red cell as abnormal. Removal of the spleen in patients with HS results in the abnormal red cells surviving almost as long as normal cells. In certain other spherocytic anemias, particularly autoimmune hemolytic anemia, splenectomy does not always improve the anemia. Not infrequently the abnormal red cell destruction continues in the liver. In a bulk flow system, HS blood shows a minimal increase in viscosity (Erslev and Atwater, 1963; Murphy, 1967) due to the increased concentration of Hb per unit volume and the abnormal shape. Studies in a filtration system (Murphy, 1967, modified from Jandl *et al.*, 1961) showed that a mixture of normal and HS cells were filtered equally well at pH 7.4, whereas at a lower pH, 6.8, HS cells were selectively held by the filter. The influence of pH on the flow properties of the HS cell probably is of significance in view of other studies of blood from the spleen. Emerson *et al.* (1956) and J. R. Murphy (unpublished observations) have demonstrated that the pH of blood from spleen pulp is significantly decreased. Direct readings of pH in the intact spleen at laparotomy, prior to ligation of vessels, have shown pH values that were 0.4 to 0.6 pH units less than the pH in either fascial spaces or lymph nodes. The lactic acid content of blood from the spleen pulp was found to be 6 to 8 times the concentration in the splenic vein. These studies indicate that there is a blood-containing space in the spleen, which is not in dynamic equilibrium with the arteriovenous system. Weiss (1963) and Weiss and Tavassoli (1970) have shown in rabbits that the microcirculatory path for a red cell in the red pulp of the spleen is not from arteriole to sinus to vein. Arterioles terminate within cords of reticulo-endothelial cells and the red cell must pass between these cord cells, through a basement membrane, and between the endothelial cells lining the sinus in order to enter the sinus. These studies of splenic structure and the metabolic environment in the spleen strongly suggest that the restricted flow and low pH are the unusual features of the microcirculation in this organ which are related to the removal and destruction of certain abnormal red cells.

The actual destruction of the HS cell in the spleen is related to the response of this cell to the splenic environment. Incubation of HS cells at pH 7.0 to 6.8 results in a more rapid deterioration of the membrane compared to normal cells. Abnormalities in cation permeability leading to increased cation content, increased cell water, and osmotic lysis of the HS cell have been thought to be related to splenic destruction (Jandl, 1965; Jacob, 1966). However, examination of cells from the spleen do not support this hypothesis in that the mean corpuscular hemoglobin concentration (MCHC) of these cells was not found to be decreased as it would be if volume were increased (Emerson *et al.*, 1956; J. R. Murphy, unpublished). LeCelle and Weed (1969) have proposed a mechanism of sequestration based on increased rigidity of the HS cell with deoxygenation. No change in deformability or viscosity with deoxygenation of HS cells could be demonstrated when the cells were studied in serum (Brereton and Murphy, 1971). Changes in the membrane, without volume changes, result in sphering and eventual osmotic lysis within the spleen.

The spleen is also thought to be partially responsible for the destruction of red cells containing Heinz bodies. The Heinz body is an inclusion body in the red cell representing abnormal denaturation of hemoglobin, and is seen with crystal violet staining. This form of hemolytic anemia can occur in normal individuals with administration of certain oxidant compounds, in patients with unstable hemoglobins, and in patients with a deficiency of the red cell enzyme, glucose-6-phosphate dehydrogenase (G-6-PD), either following the administration of certain oxidant drugs or during a variety of other conditions. Patients with G-6-PD deficiency are more susceptible to hemolysis with oxidant drugs than are normal individuals. The mechanism of cell destruction in humans with red cells containing Heinz bodies is not well worked out but is thought to be similar to animals given oxidant compounds which cause hemolysis with Heinz bodies. In these animals the spleen is thought to play a significant role with many cells containing Heinz bodies found in the spleen. The studies of Rifkind (1966) have demonstrated red cells containing Heinz bodies "trapped" in the cords of animal spleens. The appearance of these cells is such to suggest that the Heinz bodies within the cell cause the cell to be more rigid or less deformable, so that it is not able to pass through the splenic "filter." Recent studies by Ham *et al.* (1973) indicate that, at least in dogs, there are changes in the red cell, other than Heinz bodies, which are related to its destruction. They were able to demonstrate changes in the physical properties of cells independent of Heinz bodies which correlated with splenic sequestration of damaged cells.

4. *Hb CC Disease*

Hb CC disease is similar in many respects to hereditary spherocytosis. In this hemoglobinopathy there is a mild hemolytic process with splenic destruction, but probably less shortening of survival than in the usual HS patient. Patients with Hb CC disease do not have manifestations of the disease in any organs other than splenomegaly. This is in contrast to Hb SC disease which will be discussed subsequently. Charache *et al.* (1967) and Murphy (1968) have demonstrated abnormal rheological properties of the Hb CC cell which correlate with splenic sequestration. Hb CC blood has an increased viscosity and the cells are less deformable as measured in a filtration system. Although there is a mild anemia, hematocrit 33 to 37%, these patients do not have the crises similar to those seen in HS and, therefore, have not had the spleen removed. One patient who has been seen by the author has normal renal and liver functions with a normal ECG and no cardiomegaly at age 69. This disease process is an excellent example of the uniqueness of the various areas of the microcirculation and how red cells interact with the microvasculature, particularly in the spleen.

5. *Sickle Cell Anemia*

Sickle cell anemia or Hb SS disease represents the severe end of the spectrum of disease in the hemoglobinopathies. In Hb SS disease there are abnormalities in many organs or areas of the microcirculation. The disease process is thought to be related to changes in flow in the microcirculation, resulting from changes in shape and rheologic properties when the Hb SS cell is deoxygenated or sickled. The conclusive proof of this theory awaits some form of treatment which will prevent the sickling process. The manifestations of this disease, including symptoms and pathology, are consistent with both transient and/or permanent obstruction in flow in the microvasculature of different organs. The disease is characterized by hemolytic anemia, pain crisis, and the slow, progressive deterioration in function of certain organs, including the kidney, lungs, heart, liver, and brain.

The precise mechanism whereby the change in shape of the cell leads to vascular obstruction is not known. Deoxygenation of the Hb SS cell results in molecular alignment of the Hb and the sickle shape. This cell is rigid or nondeformable and results in a many fold increase in blood viscosity. Two important factors which relate to the pathophysiology are (1) the time required for the sickling process to occur and (2) the significance of permanently sickled cells. The length of time required for the change in flow properties of the cell is important in regard to where the cell is in the microvasculature when the change occurs. Observations on coronary sinus blood from patients with Hb SS disease have shown fewer sickled cells than expected at that particular pO_2 and pH (Jensen *et al.*, 1960). These studies suggested that several minutes were necessary for the sickle shape to appear at physiological pH and pO_2. *In vitro* studies of cell filtration and deoxygenation reported by Messer and Harris (1970) indicated the changes occurred in fractions of a second. They also showed changes in flow properties prior to the shape change. However, they used a chemical means of completely deoxygenating blood and were not dealing with a physiological pO_2. Thus, *in vitro* studies at a very low pO_2 show a rapid change in flow properties while *in vivo* observations suggest a slower process of sickling or possibly the presence of factors which prevent sickling. Hopefully, future studies will resolve this important point. Bertles and Milner (1968) have shown that oxygenated Hb SS blood has an increased viscosity compared to normal blood and that this increase was primarily due to the irreversibly sickled cells. Both of these factors, sickling with deoxygenation and permanently sickled cells, probably play a role in vascular obstruction and tissue anoxia which are thought to be the basic pathophysiology of Hb SS disease.

The occurrence of pulmonary vascular problems in Hb SS disease can be related to obstruction of the microvasculature in the lung by sickled cells formed in the peripheral venous system. Whether or not this is the only mechanism for the pulmonary thromboembolic problem has not been determined. The differentiation of the pulmonary infarcts and pneumonia in Hb SS disease remains a difficult clinical problem. In some patients there is the progressive development of pulmonary fibrosis and cor pulmonale (Song, 1971). A situation similar to that in the lung could occur in the portal system with sickled cells in the portal vein resulting in obstruction of the microvasculature in the liver. The degree of sickling in portal vein blood would be dependent on the oxygen utilization in the splanchnic circulation. There are a variety of pathological changes seen in the liver in Hb SS disease. In postmortem examinations of adults with Hb SS disease, hepatic necrosis or cirrhosis are common findings (Song, 1957). Recent studies of liver function and biopsy specimens (Rosenblate *et al.*, 1970) revealed abnormalities in all patients. Of particular interest was the confirmation of earlier postmortem observations of the Kupffer cells (Green *et al.*, 1953). In both postmortem and biopsy studies, the Kupffer cells were enlarged and filled with sickled red cells. Green *et al.* (1953) had suggested that these swollen Kupffer cells caused obstruction to sinousoidal blood flow. However, increases in portal vein pressure have not been demonstrated. The changes in the Hb SS cell which lead to erythropagocytosis by the Kupffer cells also have not been defined.

In other tissues the situation is less clear. Does the obstruction begin with sickling in the collecting venules, resulting in an increased viscosity and decrease in flow with retrograde obstruction in the capillary beds? Irreversibly sickled cells could result in obstruction either at the arteriolar-capillary junction or within the capillary itself. Irrespective of where the initial obstruction occurs in the microvasculature, it is not difficult to appreciate the development of a vicious cycle with obstruction leading to anoxia and a lower pH, both of which could cause further sickling and obstruction. If there were a significant diffusion of oxygen out of arterioles, as suggested by Duling and Berne (1971), and a rapid change in the flow properties of the cell, sickling could occur prior to the cells entering the capillary and thus lead to obstruction of capillaries at the arteriolar-capillary junction. The length of time required for the change in flow properties to occur is critical to this hypothesis. The observations of Duling and Berne (1971) suggest a very attractive hypothesis to explain the rather unique changes seen in the retina of patients with Hb SS, SC, or S-thalassemia disease (Goldberg *et al.*, 1971). In patients with these hemoglobinopathies there are microinfarcts and a proliferating vasculitis with neovascularization more marked around the periphery of the retina. This is particularly so in Hb SC disease. These areas of the retina receive their blood supply from long arterioles which extend out from the optic disc to the peripheral areas of the retina. Anoxia from obstruction on the arteriolar side of the capillary bed could explain the neovascularization seen in the retina. There does not seem to be any good explanation for the relative absence of capillary proliferation in other tissues in Hb SS disease. Indeed, fibrosis with scar formation, increase in collagen, and loss of normal tissue is the usual histologic picture in Hb SS disease (Song, 1971).

The target organs or the organs most often affected in Hb SS disease, in addition to lung and liver, include kidney, spleen, heart, and brain. Incapacitating dysfunction in any one or combination of these organ systems can eventually result in the patient's demise. The endocrine glands seem to be relatively free of involvement in this disease. In addition to the severe renal disease associated with Hb SS disease, hematuria is not uncommon in Hb SC disease and indivduals with Hb SA or sickle trait. Perillie and Epstein (1963) have suggested that the hyperosmolarity which occurs in the microvasculature of the kidney causes sickling. More recent studies by Ham *et al.* (1968) clearly indicate that hyperosmolarity per se does not cause sickling. Normal cells and Hb SS or Hb SA cells behave in an identical fashion in hypertonic media. The rheologic properties of these red cells in hypertonic media were similar to the properties of sickled Hb SS cells. Thus, some other factor in the microcirculation, such as low pO_2 or pH, in addition to the hypertonicity must be invoked to explain the hematuria seen in these patients with S Hb. The spleen appears to be the one tissue which shows the most change in Hb SS disease in that it is virtually destroyed by multiple infarctions by the time the patient reaches adulthood. In a few relatively young patients a large spleen which has not been infarcted can cause a more severe anemia requiring splenectomy. The low pH and pO_2 found in the spleen (Murphy, 1971) provide sufficient reason for sickling to occur in the microcirculation of the spleen, leading to cell destruction, obstruction of the microvasculature, and, ultimately, anoxic necrosis of the spleen. Robinson and Watson (1966) have suggested that the autosplenectomy in Hb SS disease could be causally related to the increased incidence of certain bacterial infections. The loss of the spleen and the degree of erythrophagocytosis in the liver suggest the possibility of reticuloendothelial blockade in this situation.

The severe anemia in Hb SS disease probably is of significant benefit to these patients in regard to blood viscosity. In the cone-plate viscometer (bulk flow system) sickling results in doubling of viscosity at a hematocrit of 20%, whereas viscosity increases six- to eightfold with sickling at a hematocrit of 40% (J. R. Murphy, unpublished). Dintenfass (1964) observed a several hundredfold increase in viscosity with sickling of packed Hb SS cells. Thus, the low hematocrit may protect these patients. Transfusion of Hb SS patients, particularly prior to surgical procedures, can lead to disastrous consequences. The combination of secondary polycythemia, chronic lung disease, and Hb SA can lead to multiple thromboembolic phenomena involving a variety of organ systems. Thromboembolic processes can occur in sickle trait individuals (Hb SA) in any situation in which the pO_2 and/or pH are sufficiently reduced to cause sickling.

6. *Hb SC Disease*

Hb SC disease is usually a less severe disease compared to Hb SS, but certainly it is not similar to the usual asymptomatic course of individuals with Hb SA. Thromboembolic manifestations and organ dysfunctions are in general less severe than in Hb SS disease. However, involvement of the hip with aseptic necrosis and retinal disturbances are relatively common. The rheologic properties of cells with Hb SC are quite different from cells with either Hb SS or SA. The viscosity of Hb SC blood when oxygenated is greater than that of Hb SS blood, but is not as high as that of Hb CC blood. The viscosity of oxygenated Hb SA blood is the same as normal. The presence of C hemoglobin has been shown (Griggs and Harris, 1956) to potentiate sickling in that Hb SC cells sickle at a higher pO_2 than Hb SA cells, but require a lower pO_2 for sickling when compared to Hb SS cells.

The manifestations of Hb SC disease during pregnancy are very similar to that of Hb SS disease. In both diseases severe anemia, thromboembolic phenomena, and fetal loss are high (Smith and Krevens, 1959). This increased severity of Hb SC disease during pregnancy strongly suggests an important role for fibrinogen in the pathophysiology of the microcirculation. The marked increase in fibrinogen which occurs in pregnancy profoundly changes the rheologic behavior of red cells in the microcirculation. Normal pregnant women at or near term have significant clumping of cells in the microvasculature of the bulbar conjunctiva. In Hb SC disease this change in the microcirculation could lead to stasis, less optimal flow, a greater degree of deoxygenation, and thus sickling. In all of the disease states involving Hb S, increases in plasma fibrinogen with inflammatory processes may be a significant factor. The precipitation of pain crises in Hb SS disease with many different infections could be related to increases in fibrinogen. Certainly prospective studies of this phenomena are in order.

V. Conclusions

It may be appropriate to conclude these remarks concerning the interrelationships of the microcirculation and hematology by reconsidering the role of the spleen in three specific congenital red cell abnormalities. The spectrum of organ system dysfunctions in different hematologic disorders clearly indicates the many unique aspects of the microcirculation in these different organs. The spleen, from a hematologist's viewpoint, probably contains one of the most unique microcirculations of any organ. In Hb CC disease there is a relatively mild shortening of the red cell life-span with splenic destruction of cells and minimal splenomegaly. In hereditary spherocytosis there is a moderate shortening of red cell survival, moderate splenomegaly, and significant clinical symptoms. Splenectomy results in the lengthening of the abnormal red cell life-span virtually to that of normal cells. In Hb SS disease the spleen is destroyed by the sickling–thrombosis–infarct process. The relationship of the microcirculation and the reticulo-endothelial system, in regards to the removal of red cells from the circulation, remains to be defined in many disease states. There is virtually no understanding of the removal of senescent normal cells. The differences between spleen and liver are demonstrated in HS. The similaries in spleen and liver RES function are evident in autoimmune hemolytic anemia and Hb SS disease.

References

Bertles, J. F., and Milner, P. F. A. (1968). Irreversibly sickled erythrocytes: A consequence of the heterogeneous distribution of hemoglobin types in sickle-cell anemia. *J. Clin. Invest.* **47,** 1731–1741.

Boggs, D. R. (1967). The kinetics of neutrophilic leukocytes in health and disease. *Semin. Hematol.* **4,** 359–386.

Brain, M. C., and Hourihane, D. O. (1967). Microangiopathic haemolytic anemia: The occurrence of haemolysis in experimentally produced vascular disease. *Brit. J. Haematol.* **13,** 135–142.

Brereton, W., and Murphy, J. R. (1973). *J. Lab. and Clin. Med.* In press.

Carr, R. E., and Henkind, P. (1963). Retinal findings associated with serum hyperviscosity. *Amer. J. Ophtholmol.* **56,** 23–31.

Charache, S., Conley, C. L., Waugh, D. F., Ugoretz, R. J., and Spurrell, J. R. (1967). Pathogenesis of hemolytic anemia in homozygous hemoglobin C disease. *J. Clin. Invest.* **46,** 1795–1811.

Chievitz, E., and Thiede, T. (1962). Complications and causes of death in polycythaemia vera. *Acta Med. Scand.* **172,** 513–523.

Cline, M. J., Solomon, A., Berlin, N. I., and Fahey, J. L. (1963). Anemia in macroglobulinemia. *Amer. J. Med.* **34,** 213–220.

Davidson, R. J. L. (1969). March or exertional Haemoglobinuria. *Semin. Hematol.* **6,** 150–161.

Duling, B. R., and Berne, R. M. (1971). Oxygen and the local regulation of blood flow: Possible significance of longitudinal gradients in anterial blood oxygen tension. *Cir. Res.* **28,** Suppl. I, 65–69.

Dintenfass, L. (1964). Rheology of packed red blood cells containing hemoglobins A-A, S-A, and S-S. *J. Lab. Clin. Med.* **64,** 594–600.

Emerson, C. P., Shen, S. C., Ham, T. H., Fleming, E. M., and Castle, W. B. (1956). Studies on the destruction of red blood cells. *Arch. Intern. Med.* **97,** 1–38.

Erslev, A. J., and Atwater, J. (1963). Effect of mean corpuscular hemoglobin concentration viscosity. *J. Lab. Clin. Med.* **62,** 401–406.

Fahey, J. L. (1963). Serum protein disorders causing clinical symptoms in malignant neoplastic disease. *J. Chronic Dis.* **16,** 703–712.

Fahraeus, R., and Lindqvist, T. (1931). The viscosity of the blood in narrow capillary tubes. *Amer. J. Physiol.* **96,** 562–568.

Ford, W. L., and Gowans, J. L. (1969). The traffic of lymphocytes. *Semin. Hematol.* **6,** 67–83.

French, J. E. (1971). Atherogenesis in thrombosis. *Semin. Hematol.* **8,** 84–94.

Gilinson, P. J., Jr., Dauwalter, C. R., and Merrill, E. W. (1963). A rotational viscometer using an AC torque to balance loop and air bearing. *Trans. Soc. Rheol.* **7,** 319–331.

Goldberg, M. F., Charache, S., and Acacio, I. (1971). Ophthalmologic manifestations of sickle cell thalassemia. *Arch. Interol. Med.* **128,** 33–39.

Green, T. W., Conley, C. L., and Berthrong, M. (1953). The liver in sickle cell anemia. *Bull. Johns Hopkins Hosp.* **92,** 99–127.

Griggs, R. C., and Harris, J. W. (1956). The biophysics of the variants in sickle cell disease. *Arch. Intern. Med.* **97,** 315–326.

Ham, T. H., Dunn, B., Kellermeyer, R. W., and Murphy, J. R. (1973). *J. Lab. and Clin. Med.* To be published.

Ham, T. H., Dunn, R. F., Sayre, R. W., and Murphy, J. R. (1968). Physical properties of red cells as related to effects *in vivo.* I. Increased rigidity of erythrocytes as measured by viscosity of cells altered by chemical fixation, sickling and hypertonicity, *Blood* **32,** 847–861.

Hecht, H. H. (1966). A physiological classification of cor pulmonale. *Med. Clin. N. Amer.* **50,** 37–49.

Jacob, H. S. (1966). Abnormalitits in the physiology of the erythrocyte membrane in hereditary spherocytosis. *Amer. J. Med.* **41,** 734–743.

Jandl, J. H. (1965). Leaky red cells. *Blood* **26,** 367–382.

Jandl, J. H., Simmons, R. L., and Castle, W. B. (1961). Red cell filtration and the pathogenesis of certain hemolytic anemias. *Blood* **18,** 133–148.

Jensen, W. N., Rucknagel, D. L., and Taylor, W. J. (1960). *In vivo* study of the sickle cell phenomenon. *J. Lab. Clin. Med.* **56,** 854–865.

Knospe, W. H., and Crosby, W. H. (1971). Aplastic anemia: A disorder of the bone marrow sinusoidal microcirculation rather than stem cell failure. *Lancet* **1,** 20–22.

LaCelle, P. L. (1970). Alteration of membrane deformability in hemolytic anemias. *Semiol. Hematol.* **7,** 355–371.

LaCelle, P. L., and Weed, R. I. (1969). Abnormal membrane deformability—a model for the hereditary spherocyte. *J. Clin. Invest.* **48,** 48a.

Lenfant, C., and Sullivan, K. (1971). Adaptation to high altitude. *N. Engl. J. Med.* **284,** 1298–1309.

Lertzman, M., Frome, B. M., Israels, L. G., and Cherniack, R. M. (1964). Hypoxia in polycythemia vera. *Ann. Intern. Med.* **60,** 409–417.

LoBuglio, A. F., Cotran, R. S., and Jandl, J. H. (1967). Red cells coated with immunoglobulin G: Binding and sphering by mononuclear cells in man. *Science* **158,** 1582.

McClugage, S. G., McCuskey, R. S., and Meinke, H. A. (1971). Microscopy of living bone marrow *in situ.* II. Influence of the microenvironment of hemopoiesis. *Blood* **38,** 96–107.

Mackenzie, M. R., Fudenberg, H. H., and O'Reilly, R. A. (1970). The hyperviscosity syndrome. I. In IgG myeloma the role of protein concentration and molecular shape. *J. Clin. Invest.* **49,** 15–20.

Marchesi, V. T., and Florey, H. W. (1960). Electron micrographic observations on the emigration of leucocytes. *Quart. J. Exp. Physiol. Cog. Med. Sci.* **45,** 343–348.

Marchesi, V. T., and Gowans, J. L. (1964). The migration of lymphocytes through the endothelium in lymph nodes: An election microscope study. *Proc. Roy. Soc., Ser. B* **159,** 283–290.

Merrill, E. W., Cokelet, G. C., Britten, A., and Wells, R. (1963). Non-Newtonian rheology of human blood: Effect of fibrinogen deducted by subtraction." *Circ. Res.* **13,** 48–55.

Messer, M. J., and Harris, J. W. (1970). Filtration characteristics of sickle cells: Rate of alteration of filterability after deoxygenation and reoxygenation, and correlations and sickling and unsickling. *J. Lab. Clin. Med.* **76,** 537–547.

Monge, C., Lozano, R., and Whittembury, J. (1965). Effect of blood-letting on chronic mountain sickness. *Nature (London)* **207,** 770.

Murphy, J. R. (1967). The influence of pH and temperature on some physical properties of normal erythrocytes and erythrocytes from patients with hereditary spherocytosis. *J. Lab. Clin. Med.* **69,** 758–775.

Murphy, J. R. (1968). Hemoglobin CC disease; rheological properties of erythrocytes and abnormalities in cell water. *J. Clin. Invest.* **47,** 483–1495.

Nicolau, C. T., Teitel, P., Fotino, M., Butoianu, E., and Targar, S. (1964). Alterations of erythrocyte plasticity in blood diseases (a three years' clinical experience with the erythrocyte filterability test [E. F. T.]) *Sangre* **9,** 282–288.

Penaloza, D., and Sime, F. (1971). Chronic cor pulmonale due to loss of altitude acclimatization (chronic mountain sickness). *Amer. J. Med.* **50,** 728–743.

Perillie, P. E., and Epstein, F. H. (1963). Sickling phenomenon produced by hypertonic solutions: A possible explanation for hyposthenuria and sicklemia. *J. Clin. Invest.* **42,** 570–580.

Rand, R. P., and Burton, A. C. (1964). Mechanical properties of the red cell membrane. I. Membrane stiffness and intracellular pressure. *Biophys. J.* **4,** 115–135.

Replogle, R. L., and Merrill, E. W. (1970). Experimental polycythemia and hemodilution. *J. Thorac. Cardiov. Surg.* **60,** 582–588.

Rifkind, R. (1966). Destruction of injured red cells *in vivo*. *Amer. J. Med.* **41,** 711–723.

Robinson, M. G., and Watson, R. J. (1966). Pneumoncoccal meningitis in sickle cell anemia. *N. Engl. J. Med.* **274,** 1006–1008.

Rodbard, S. (1971). Local regulation of blood flow, *Cir. Res.* **28,** Suppl. I, 2–8.

Rosenblate, H. J., Eisenstein, R., and Holmes, A. W. (1970). The liver in sickle cell anemia. A clinical-pathologic study. *Arch. Pathol.* **90,** 235–245.

Rosenblum, W. I., and Asofsky, R. M. (1968). Factors affecting blood viscosity in macroglobulinemic mice. *J. Lab. Clin. Med.* **71,** 201–211.

Scott, J. B., and Radawski, D. (1971). Role of hyperosmolarity in the genesis of active and reactive hyperemia. *Circ. Res.* **28,** *Suppl. I,* 26–32.

Song, J. (1971). "Pathology of Sickle Cell Disease." Thomas, Springfield, Illinois.

Song, Y. S. (1957). Hepatic lesions in sickle cell anemia. *Amer. J. Pathol.* **33,** 331–351.

Smith, E. W., and Krevins, J. R. (1959). Clinical manifestations of hemoglobin C disorders. *Bull. Johns Hopkins Hosp.* **104,** 17–43.

Stamatoyannopoulos, G., Bellingham, A. J., Lenfant, C., and Finch, C. A. (1971). Abnormal hemoglobins with high and low oxygen effinity. *Annu. Rev. Med.* **22,** 221–234.

Torrance, J., Jacobs, P., Restrepo, A., Eschbach, J., Lenfant, C., and Finch, C. A. (1970). Intraerythrocytic adaptation to anemia. *N. Engl. J. Med.* **283,** 165–169.

Troup, S. B., Reed, C. F., Marinetti, G. V., and Swisher, S. N. (1960). Thromboplastic factors in platelets and red blood cells: Observations on their chemical nature and function *in vitro* coagulation. *J. Clin. Invest.* **39,** 342–351.

Waldenstrom, J. (1944). Inapient myelomatosis or "essential" hyperglobulinemia with fibrogenopenia—A new syndrome? *Acta Med. Scand.* **117,** 216–247.

Weisman, R., Ham, T. H., Hinz C. F., and Harris, J. W. (1955). Studies of the role of the spleen in the destruction of erythrocytes. *Trans. Ass. Amer. Physicians* **58,** 131–140.

Weiss, L. (1963). The structure of intermediate vascular pathways in the spleen of rabbits. *Amer. J. Anat.* **113,** 51–91.

Weiss, L., and Tavassoli, M. (1970). Anatomical hazards to the passage of erythrocytes through the spleen. *Semin. Hematol.* **7,** 372–380.

Woodson R. D., Torrance, J. D., Shappell, S. D., and Lenfant, C. (1970). The effect of cardiac disease on hemoglobin-oxygen binding, *J. Clin. Invest.* **49,** 1349–1356.

Zweifach, B. W. (1961). "Functional Behaviour of the Microcirculation." Thomas, Springfield, Illinois.

14 INTRAVASCULAR COAGULATION AS A CLINICAL PROBLEM: CONSUMPTION-COAGULOPATHIES

FRANZ RODRÍGUEZ-ERDMANN, M.D.

I. Introduction

The recognition of acquired bleeding tendencies as a result of depletion of circulating clotting factors is not new, but the precise physiopathology and clinical relevance is still a matter of discussion. Many of its manifestations were initially considered a paradox. Through the experiences accrued from many schools and disciplines, our knowledge has crystallized in the concept that in the "consumption-coagulopathies," both thrombosis and hemorrhagic diathesis—otherwise considered diametrically opposed conditions—belong to the same clinical entity.

In this chapter, reference is made to some mechanisms which lead to intravascular fibrin deposition as well as to disarrangements of the coagulation system.

II. Physiologic and Experimental Basis of Intravascular Coagulation

The clotting mechanism is a complex system in which a series of proteins and lipids interact with platelets, leading to its ultimate physiologic purpose: maintaining the blood within its vascular compartment. With vascular damage, this physiologic role is achieved through two mechanisms. An initial process, which is known as *hemostatic,* leads to the formation of a platelet plug. The second, *coagulation* per se, leads to the formation of fibrin which "seals off" the platelet clump. As vascular healing takes place, fibrin is removed by a special enzymatic system called the fibrinolytic mechanism.

Although the coagulation system is controlled by a variety of inhibitors so that only focal clotting at sites of vascular damage takes place, under certain conditions the coagulation mechanism may be activated ubiquitously, leading to diffuse intravascular fibrin deposition and to an abnormal circulating blood which may have more characteristics of serum than plasma (*vide infra*). If this condition is not fulminating, the fibrinolytic mechanism may be activated, sometimes so briskly that it overcasts the primary (clotting) process.

A. Brief Review of the Coagulation System

The areas of hemostasis, coagulation, and fibrinolysis have been well reviewed, and only certain points will be emphasized here.

The coagulation system centers around the process in which prothrombin is activated to thrombin, the enzyme which in turn will allow fibrinogen to polymerize to fibrin. There are two known pathways by which the prothrombin is activated. The *intrinsic system* requires only a foreign surface to trigger the concotany of events in which platelets and the hemophilic factors play an important role. The *extrinsic mechanism* requires the addition of tissue fluid (thromboplastin) to rapidly activate the clotting system by circumventing the time-consuming chain of events of the intrinsic pathway. Figure 1 depicts the pathways.

It is obvious that certain changes occur in the plasma as it changes to its clotted form, serum. As prothrombin is activated to thrombin and as fibrinogen is converted to fibrin, their initial levels fall, or more accurately, these factors are *consumed* as plasma becomes serum. Thrombin also has a direct action on factors V, VIII, and XIII and on platelets, thus their values are lower in serum than in the original plasma. Figure 2 shows these changes schematically. It should be noted that the conversion of fibrinogen to fibrin is a much better understood process than any of the other steps

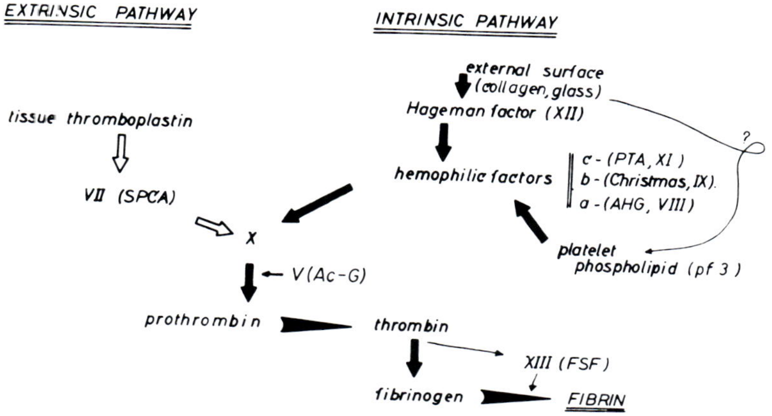

Fig. 1. Diagrammatic representation of the clotting system.

shown in Fig. 1. It consists of one nonenzymatic and two enzymatic steps. First, thrombin removes two small peptides from fibrinogen, which is then called fibrin monomere. Fibrin monomeres then undergo the nonenzymatic step of polymerization. The third step requires the action of factor XIII which through transamidation converts the loose bindings between the

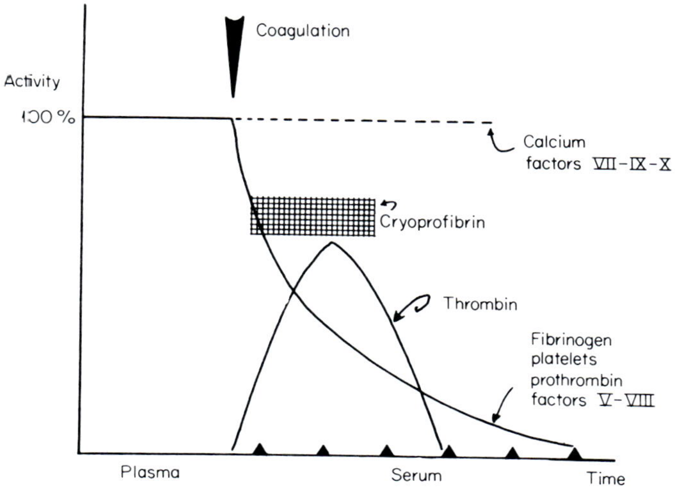

Fig. 2. Schematic representation of clotting activities when blood coagulates. While plasma is converted into serum, the activity of some clotting factors decreases (consumption). (From Rodríguez-Erdmann, 1965a.)

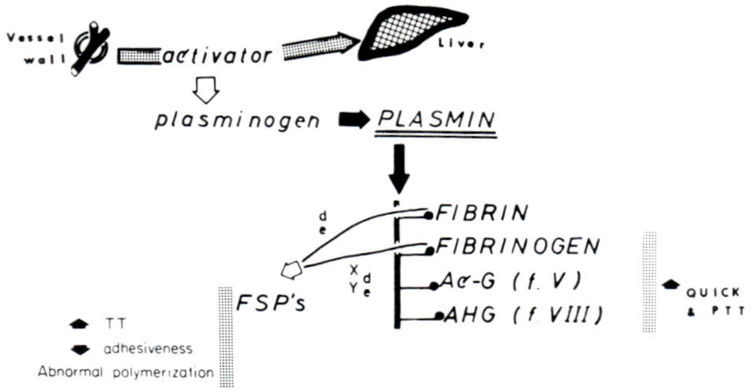

Fig. 3. Schematic representation of the fibrinolytic system.

fibrin monomeres into a stable bond. The early products of the polymerized fibrin may be soluble and, thus, found in circulating blood.

The mechanism of removal of fibrin is represented in Fig. 3. In a simplistic way it can be stated that plasminogen is—as prothrombin is for coagulation—the center of fibrinolysis. Its activation occurs mainly through the short-lived *activator* which comes from the vessel wall and is cleared by the liver. It would appear from a teleological viewpoint that *fibrin* is the primary target of plasmin and that the action on *fibrinogen* is, in view of their molecular similarity, an incidental one. However, the recent studies on the biological activities of the bioproducts of fibrinogen digestion by plasmin (from here on referred to as fibrinogen degradation products, FDP's) have shown that it is not incidental, but rather it fulfills a specific role. The "earlier" (large) split products (X, Y) have antithrombin activity and the "late" (small) ones (d, e) have the property of interfering with polymerization. Figure 4 illustrates the point: fibrinolysis interferes with

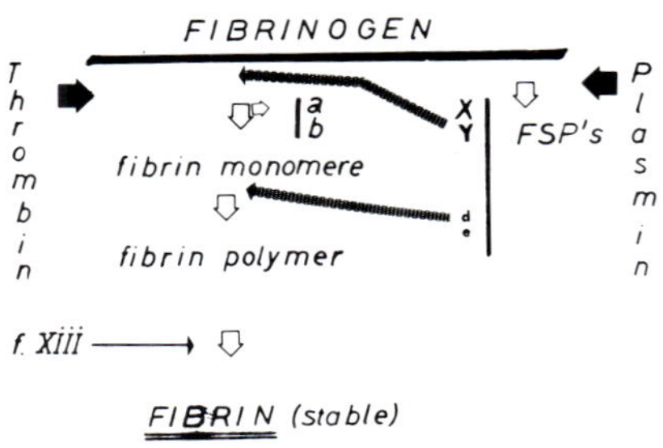

Fig. 4. Diagrammatic representation of the actions of thrombin and plasmin on fibrinogen. Note how the fibrinogen-split products (FSP's) interfere with the thrombin action (X,Y) and with polymerization (d,e).

TABLE I

NOMENCLATURE AND SOME PROPERTIES OF THE COAGULATION FACTORS

Clotting factor and alternate name		Found in Plasma	Found in Serum	Ba SO_4 adsorbable?	Vitamin K dependent ?
I	Fibrinogen	Y[a]	N[a]	N	N
II	Prothrombin	Y	N	Y	Y
III	Thromboplastin	N	—	N	N
IV	Calcium	Y	Y	N	N
V/VI	Ac-G, labile factor	Y	N	N	N
VII	SPCA, stable factor, convertin, autoprothrombin I	Y	Y	Y	Y
VIII	AHG, AHF, hemophiliac factor A, platelet cofactor I	Y	N	N	N
IX	Christmas factor, PTC, hemophilic factor B, autoprothrombin II, platelet cofactor II	Y	Y	Y	Y
X	Stuart–Prower factor, autoprothrombin C	Y	Y	Y	Y
XI	PTA, hemophilic factor C	Y	Y	N	N
XII	Hageman factor	Y	D[a]	N	N
XIII	FSF	Y	D	N	N

[a] Y, yes; N, no; D, decreased.

further deposition of fibrin and, thus, is a mechanism of defense against coagulation. It should also be remembered that plasmin acts on factors V and VIII, thus interfering at an earlier stage of the clotting concotany. Table I summarizes nomenclature and some properties of the coagulation factors.

B. EXPERIMENTAL MODEL OF INTRAVASCULAR COAGULATION: SANARELLI-SHWARTZMAN PHENOMENON

The Sanarelli–Shwartzman phenomenon (SSP, indiscriminately referred to as generalized Shwartzman reaction) is that reaction observed in rabbits which has provided great insight into the physiopathology of the consumption-coagulopathies, and, thus, a brief review of the phenomenon appears mandatory.

If a rabbit receives two intravenous injections of endotoxin within a 24-hr period, the animal will develop shock, hemorrhagic diathesis, and may die either early (some in 8–15 hr) in shock or at a later phase (30–70 hr) in renal failure. The morphologic substrate (Fig. 5) is characterized by ischemic necrosis and hemorrhages of various organs, as well as right ventricular dilatation and liver congestion. Histologically, intravascular fibrin deposition may be ubiquitous but more pronounced in the glomerula, plexus choroideus, lungs, adrenals, and liver.

Although not yet absolutely clarified, the pathogenesis of this reaction was greatly illuminated by the observation that heparin given after the second endotoxin injection blocks the deposition of fibrin and, thus, modifies the fatal outcome of the reaction. This denotative finding brought attention to the clotting mechanism and resulted in the observation that shortly after the second endotoxin injection the circulating plasma acquired "serum" qualities (*vide supra*). In this basic observation lies the nature of the hemorrhagic diathesis and the concept of the consumption-coagulopathies.

Why are two injections of endotoxin required to elicit an SSP? It has been demonstrated that the first endotoxin injection blocks the phagocytic (granulopectic) activity of the RES. Both endotoxin and clotting by-products are removed from circulation by the RES, however, the amount that can be phagocytized is limited. For a given period of time, the RES will appear "engulfed" morphologically (Fig. 6) and will not be able to remove additional circulating endotoxin or clotting by-products so that they will be able to exert their deleterious actions. These effects can be summarized in three main groups (Fig. 7). Activation of the clotting mechanism is first. Endotoxin does not activate prothrombin directly, but acts on an earlier stage of the intrinsic mechanism. Although it is possible that endotoxins of different origins operate in various ways, it is currently thought that they activate the Hageman factor as well as release the lipid procoagulant from the platelets (platelet factor 3). Further, endotoxins have been proven to have vasotonic effects, and the response and effects of adrenergic blockers are currently under investigation. Last, recent electron microscopic studies have shown endothelial damage. "Sloughed" endothelial cells have been found in circulation even when the animal had been anticoagulated. The exposure of subendothelial collagen to circulation would promote coagulation.

The first endotoxin injection, which indeed "prepares" the animal, can

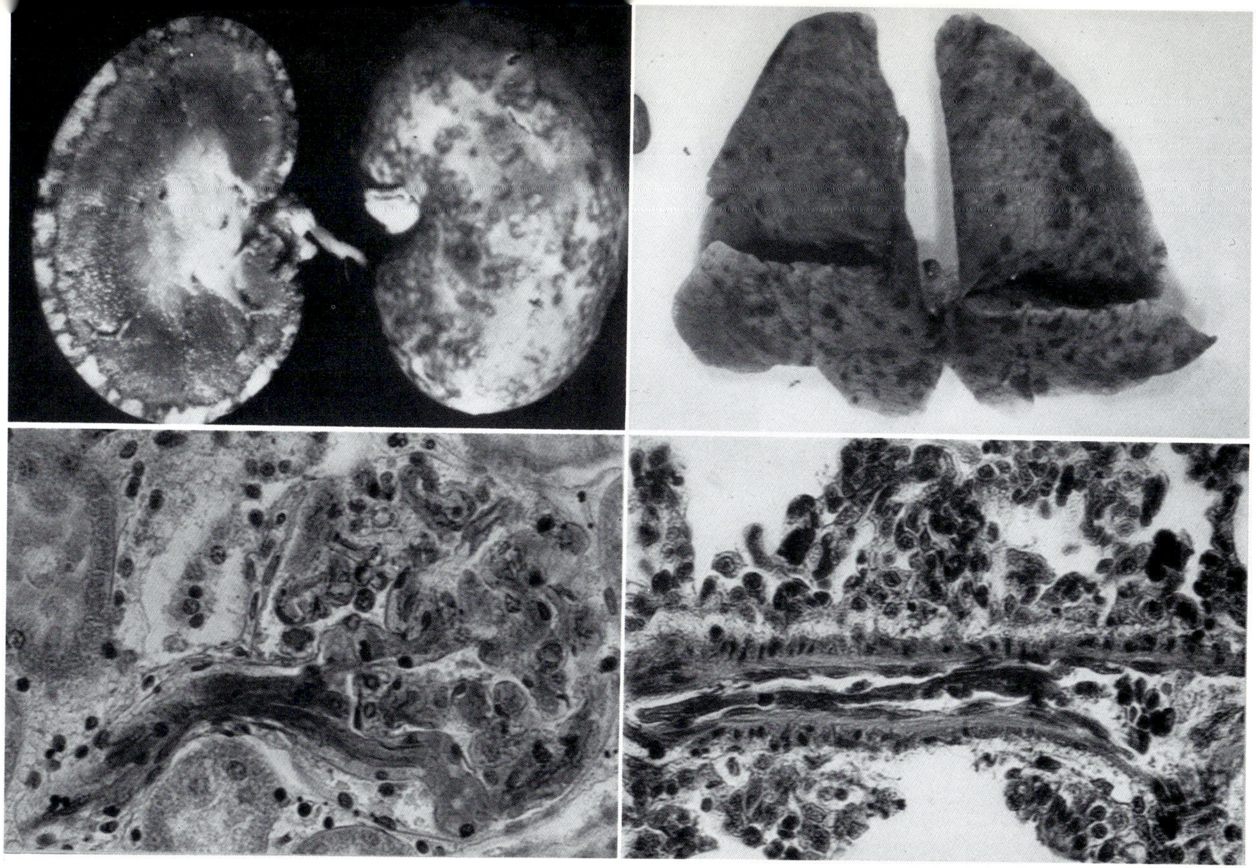

Fig. 5. Morphological findings in the Sanarelli–Shwartzman phenomenon of the rabbit. Upper pictures: intracapillary deposition of fibrin in a lung vessel (left) and glomerulum (right). (Goldner–trichrome, 720× and 360×, respectively.) Lower pictures: corresponding gross findings in lungs and kidney.

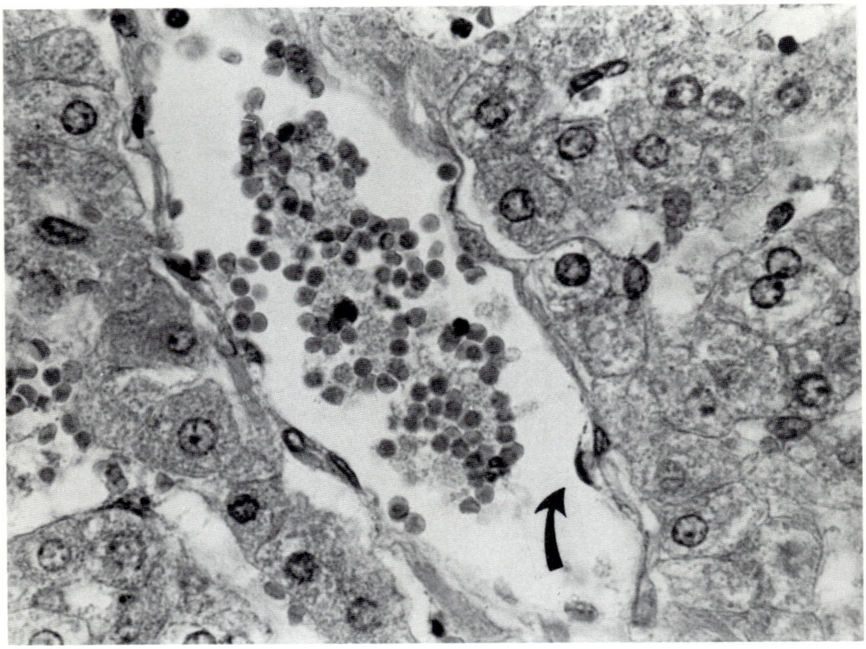

Fig. 6. Hepatic vein showing platelet clump. Note "engorged" Kupfer cell (arrow). (H & E, 720×.)

be substituted by known ways of depressing the RES function (Thorotrast, denaturated protein, etc., see Table II). The second endotoxin injection, sometimes referred to as "provocative," may be replaced by any potent procoagulant (Table II). The combination of a "blocking" agent and an effective procoagulant, as well as prolonged procoagulant stimulation, may be enough to elicit an SSP. Another interesting feature is the observation that a pregnant rabbit requires only one injection of endotoxin; the nature of the pregnancy-induced "preparation" remains to be elucidated.

The varied susceptibility of different animal species to develop the SSP is an observation of major import. Rabbits are the ideal lieges, while dogs do not develop an SSP. This species difference has been correlated with the animal's ability to enhance fibrinolysis; the dog reacts briskly with systemic fibrinolysis, while the rabbit elicits only a weak focal fibrinolysis. However, if a rabbit undergoing the SSP is treated with streptokinase (a fibrinolytic activator), the deposited fibrin will be removed and the animal survives.

TABLE II

METHODS OF SUBSTITUTION FOR ENDOTOXIN INJECTIONS[a]

First endotoxin injection[b] Preparation	Second endotoxin injection[c] Provocation
Thorotrast	Biothrombin
Carbon colloid	Platelet factor 3
Fat infusion	Autoprothrombin C
Radiation	(Fibrin[d])
Resin thrombin	

[a] Modified from Rodríguez-Erdmann and Naimi, 1967.
[b] Viz. impairment of RES function.
[c] I.e., activation of clotting.
[d] Fibrin is included in the table because it is the final product of coagulation even though it has no procoagulant activity per se.

The flow disturbances encountered after the fibrin has been deposited in the capillary bed have been interpreted by Hardaway as the *primum movens* in the pathogenesis of irreversible shock. Repercussions of the physical presence of fibrin within the vessels are not only manifested by impaired blood flow, but also by trauma to the red cells. Figure 8A depicts morphological observations made in rabbits undergoing experimental intravascular coagulation, and in Fig. 8B, the peripheral smear shows traumatized ery-

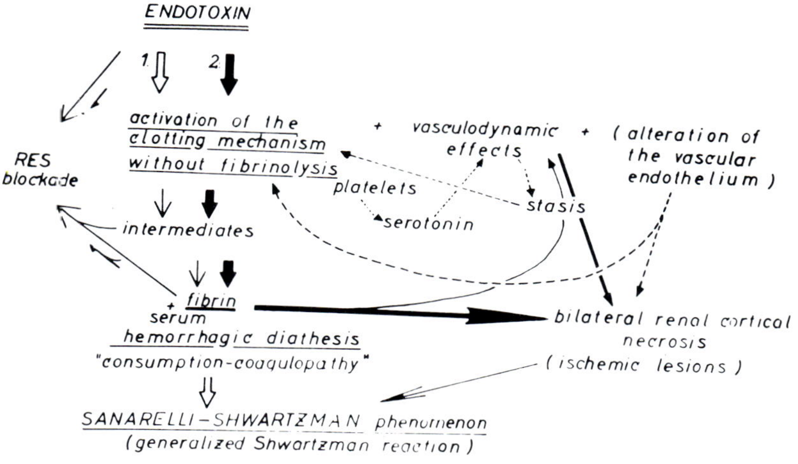

Fig. 7. Schematic representation of the mechanisms involved in the pathogenesis of the Sanarelli–Shwartzman phenomenon of the rabbit. See text.

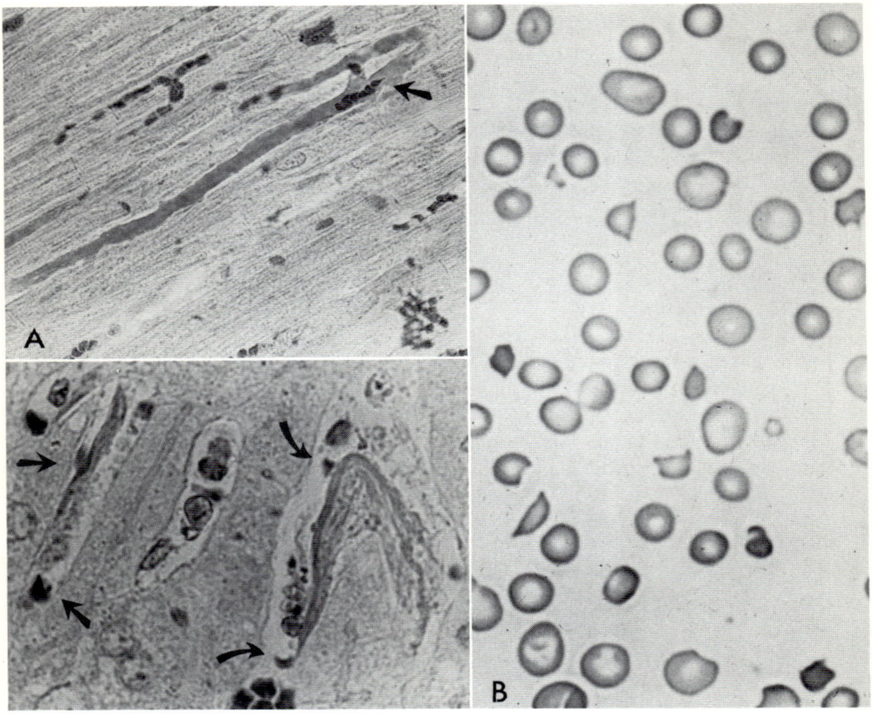

Fig. 8. (A) Intravascular fibrin deposition in myocardium and liver in an animal undergoing an experimental syndrome of diffuse intravascular coagulation (Goldner-trichrome, heart × 500; liver, × 720). Note distorted red blood cells (arrows). (B) Peripheral blood smear demonstrating pronounced red blood cell fragmentation. (From unpublished material abstracted in Rodríguez-Erdmann, 1968.)

throcytes. Bull *et al.** were able to demonstrate *in vitro* red cell fragmentation by passing blood through a fibrin mesh (Fig. 9).

III. Clinical Entities

Any mechanism leading to the ubiquitous activation of the clotting system may produce a picture with characteristics similar to those discussed above. Figure 10 depicts possible trigger pathways of clinical entities which have been associated with intravascular activation of the clotting mechanism. Since stasis is known to play an important role in pathological clotting, intravascular coagulation may be seen in certain giant vascular

* Author's preference for *et alii* was overruled by editor so that use of *et al.* would be consistent throughout treatise.

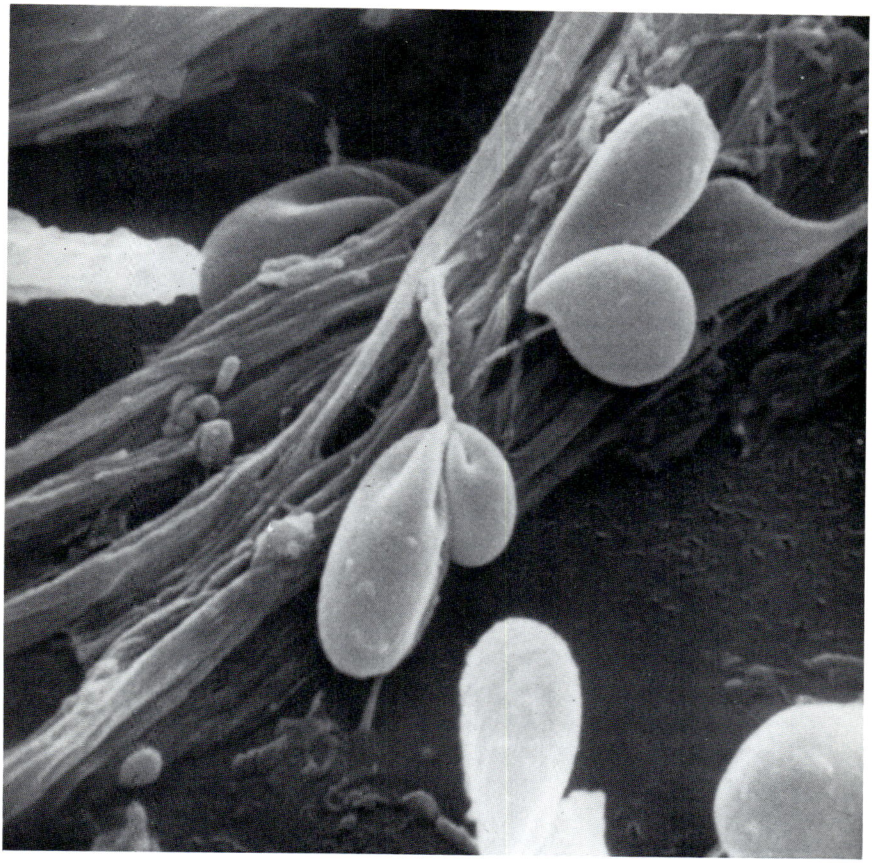

Fig. 9. Erythrocytes trapped in fine fibrin strands. Scanning electron microscopic view prepared by and reproduced through the generosity of Dr. Brian S. Bull (University of Loma Linda School of Medicine) and with permission of the Editor of *Blood* (Bull and Kuhn, 1970).

malformations as well. The following classification of these clinical entities is proposed:

1. Syndromes which may be identified as human equivalents of the experimental generalized Shwartzman reaction.
2. Clinical entities in which thromboplastic material enters into circulation.
3. Giant vascular malformations.
4. Syndromes of mixed or poorly understood etiology and pathogenesis.

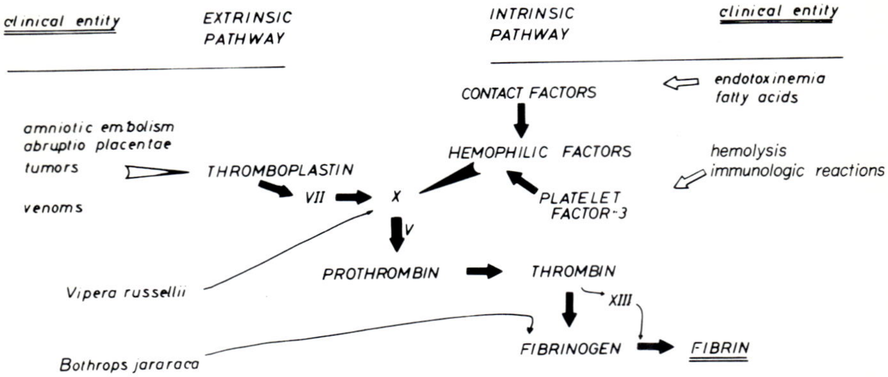

Fig. 10. Possible pathways of intravascular activation of the clotting mechanism in certain clinical entities. Bold arrows represent the clotting concotany. Open arrows depicit sites where the clotting mechanism is activated in the given clinical entities. The sites of action of the venoms of *Vipera rusellii* and *Bothrops jararaca* are shown by their respective arrows.

Group 1

Syndromes in which *endotoxin* is supposed to be liberated into circulation may be associated with a foudroyant clinical picture, whereby coaguloanalytical as well as pathological findings resemble the generalized Shwartzman reaction. Septic abortion, Waterhouse–Friderichsen syndrome and, in general, any gram-negative septicemia are among the entities which have been commonly identified as "human equivalents" of the experimental generalized Shwartzman reaction. Even though detailed studies of RES function and trigger mechanism in these clinical entities have not been performed, the similarity provides a plausible working hypothesis. The operative mechanisms would be similar to those discussed in the experimental section *(vide supra)*. However, it should be remembered again that extrapolation of knowledge obtained from experimental material into human pathology can only be accepted *cum grano salis.*

Group 2

Thromboplastic material may enter the circulation either by "autoinfusion" of tissue thromboplastin or by injection from an exogenous source (such as viper bites). These latter entities are not common in our environment but have awakened great interest because of the pharmacological potential of the venoms.

That tissue juice containing thromboplastic activity may gain access into circulation can be easily visualized in trauma, tumors (especially promyelocytic leukemias), and certain obstetric entities such as *abruptio placentae* and amniotic fluid embolization. It should be noted that the thromboplastic activity of the amniotic fluid is low, however, it may carry elements (hair, meconium, etc.) which can impair the flow in the pulmonary bed, leading thus to acute *cor pulmonale.*

GROUP 3

Giant vascular malformations such as hemangiomas, cavernomas, and aneurysms have been associated with severe alterations in the hemostatic mechanism, namely hypofibrinogenemia, thrombocytopenia, "deficiencies" of other clotting factors, and different degrees of fibrinolytic response. The association of hemangiocavernoma with consumption-coagulopathy has been referred to as Kasabach–Merritt syndrome, and that with *naevus flammeus,* Klippel–Trénaunay syndrome. Often large phleboliths are found in the first syndrome (Fig. 11). Also of interest are large aortic aneurysms which may contain, as in one case observed by the author, a huge fibrin clot weighing over 1 kg. Stasis may well be the most important factor in the activation of the coagulation system (perhaps within the frame of an alteration which Lasch has termed *latent-coagulation*). The precise mechanism remains, however, to be elucidated.

GROUP 4

Mixed clinical entities comprising *shock* (stasis), *infection* (gram-negative septicemia), and/or *trauma* (antoinfusion of thromboplastic material) can be readily visualized as being more than theoretical possibilities. Further, conditions in which the pathogenesis of the intravascular activation of the coagulation system is not clear are mentioned below:

Pneumoccocal septicemia in asplenic patients
Hemolytic crisis (*falciparum* malaria, favism)
Mismatched transfusions (platelet lysis, hemolysis, antibody–antigen complexes)
Rickettsial infections (vascular bed damage?)
Extracorporeal circulation (hemolysis, Hageman activation, etc.)
Acidosis, congenital cardiopathies
Heat stroke, malignant hyperthermia
Fat embolization (activation of the "contact" factors?)
Purpura fulminans (or *purpura necroticans*)

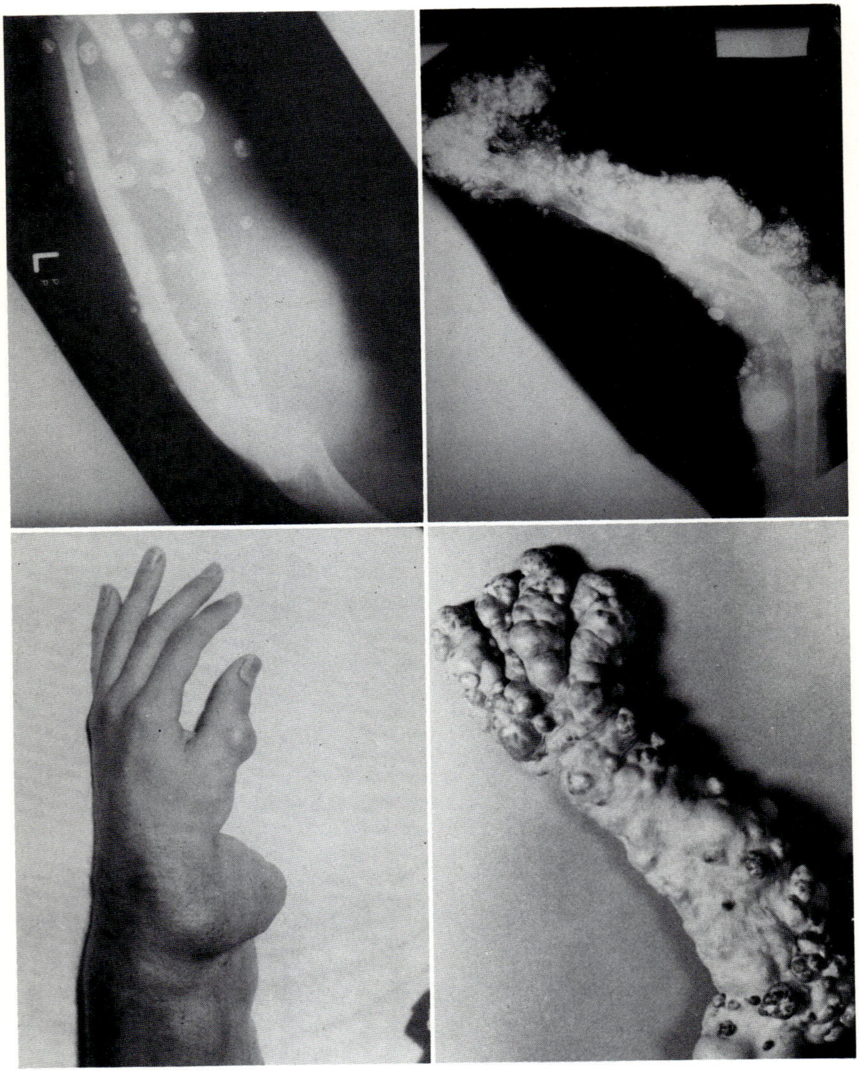

Fig. 11. Congenital giant hemangiomata (Kasabach–Merritt syndrome) with their corresponding roentgenograms (left, female, 78 years old; right, male, 20 years old).

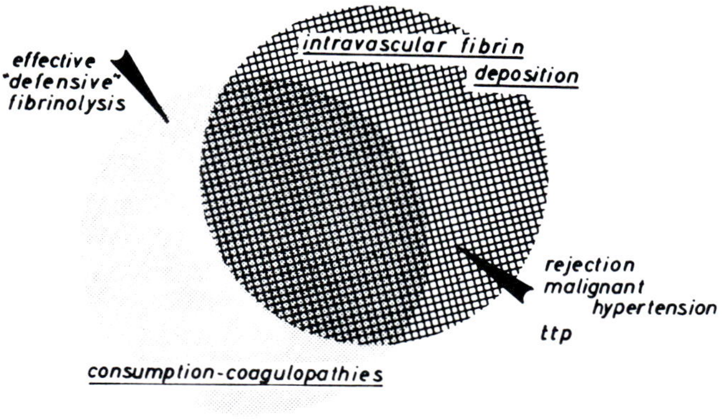

Fig. 12. Diagrammatic representation of the overlap between consumption-coagulopathies and entities with intravascular fibrin deposition. While consumption-coagulopathies may lack histological proof of fibrin deposition, some entities having intravascular deposition may lack systemic proof of activation of the coagulation system.

IV. Clinical Aspects

It is apparent from the above introduction that the medical manifestations of the endless list of potential clinical entities is as wide and long as the list itself, and as a rule of thumb it is suggested that the diagnosis of intravascular coagulation be considered in such clinical entities as thrombocytopenia, unexplained bleeding, shock, infection, or renal failure. However, it should be emphasized that a patient with a consumption-coagulopathy may present perhaps one or more of the above signs.

Does the morphological finding of intravascular fibrin represent a consumption-coagulopathy? Since the term consumption-coagulopathy implies a *ubiquitous* manifestation of the activation of the clotting mechanism, the answer is no. Thus, *focal fibrin deposition* [as seen in infections, rejection, and perhaps, also, vasculitis such as thrombotic thrombocytopenic purpura (TTP)] may lack systemic manifestations of clotting activation. On the other hand, overt consumption-coagulopathies need not have fibrin in postmortem material. See Fig. 12.

A. Diagnosis

The diagnosis is primarily made by thinking of the possible etiopathogenesis at bedside, but it *must* be corrobated in the laboratory. By and large, the coaguloanalytical findings will be those of "serum" in circula-

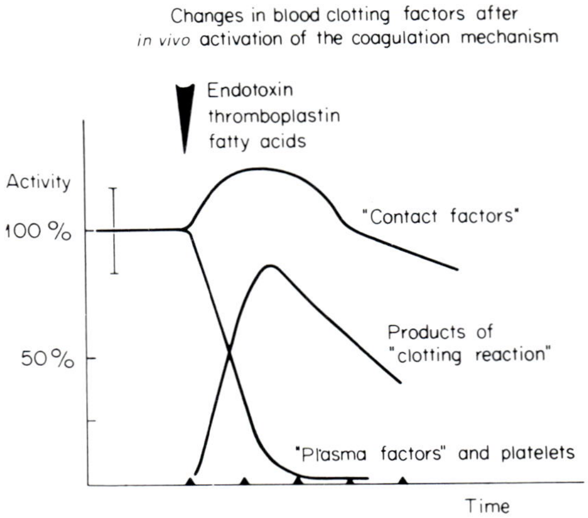

Fig. 13. Schematic representation of the theoretical behavior of clotting factors in a consumption-coagulopathy (see text and compare with Fig. 2).

tion. However, in view of the acuteness of some clinical conditions and the mildness or chronicity of others, the findings cannot be defined in one table. Simplicity not withstanding, we find Fig. 13 useful. It shows the changes to be expected, providing one takes into consideration the time component, the fact that in chronic and intermittent states the coagulation mechanism (in view of its dynamic state) may be in a compensated state, and, last, that the percentage of consumption of certain factors may be a relative one. For example, factor VIII, being an acute phase reactant, may in a given state be very elevated (300-800%) and appear in the corresponding consumption-coagulopathy to be in normal range (perhaps 80–150%), but representing indeed a "consumed" value. Fibrinogen behaves similarly, and its values may be found high in uncomplicated infections, pregnancy, etc. Platelets deserve special mention since thrombocytopenia is indeed a *conditio sine qua non* of intravascular clotting (*vide supra*). We know of three cases of myeloproliferative diseases in which the platelet count appeared to be "normal," however it had previously been elevated in these instances and, thus, the "normal" value was only an expression of consumption.

Great interest has arisen in what we proposed to refer to as "*products of clotting reaction.*" These are intermediate products of the coagulation system and are represented mainly by the fibrin monomere or soluble fibrin monomeres, which can be interpreted as products of partial exposure of fibrinogen to thrombin. Although measurement of these products may in the future afford the best means of establishing the diagnosis of intravascular coagulation, the methods thus far described are, for the most part, either too complicated or not specific enough. This is the case of the ethanol-gelation test, the search for cryoprofibrin, and the protamine paracoagulation test, which in spite of the enthusiastic reports of their introducers, have not lived up to their expectancies in the hands of other specialists.

The activation of the clotting system almost always elicits, even if not overtly, a fibrinolytic response, which can be indirectly assessed by the presence of fibrin-split products. Since it is not within the scope of this review to analyze the methods of their determination, reference will be made only to the fact that they are not diagnostic of intravascular clotting, since they are also present in fibrinolytic states, including focal fibrinolysis as in hematomata, pulmonary embolization, certain collagen diseases, and, due to technical reasons, they also appear to be present in dysfibrinogenemic states.

From this discussion it can be stated that at the present time *there is not a single test which is specific or reliable enough* to establish by itself the diagnosis of intravascular coagulation. The diagnosis can be best established by a combination of factor determinations, taking into consideration that the clotting mechanism is not a static but a dynamic system.

B. Differential Diagnosis

The differential diagnosis of the consumption-coagulopathies comprises syndromes which have long been recognized, and thus classically have been termed acquired hypofibrinogenemias. The historical reason for this terminology is obvious, since methods for the determination of fibrinogen were available early in the century, while reliable platelet counting appeared decades later and analytical clotting methods are indeed newcomers. Until recently, the known acquired hypofibrinogenemic states were only few in number and were mainly identified with the syndromes of intravascular coagulation. Recently, other entities have been added. The following classification is proposed:

1. Consumption-coagulopathies *(vide supra)*
2. Fibrinolytic states
   a. Primary or *proteolytic* states of which five entities have been identified: (a) hepatic disease; (b) drugs; (c) tumors (?); (d) dissecting aneurysms, and (e) "idiopathic."
   b. Secondary or *defensive* fibrinolysis comprises states identical to group A, however an effective defensive fibrinolysis is present.

TABLE III

BASIS FOR THE DIFFERENTIAL DIAGNOSIS IN ACUTELY ACQUIRED COAGULOPATHIES

	Consumption-coagulopathies	Proteolytic states (uncomplicated)	Nonconsumptive coagulopathies
Platelets	Decreased	Normal	Decreased (? always)
Fibrinogen	Decreased	Decreased	Decreased
Prothrombin	Decreased	Normal	Decreased
Factor V	Decreased	Decreased	Decreased
Factor VIII	Decreased (?normal)	Decreased (normal)	Decreased or high level
FSP's[a]	Present	Elevated	Absent or low titer
Cryoprofibrin	Present	Absent	Absent

[a] Molecules immunologically similar to fibrinogen.

3. Acute and severe liver failure, with the lack of protein synthesis, may lead to a coaguloanalytical picture sometimes difficult to differentiate from an acute consumption-coagulopathy. In order to stress the diagnostic difficulties, we have proposed the term *"nonconsumptive coagulopathy."*
4. Hypofibrinogenemia is associated with the use of asparaginase, a drug used in chemotherapy. Its nature remains to be elucidated.
5. Dysfibrinogenemia has been described both in association with hepatoma and as an experimental condition after the use of arvin, a pit viper venom.

The first three conditions are indeed frequently encountered in a hospital environment; not so the last two, which are more clinical curiosities than medical problems. A guideline for the differential diagnosis of these first three entities is depicted in Table III.

C. TREATMENT

Since one can visualize that the alterations in these syndromes are the direct consequence of the action of thrombin, an immediately acting antithrombin, such as heparin, seems to be the drug of choice. However, it must be emphatically stated that the activation of the clotting mechanism is either an intermediate link or a manifestation of a sometimes very complicated condition, and so heparin therapy may not be the only indicated treatment. One should focus on the basic problem of the disease in question.

For practical purposes one may conceive of two groups of consumption-coagulopathies: (1) acute course, in which perhaps the more severe require anticoagulation and this only during a short period since beyond the lapse in which the trigger mechanism is operative anticoagulation would be of no benefit. (2) chronic or intermittent course, in which the trigger stimulation is long-acting and, thus, heparin should be given for longer periods.

It should be noted that in cases presenting secondary fibrinolysis, this reaction should be recognized as a *defensive reaction* of the organism and not blocked since it may lead to further deposition of fibrin and alterations in the microcirculation. A glance at Fig. 4 should clarify this.

It should also be briefly mentioned that restitution of fibrinogen may be a hazardous affair since it may only increase the available clottable substance and worsen the clinical picture. Some authors have postulated that the use of fibrinogen may not be dangerous *if* heparin is given simultaneously. The rationale is vague since adequate heparinization (thus blocking the thrombin activity) makes the presence of fibrinogen superfluous.

D. Epiphenomena

The presence of "microangiopathic" components in the peripheral smear of the animal undergoing the generalized Shwartzman reaction has been established (Fig. 8B). In certain syndromes of intravascular coagulation, similar findings may be found. Since this morphological finding has unfortunately been given diagnostic value by some authors, the following observations are in order:

(a) As stated above, not all proven consumption-coagulopathies have helmet cells in the smear. In a study by Jacobson and Jackson, less than half of the proven cases showed helmet cells.

(b) On the other hand, many entities not related to the consumption-coagulopathies present helmet cells. As a matter of fact, helmet cells are a "constant" (normal?) finding in senility, thus losing any diagnostic value. In an unpublished observation we could demonstrate that the percentage of helmet cells increases with age. Helmet cells are extremely rare in childhood and are, as stated above, a rather regular finding at an advanced age, especially if hypertension or atherosclerosis is present.

(c) The term "microangiopathic" is misleading if applied to all the hemolytic anemias with increased helmet cells in the smear. Where is the microangiopathy in a prosthetic valve inducing hemolysis? It seems better to term these entities as "traumatic hemolytic anemias." Table IV depicts its tentative classification.

TABLE IV

TRAUMATIC HEMOLYTIC ANEMIAS: ATTEMPT AT CLASSIFICATION[a]

1. In association with thrombocytopenia
   - Consumption-coagulopathies
   - Entities of uncertain etiology
     - TTP[a]
     - HUS[b]
2. Thrombocytopenia not obligatory ("microangiopathic" in proper sense)
   - Rejection
   - Vasculitis (SLE)[c]
   - Malignant hypertension
3. In association with valvular heart disease (with or without prosthesis) ("macroangiopathic" in proper sense)
4. Various
   - Normal, aged population
   - Anemias with severe poikilocytosis (combined factors)

[a] Modified from Rodríguez-Erdmann, 1971.
[b] Thrombotic thrombocytopenic purpura.
[c] Hemolytic uremic syndrome.
[d] Systemic lupus erythematosus.

A review of the topic of intravascular coagulation may not be concluded without mentioning that there are some systems in the organism which may play a very important role in the pathogenesis of intravascular coagulation, The role of the RES has already been alluded to. The role played by the complement is uncertain and that of the kallikrein enzyme system has yet to be elucidated. It appears that very strong ties and interrelations exist between clotting (Hageman factor) and these two systems.

Selected References

Abildgaard, C. (1969). Recognition and treatment of intravascular coagulation. *J. Pediat.* **74,** 163–176.

Bachmann, F. (1969). Disseminated intravascular coagulation. *Dis. Mon.,* (December). Yearbook Publisher, Chicago, Illinois.

Baille, Y., Blanc, T., Monties, J. R., Goud, A., and Henry, E. (1970). Syndrome de coagulation intravasculaire diséminée chronique et cardiopathie congénitale cyanogène. *Presse Med.* **78,** 1571–1574.

Brain, M. C. (1969). Microangiopathic hemolytic anemia. *N. Engl. J. Med.* **281,** 833–835.

Brodsky, I., and Siegel, N. (1970). The diagnosis and treatment of disseminated intravascular coagulation. *Med. Clin. N. Amer.* **54,** 555–565.

Bull, B. S., and Kuhn, I. N. (1970). The production of schistocytes by fibrin strands. *Blood* **35,** 104–111.

Corrigan, J. C., and Jordan, C. M. (1970). Heparin therapy in septicemia with disseminated intravascular coagulation. *N. Engl. J. Med.* **283,** 778–782.

Fletcher, A. P., and Sherry, S. (1966). Thrombolytic agents. *Annu. Rev. Pharmacol.* **6,** 89–106.

Fletcher, A. P., Alkjaersig, N., and Sherry, S. (1962). Pathogenesis of the coagulation defect developing during pathological plasma proteolytic ("fibrinolytic") states. *J. Clin. Invest.* **41,** 896–916.

Hardaway, R. M. (1966). "Syndromes of Disseminated Intravascular Coagulation." Thomas, Springfield, Illinois.

Hjort, P. F., and Rapaport, S. I. (1965). The Shwartzman reaction: Pathogenetic mechanism and clinical manifestations. *Annu. Rev. Med.* **16,** 135–168.

Jacobson, R. J., and Jackson, D. P. (1970). Microangiopathic hemolytic anemia in defibrination syndromes. *Ann. Intern. Med.* **72,** 794. (absts.)

Lasch, H. G. (1959). Untersuchungen zur Dynamik im System der Blutgerinnungsfaktoren (Latente Gerinnung in der Blutbahn). Habilitationsschrift, University of Heidelberg.

Lasch, H. G., Kreckl, H., Rodríguez-Erdmann, F., Sessner, H. H., and Schütterle, G. (1961). Verbrauchskoagulopathien (Pathogenese und Therapie). *Folia Haematol. (Frankfurt am Main)* [N. F.] **6,** 325–330.

McKay, D. G. (1965). "Disseminated Intravascular Coagulation." Harper, New York.

Marder, V. J., Shulman, N. R., and Carroll, W. R. (1969). High molecular weight derivatives of human fibrinogen produced by plasmin, I and II. *J. Biol. Chem.* **244,** 2111–2119 and 2120–2124.

Merskey, C. (1968). Diagnosis and treatment of intravascular coagulation. *Brit. J. Haematol.* **15,** 523–526.

Nussenzweig, V., Seligmann, M., Pelmont, J., and Grabar, P. (1961). Les produits de degradation du fibrinogène humain par la plasmine. *Ann. Inst. Pasteur, Paris* **100,** 377–389.

Pechet, L. (1965). Fibrinolysis. *N. Engl. J. Med.* **273,** 1024–1034.

Pitney, W. R. (1971). Disseminated intravascular coagulation. *Semin. Hematol.* **8,** 65–83.

Rodríguez-Erdmann, F. (1965a). Bleeding due to increased intravascular blood coagulation. Hemorrhagic syndromes caused by consumption of blood-clotting factors: Consumption-coagulopathies. *N. Engl. J. Med.* **273,** 1370–1378.

Rodríguez-Erdmann, F. (1965b). Pathogenesis of bilateral renal cortical necrosis: Its production by means of exogenous fibrin. *Arch. Pathol.* **79,** 615–618.

Rodríguez-Erdmann, F. (1968). Experimental *in vivo* production of helmet-cells *Fed. Proc., Fed. Amer. Soc. Exp. Biol.* **27,** 500.

Rodríguez-Erdmann, F. (1971a). Conceptos actuales sobre el diagnóstico y tratamiento de los síndromes de coagulación intravascular: Coagulopatías por consumo. *Sangre* **16,** 141–150.

Rodríguez-Erdmann, F. (1971b). Anemias traumático-hemolíticas. Memorias XII. Jornada. Agrup. Mex. Est. Hematol. México, D.F. p. 190–191.

Rodríguez-Erdmann, F., and Naimi, S. (1967). Studies on the pathogenesis of the generalized Shwartzman reaction. IV. Production of a Shwartzman-like phenomenon with autoprothrombin-C. *Thromb. Diath. Haemorrh.* **17,** 156–164.

Rodríguez-Erdmann, F., Button, L., Murray, J. E., and Moloney, W. (1971a). Kasabach-Merritt syndrome: Coaguloanalytical observations. *Amer. J. Med. Sci.* **261,** 9–15.

Rodríguez-Erdmann, F., Carpenter, C. B., and Galvanek, E. G. (1971b). Experimental dysfibrinogenemia: *In vivo* studies with Arvin. *Blood* **37,** 664–674.

Saint-Martin, J., Huault, G., Josso, F., Joly, J. B., Kachaner, J., and Feron, J. F. (1971). Coagulopathies de consumation chez le nouveau-né. *Arch. Fr. Pediat.* **28,** 17–36.

Seaman, A. J. (1970). The recognition of intravascular clotting: The plasma protamine paracoagulation test. *Arch. Intern. Med.* **125,** 1016–1021.

Selye, H. (1966). "Thrombohemorrhagic Phenomena." Thomas, Springfield, Illinois.

Sherry, S. (1968). Fibrinolysis. *Annu. Rev. Med.* **19,** 247–268.

Sherry, S. (1968). Fibrinolytic agents. *Dis.-Mon.,* (May). Yearbook Publisher, Chicago, Illinois.

Simone, J. V. (1970). Disseminated intravascular coagulation. *Advan. Intern. Med.* **15,** 339–355.

Streif, F., Peters, A., and Alexander, P. A. (1968). Difficultés du diagnostic biologique du syndrome de coagulation intravasculaire disséminée. *Nouv. Rev. Fr Hematol.* **8,** 104–110.

Teger-Nilsson, A. C. (1968). Studies on tissue thromboplastin, thrombin and fibrinopeptides in intravascular coagulation, *Acta Physiol. Scand., Suppl.* **319.**

15 NEOPLASIA AND THE MICROCIRCULATION

SUMNER WOOD, JR., M.D.

I. Introduction

The biologic behavior of cancer cells may be described by four fundamental features: growth, invasion, spread, and, occasionally, inappropriate function. The microvascular system of the body is intimately related and concerned with each of these fundamental features.

There is one general principle which seems to apply whether one is dealing with autochthonous or transplanted tumors, primary or metastatic in origin. This concept is that (except for angiomas and angiosarcomas) the vessels of tumors originate from the blood vessels or microvascular system of the host and generally consist of a single layer of endothelial cells resembling capillaries. The newly formed vessels in malignant tumors are usually small and simple in structure; and in rapidly growing tumors they consist of little more than irregular channel lined by endothelium only or by naked tumor cells. These general observations have been confirmed by electron microscopy (Warren, 1967; Warren and Shubik, 1966).

Extensive studies of the biology of cancer cells of many different types have shown, however, that the growth characteristics of the cells are not in any significant sense the feature that clearly distinguishes the malignant from the normal, nor is there a uniform pattern of abnormal growth (Baserga, 1971). The two biological characteristics which *most* distinguish cancer cells from normal cells are their ability to *invade* surrounding tissues and *spread* (Wood and Sträuli, 1973).

II. Growth

There are endless variations in the growth rates of different tumors, in their local invasiveness, and in their routes and sites of metastasis via the microcirculation (Wood and Sträuli, 1973). Although multiplication of neoplastic cells may proceed more rapidly than that of normal cells, this property alone does not imply malignancy of a tissue (Baserga, 1971); indeed, the generation times of cells during embryogenesis, regeneration of the liver, or normal replacement of intestinal mucosa is shorter than that of the majority of tumor cells. Recently, Tannock (1970) has described the cytokinetics of capillary endothelium in mammary tumors of mice and found that the mean generation time of endothelial cells within tumors is generally longer than that of the tumor cells. Thus, these tumor cells divide more rapidly than do the capillary endothelial cells within the tumor.

III. Invasion

The mechanisms of invasion are complex, subject to much speculation, and promising as a field for future research endeavors that may have major therapeutic significance and importance (Leighton, 1969). As an essential prerequisite for metastasis formation, the invasive characteristics of malignant cells may be related to one or more of the following properties: (1) enzymatic or lytic factors that modify the stroma, (2) tissue pressure created by cellular multiplication, or (3) locomotion (Wood *et al.,* 1967). The microvascular system plays an intimate role in each of these concepts.

A. Enzymatic or Lytic Factors That Modify the Stroma

Active infiltration of stroma and blood vessels by malignant cells possibly proceeds by the tumor elaborating at its growing margin lytic substances that destroy surrounding tissues. In this connection, recent microchemical (Sylvén, 1967b) or histochemical methods (Burstone, 1956) have demonstrated proteolytic enzymes within or around tumor cells in areas of invasion. In addition, the membranes of cancer cells may be altered, thus permitting the more facile entry or egress of small and large molecules (Sylvén, 1967b; Wallach, 1969). Sylvén (1967a, 1970; Sylvén and Holmberg, 1965) has reported complex and highly interesting data on on the microinvasion of cancer in animals, including the possible role of a small polypeptide and cathepsin B in invasion and local destruction of adjacent tissues. The role of these products in the systemic dissemination or clinical cachexia of cancer is not as yet clear.

B. Tissue Pressures Created by Cellular Multiplication

The division of tumor cells leads to expansive growth, pressure atrophy of surrounding tissues, and the formation of a capsule, but does not contribute significantly to invasion of stroma or blood vessels per se (Wood and Sträuli, 1973). For example, malignant cells invade even when they grow very slowly. Although the nonneoplastic invasion of neutrophils *in vivo* is not accompanied by cellular division *in situ*, invasion by normal chorionic tissue, though proliferative in nature, characteristically is self-limiting. Thus, the growth of tumor cells affords the tissue pressure and cell mass necessary for invasion of blood vessels and surrounding tissue by providing new tissue, but the actual mechanisms of invasion apparently involve other factors (Florey, 1970), including the lytic factors mentioned above and the cellular locomotion described in the next section.

C. Locomotion

Using *in vivo* cinemicrographic techniques in the rabbit ear chamber, we have directly documented the locomotion of individual V2 cancer cells in tissues of the living rabbit (Wood *et al.*, 1967). These data significantly explain one of the most important, interesting, and fundamental aspects of cancer—namely, the ability of the cancer cell to move, to invade adjacent, normal tissue, and to metastasize to local or distant areas of the body by the lymphatic or microvascular system. It is important to emphasize that, so far as is known to date, the locomotion of individual cancer cells *in vivo,* like the motility of leukocytes *in vivo,* is random, nondirectional, and complex (Thornes *et al.*, 1968; Wood *et al.*, 1968; Wood, 1971).

Another factor contributing to the increased motility *in vivo* of cancer cells is their decreased cohesiveness in comparison with normal cells (Weiss, 1967), a property which may be of importance in enabling the cells to detach themselves from the main mass, of clinical significance in making possible their detection by methods of exfoliative cytology, and of prognostic significance in terms of their ability to invade or enter blood vessels and spread to distant portions of the body. The act of locomotion

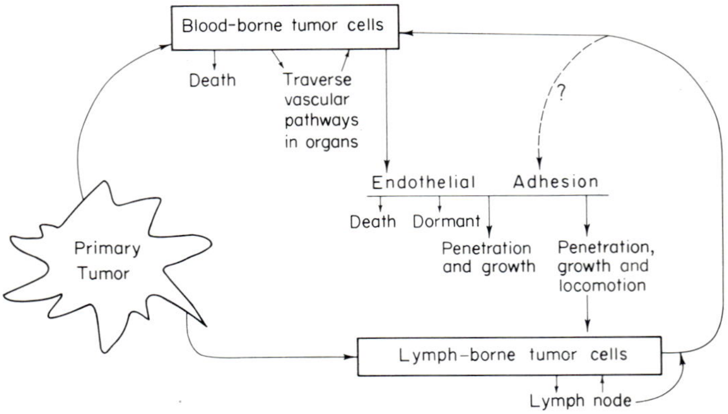

Fig. 1. Diagram of the relationships between the intravascular and intralymphatic spread of embolic cancer cells.

of individual cancer cells, as well as groups of cancer cells, may explain their active invasion and spread in tissues of the living animal and may be of significant value in testing new methods for controlling the invasion and spread of cancer (Thornes *et al.*, 1968; Wood, 1971).

IV. Metastasis

Tumors spread by two mechanisms: (1) direct extension and (2) metastasis. As direct extension is self-explanatory, only metastasis will be discussed. The occurrence of metastasis is the most decisive factor determining the choice of treatment and the success of therapy (Cole *et al.*, 1961). The two routes by which tumor cells spread and form metastasis are vascular and lymphatic (see Fig. 1). Since we know relatively little about the precise events in the lymphatic dissemination of cancer (Sträuli, 1970), our discussion will be based primarily upon present knowledge of the microvascular spread of cancer.

V. Vascular Spread of Cancer

The occurrence of direct venous invasion and hematogenous transport of tumor cells is being recognized with increasing frequency. Venous invasion is demonstrated in about 40% of resected carcinomas of the rectosigmoid, 70% of lung cancers, and in 80% of gastric cancers. Manipulation or operative trauma may increase the number of cells released from the primary tumor into blood vessels and lymphatics (Cole *et al.*, 1961). The prognostic significance of finding tumor cells in the blood is not as yet established. Tumor cell embolism does not necessarily mean metastasis formation in patients since many patients with venous invasion and circulating tumor cells have survived for many years after surgical excision of the primary growth. Experimental studies have revealed that a large number of tumor cells must be injected into the blood stream to produce a single metastasis.

Examined *in vivo* in the rabbit ear chamber, metastasis formation in the microvascular system has been recorded from a minimum of three V2 carcinoma cells, generally six to ten (Wood, 1958; Wood *et al.*, 1961). In this connection, in the microcirculation it is interesting to note that a single adhesive tumor cell alone has *not* as yet been observed to produce a metastatic nodule (Wood, 1971). The most important feature of the intravascular behavior of tumor cells is selective, firm adhesion to vascular endothelium of a small postcapillary venule (Fig. 1). Such cells may perish, remain dormant (G_0), or initiate the formation of a blood clot composed predominately of fibrin, thus altering capillary endothelium and attracting neutrophils that penetrate between the endothelial cells. Subsequently, the cancer cells may move through the capillary endothelial cells and into the perivascular connective tissue within which the cells proliferate, thereby producing a metastasis.

Once in the perivascular connective tissue, the active locomotion of V2 cancer cells results in the entry of tumor cells into adjacent, minute, delicately walled afferent lymphatics (Wood, 1971); this event may occur within 6 hrs after the cancer cells arrive in the region of the capillaries (Wood, 1958). The *in vivo* data directly document the intimate relationships which exist between the vascular and lymphatic systems in the spread of cancer (Fisher and Fisher, 1966) (Fig. 1). These fundamental events warrant confirmation in future research endeavors, extending them to the study of other tumor–host systems to determine the general nature of these present conclusions.

Many *experimental* factors have been studied which are capable of significantly altering the rate of metastasis formation from blood-borne tumor cells (Wood *et al.*, 1961) (Table I). Certain of these, such as hormones and anticoagulants, warrant special consideration since they could conceivably be endogenous regulators of the cell–host equilibrium under natural conditions.

Based on our analyses of the behavior of tumor cells and their components, interreactions, and environments in the microcirculation of the

TABLE I

EXPERIMENTAL FACTORS THAT ALTER THE FREQUENCY OF METASTASES DEVELOPING FROM BLOOD-BORNE TUMOR CELLS [a]

Increased Metastases	Decreased Metastases
Duration of tumor growth	Heparin
Rate of tumor growth	Warfarin or Dicumarol
Pregnancy	Fibrinolytic agents (plasmin)
Stress	Adrenal steroids (glucocorticoids)
Adrenocorticotropic hormone (ACTH)	Radiation
Adrenal steroids (glucocorticoids)	Chemotherapeutic agents
Growth hormone (GH)	
Trauma (including biopsy and massage)	
Large doses of viable tumor cells	
Dead tumor or normal cells	
Alimentary hyperlipemia	
Protamine	
Temperature	
Advanced tumor growth	
Radiation	
Chemotherapeutic agents	

[a] For references and details, see Wood *et al.* (1961).

rabbit ear chamber, we suggested that factors may enhance metastasis formation from blood-borne tumor cells if they increased leukocytic sticking or produced potential hypercoagulability, and provided these agents were without direct or lethal effect upon tumor cells. On the other hand, agents that diminish metastasis formation from blood-borne tumor cells were characterized as factors which reduced endothelial stickiness, detached adhesive cells, retarded intravascular coagulation, or exerted a direct, lethal effect on cancer cells (Wood, 1968; Wood *et al.*, 1961).

Recently, the role of Triton, WR1339, a nonionic detergent, in the prevention of experimental metastases in mice has been described (Franchi *et al.,* 1971; Rosso *et al.,* 1969). These and similar studies (Gasic *et al.,* 1968; Gastpar, 1970) indicate the expanding awareness of and interest in new chemotherapies to control the invasion or dissemination of cancer in the microvascular system, and may lead to improved and different modes for the therapy of cancer when appropriately combined with surgery or irradiation.

Recently, contradictory results have been reported on the endothelial sticking and emigration of tumor cells and leukocytes. A purified protein, free of nucleoprotein, thermolabile, and free of proteolytic activity, which causes endothelial adhesion and emigration of intravascularly injected tumor cells in rats, has been isolated from human and animal tumors (Ozaki *et al.,* 1971). Moreover, this specific protein factor fails to elicit a significant degree of increased microvascular permeability or increased emigration of leukocytes *in vivo.* It has been shown that factors including histamine and bradykinin, which alter endothelial vascular permeability or cause emigration of polymorphonuclear leukocytes, fail to enhance capillary endothelial adhesion or emigration of injected tumor cells (Ozaki *et al.,* 1971). These new observations require confirmation, but at present suggest the important role of specific substances as mediators of the capillary endothelial adhesion within blood vessels, emigration from the microvascular system, and invasion of tumor cells.

VI. Neovascularization

Once V2 tumor cells have reached the perivascular connective tissue, an event which occurs within 2 to 3 hr after initial arrival in the region of the postcapillary venules, growth occurs, and as early as 18 hr, minute, delicate new blood vessels originate from postcapillary venules and grow to nourish the developing tumor nodule (Wood, 1958; Wood *et al.,* 1961). At the same time, capillary endothelial proliferation results in the reestablishment of intact endothelium at the sites of earlier penetration by cancer cells (Wood, 1958; Wood *et al.,* 1961). Within preexisting and newly formed capillaries in the region of the tumor, however, there is an increase in leukocytic sticking to the poorly defined capillary vascular endothelium within or adjacent to a growing tumor. This event is associated with an increased microvascular permeability (Wood, 1968).

Between 48 and 72 hr, new capillaries extended completely through the V2 tumor focus in the rabbit ear chamber (Wood, 1958, 1968). Blood flow within these vessels was slow, the vessels were of small caliber, and the vessels exhibited numerous anastomosing channels or loops resulting in an *inefficient vascular perfusion.* The capillary endothelium was poorly defined within and about growing tumor cells. After three days, the laterally expanding tumor obsecured and ultimately destroyed by gradual obstruction and eventual obliteration preexisting and newly formed microvessels. Liquefaction necrosis occurred in the central area of the tumor. Tumor cells continued to grow laterally and progressively. Abundant new capillaries grew centrifugally. A narrow zone (100 to 200 μm in thickness) at the periphery of the tumor remained well vascularized by the above-described, newly formed microvessels with poorly defined endothelial sur-

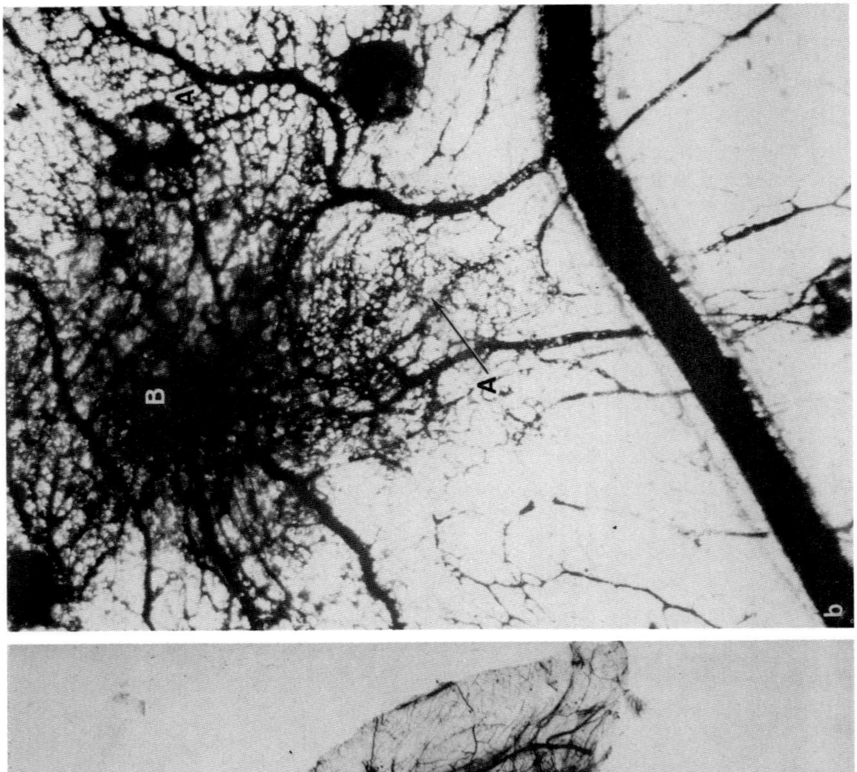
A
A
B
b
A
A
B
A
A
a

faces, increased leukocytic sticking, and increased capillarly permeability. In contrast, the microsvascular system in the connective tissue adjacent to the tumor had sharply defined endothelium along which leukocytes rolled in a normal fashion. The central area of the enlarged, growing tumor became necrotic. After 2 weeks, metastatic tumor was found in the cervical lymph nodes and lungs.

The precise mechanisms by which malignant cells are able to provide a continued microvascular proliferation remain important (Fig. 2), although recent preliminary observations suggest that experimental or human tumor cells may secrete a diffusable factor (Ehrmann and Knoth, 1968; Folkman *et al.*, 1971; Gitterman and Luell, 1969; Greenblatt and Shubik, 1968). Folkman has named this biological material "Tumor Angiogenesis Factor" (TAF), a heat-labile, RNA-containing protein, separable from human and animal tumors. TAF is reported to be mitogenic for capillary endothelial cells and may be responsible for formation of new capillaries, apparent within 18 hr (Folkman *et al.*, 1971; Folkman, 1971), the same time as reported above for the formation of new blood vessels *in vivo* from preexisting capillaries in the rabbit ear chamber containing V2 cancer cells (Wood *et al.*, 1961; Wood, 1968). Future studies of the production, properties, and inhibition of TAF-like substances may reveal significant new approaches to both the diagnosis and control of tumor growth in primary and metastatic sites.

Fig. 2. *Transfilter* induction of *neovascularization* on the chorioallantoic membrane (CAM) of embryonated chick eggs by human epidermoid carcinoma (H. Ep. #3) (Toolan). A portion of the CAM of a 10-day-old chick embryo was "dropped" by separating it from the normally adhering shell membrane. This creates an artificial air space. A part of the shell and shell membrane over the artificial air space are removed. Through this "window" a Millipore filter (1 cm^2, 25 μm thick, 0.45-μm pore size) is placed on the CAM; a 1 mm^3-fragment of H. Ep. #3 tumor is implanted on the upper surface of the filter. The window is sealed with cellophane tape. After 3 days of incubation of eggs at 38°C, Pelikan India Ink was injected intravenously to outline the blood vessels. (a) Portion of the CAM below the artificial air space after removal of the filter and tumor fragment. The CAM has thickened at the margin of the filter (A). Within the region previously occupied by the filter there is an area of intense neovascularization (B) induced by the tumor implant across the membrane (26×). (b) Details of neovascularized area showing fine network of newly formed blood vessels (A). The central region is obscured by the extravasation of ink (B) through the delicate, fragile newly formed blood vessels (180×). (Photographs generously supplied by Charles O. Gitterman, Ph.D.; see Gitterman and Luell, 1969, for more details.)

VII. Latency and Organ Selectivity

The mechanisms responsible for the latency (or dormancy, G_0) and organ selectivity of metastasis are at present unknown. Some of these may be explained by pecularities of the microvascular system. For example, we do not as yet understand why certain carcinomas, such as those of the thyroid, breast, prostate, lung, or kidney in particular, may develop as metastatic foci in bones (Wood and Sträuli, 1973). Are there peculiar receptor-sites in the capillary endothelium of the bones that attract embolic tumor cells from the above-mentioned bone-seeking primary tumors?

VIII. Systemic Effects

The inappropriate functions of tumors may be of importance in understanding the systemic effects of cancer (Wood and Sträuli, 1973). In considering the intravascular behavior of tumor cells in advanced cancer, we wish to point out that in rabbits with advanced V2 cancer grown at a remote site (thigh), the microcirculation of the ear chamber does not present the textbook picture of a normal microvascular system (Wood *et al.*, 1961). The abnormalities chiefly involve an increased sticking of leukocytes to vascular endothelium. The mechanisms responsible for this alteration are unknown, although this state may favor the increased endothelial adhesion of embolic cancer cells, and explain, at least in part, the increased occurrence of metastatic tumor associated with advanced cancer. In addition, in the later stages of the remote growth of V2 cancer cells in rabbits, circulating platelets assumed various elongated and atypical forms consistent with platelet activation (Wood *et al.*, 1961). The significance of this alteration is unclear. In 1912, Lubarsch proposed that circulating tumor cells regularly perished within the microvascular system and that a "toxin" was freed that prepared the vascular endothelium for the implantation of later blood-borne cancer cells. He concluded that the formation of metastases would thereby be a consequence of "autointoxication."

IX. Conclusions

With the increased precision of the biological, biochemical, and biophysical evaluations of tumor factors described above for the invasion, vascular adhesion, endothelial penetration, and neovascularization of certain tumors, a more definitive role of the products or contents of tumor cells is emerging which may be of enduring value of understanding the mechanisms of neoplastic invasion and metastasis formation, and in developing new concepts for the diagnosis and management of primary and metastatic tumors. In each of these important endeavors, the essential and intimate role of the microvascular system may profitably and properly be considered as an integral part of our understanding of the complex phenomena of neoplasia.

References

Baserga, R. (1971). "The Cell Cycle and Cancer." Dekker, New York.

Burstone, M. S. (1956). Histochemical demonstration of proteolytic activity in human neoplasms. *J. Nat. Cancer Inst.* **16,** 1149–1161.

Cole, W. H., McDonald, G. O., Roberts, S. S., and Southwick, H. W. (1961). "Dissemination of Cancer. Prevention and Therapy." Appleton, New York.

Ehrmann, R. L., and Knoth, M. (1968). Choriocarcinoma: Transfilter stimulation of vasoproliferation in the hamster cheek pouch—studied by light and electron microscopy. *J. Nat. Cancer Inst.* **41,** 1329–1341.

Fisher, B., and Fisher, E. R. (1966). The interrelationship of hematogenous and lymphatic tumor cell dissemination. *Surg., Gynecol. Obstet.* **122,** 791–798.

Florey, L. (1970). General Pathology, 4th Ed., Saunders, Philadelphia, Pennsylvania.

Folkman, J. (1971). Tumor angiogenesis: Therapeutic implications. *N. Engl. J. Med.* **285,** 1182–1186.

Folkman, J., Merler, E., Abernathy, C., and Williams, G. (1971). Isolation of a tumor factor responsible for angiogenesis. *J. Exp. Med.* **133,** 275–288.

Franchi, G., Morasca, L., Reyers-Degli-Innocenti, I., and Garattini, S. (1971). Triton WR 1339 (TWR), an inhibitor of cancer dissemination and metastases. *Eur. J. Cancer* **7,** 533–544.

Gasic, G. J., Gasic, T. B., and Stewart, C. C. (1968). Antimetastatic effects associated with platelet reduction. *Proc. Nat. Acad. Sci. U. S.* **61,** 46–52.

Gastpar, H. (1970). Stickiness of platelets and tumor cells influenced by drugs. *In* "Platelet adhesion and aggregation in thrombosis: Countermeasures." Transactions of the Eighteenth Annual Symposium on Blood (E. F. Mammen, G. F. Anderson, and M. I. Barnhart, eds.), pp. 291–303. Schattauer, Stuttgart.

Gitterman, C. O., and Luell, S. (1969). Transfilter induction of vascular proliferation on the chorio-allantoic membranes of embryonated eggs. *Proc. Amer. Ass. Cancer Res.* **10,** 29.

Greenblatt, M., and Shubik, P. (1968). Tumor angiogenesis: Transfilter diffusion studies in the hamster by the transparent chamber technique. *J. Nat. Cancer Inst.* **41,** 111–124.

Leighton, J. (1969). Propagation of cancer: Targets for future chemotherapy. *Cancer Res.* **29,** 2457–2465.

Lubarsch, O. (1912). Die Bedeutung des Traumas für Entstehung und Wachstum krankhafter Gewächse. *Med. Klin.* (*Munich*) **8,** 1651–1654.

Ozaki, T., Yoshida, K., Ushijima, K., and Hayashi, H. (1971). Studies on the mechanisms of invasion in cancer. II. *In vivo* effects of a factor chemotactic for cancer cells. *Int. J. Cancer* **7,** 93–100.

Rosso, R., Donelli, M. G., Franchi, G., and Garattini, S. (1969). Effect of Triton WR 1339 on cancer dissemination and metastases. *Eur. J. Cancer* **5,** 77–78.

Sträuli, P. (1970). The barrier function of lymph nodes. A review of experimental studies and their implications for cancer surgery. *In* "Surgical Oncology" (F. Saegesser and J. Pettavel, eds.), pp. 161–176. Huber, Bern.

Sylvén, B. (1967a). Some factors relating to the invasiveness and destructiveness of solid malignant tumours. *In* "Mechanisms of Invasion in Cancer" (Denoix, ed.), UICC Monogr. Ser. Vol. 6, pp. 48–60. Springer-Verlag, Berlin.

Sylvén, B. (1967b). Biochemical factors accompanying growth and invasion. In "Endogenous Factors Influencing Host-Tumor Balance" (R. W. Wissler, T. L. Dao, and S. Wood, Jr., eds.), pp. 267–276. Univ. of Chicago Press, Chicago, Illinois.

Sylvén, B. (1970). Metastatic spread of tumors. *In "Oncology, 1970, Vol. 1,"* (R. L. Clark, R. W. Cumley, J. E. McCay and M. E. Copeland, eds.), pp. 411–416, Yearbook Medical Publishers, Chicago, Illinois.

Sylvén, B., and Holmberg, B. (1965). On the structure and biological effects of a newly-discovered cytotoxic polypeptide in tumor fluid. *Eur. J. Cancer* **1,** 199–202.

Tannock, I. F. (1970). Population kinetics of carcinoma cells, capillary endothelial cells and fibroblasts in a transplanted mouse mammary tumor. *Cancer Res.* **30,** 2470–2476.

Thornes, R. D., Edlow, D. W., and Wood, S., Jr. (1968). Inhibition of locomotion of cancer cells *in vivo* by anticoagulant therapy. 1. Effects of sodium warfarin on V2 cancer cells, granulocytes, lymphocytes and macrophages in rabbits. *Johns Hopkins Med. J.* **123,** 305–316.

Wallach, D. F. H. (1969). Generalized membrane defects in cancer. *N. Engl. J. Med.* **280,** 761–767.

Warren, B. A. (1967). *In vivo* and electron microscopic study of vessels in two transplantable tumours in the hamster. *Bibl. Anat.* **9,** 412–417.

Warren, B. A., and Shubik, P. (1966). The growth of the blood supply to melanoma transplants in the hamster cheek pouch. *Lab. Invest.* **15,** 464–478.

Weiss, L. (1967). "The Cell Periphery, Metastasis, and Other Contact Phenomena." North-Holland Publ., Amsterdam.

Wood, S., Jr. (1958). Pathogenesis of metastasis formation observed *in vivo* in the rabbit ear chamber. *AMA Arch. Pathol.* **66,** 550–568.

Wood, S., Jr. (1968). Studies on the behavior of V2 cancer cells *in vivo. In* "Prognostic Factors in Breast Cancer" (A. P. M. Forrest and P. B. Kunkler, eds.), pp. 267–274. Livingstone, Edinburgh.

Wood, S., Jr. (1971). Mechanisms of establishment of tumor metasteses. *In* "Pathobiology Annual (H. L. Ioachim, ed.), pp. 281–308. Appleton, New York.

Wood, S., Jr., and Sträuli, P. (1973). Tumor invasion and metastasis. *In* "Cancer Medicine" (J. F. Holland and E. Frei, III, eds.). Chapter II–3, pp. 110–120. Lea & Febiger, Philadelphia, Pennsylvania.

Wood, S., Jr., Holyoke, E. D., and Yardley, J. H. (1961). Mechanisms of metastasis production from blood-borne cancer cells. *Proc. Can. Cancer Res. Conf.* **4,** 167–223.

Wood, S., Jr., Baker, R. R., and Marzocchi, B. (1967). Factors influencing the spread of cancer: Locomotion of normal and malignant cells *in vivo. In* "Endogenous Factors Influencing Host-Tumor Balance" (R. W. Wissler, T. Dao, and S. Wood, Jr., eds.), Chapter 16, pp. 223–237. Univ. of Chicago Press, Chicago, Illinois.

Wood, S., Jr., Baker, R. R., and Marzocchi, B. (1968). *In vivo* studies of tumor behavior: Locomotion of and interrelationship between normal cells and cancer cells. *In* "The Proliferation and Spread of Neoplastic Cells," pp. 495–510. Williams & Wilkins, Baltimore, Maryland.

16 THE MICROCIRCULATION OF THE BRAIN, RETINA, AND BULBAR CONJUNCTIVA

F. A. ELLIOTT, M.D.

This chapter is mainly concerned with the microvasculature of the brain and bulbar conjunctiva. No attempt will be made to describe the microcirculation of the spinal cord or peripheral nerves, or to discuss the familar role of the fine vessels in infections, collagen diseases, fat embolism, and air embolism.

I. Anatomic and Physiologic Considerations

The ultimate purpose of the cardiovascular system is to maintain blood flow through capillaries in response to the metabolic needs of the tissues. The microcirculation cannot be considered apart from the macrocirculation, since both the arterial input and the venous outflow exercise a decisive influence on what happens in the capillaries. In the brain, as elsewhere, capillary flow can be compromised by a severe fall of systemic blood pressure, structural stenosis of arteries, spasm of arterioles (in hypertensive encephalopathy), spasm of arteries (following subarachnoid hemorrhage), obstruction of capillaries, elevated venous pressure (from venous thrombosis and congestive cardiac failure), and rheologic factors which decrease the flow properties of the blood through the micovasculature.

Neurons are exquisitely sensitive to oxygen lack and to hypoglycemia, so that dysfunction is produced by lesser degrees of circulatory failure than affect other organs. This vulnerability is offset, to some degree, by certain anatomic arrangements and physiologic mechanisms which help to maintain steady perfusion.

The maintenance of cerebral blood flow is facilitated by the Circle of Willis which provides a unique anastomotic system between the carotid and vertebral-basilar systems. It is also helped by the anastomoses which exist between pial microvessels. The latter link the terminal cortical branches of the anterior, middle, and posterior cerebral arteries. A sudden and prolonged fall of blood pressure can lead to bilateral cortical and subcortical infarction in these "watershed" areas. In the presence of carotid stenosis on one side, a lesser degree of circulatory failure will cause softenings on that side only. Similarly, prolonged hypoglycemia can cause focal impairment of function through its preferential impact on an area of brain which is supplied by a stenosed artery. In these examples, it is the failure of capillary perfusion that causes the damage.

Although the intracranial arteries and arterioles possess a nerve supply, it seems to play a minor role in the control of the cerebral circulation (Reivich, 1971). This protects the cerebral vessels, to some extent, from abrupt vasoconstrictor and vasodilator impulses originating in the central nervous system.

Second, the small cerebral arteries possess a marked capacity for autoregulation when exposed to a rapid rise or a rapid fall of systemic blood pressure (Harper, 1966; Reivich, 1971). They contract when the pressure rises, and dilate when it falls, thus helping to maintain constant flow within a range of mean arterial blood pressure between 50 to 170 mm Hg. Autoregulation is apt to fail when the mean arterial pressure falls below 50 mm Hg or rises above 250 mm Hg. It can also be impaired by head injury, high intracranial pressure, and arteriosclerosis in elderly subjects. It is likely, but unproved, that the fleeting dizziness, lightheadedness, and amaurosis, sometimes experienced by arteriosclerotic individuals in response to physical and mental shocks or a sudden change of posture, may be the result of impaired autoregulation. This possibility has to be kept in mind when considering the causes of transient cerebral symptoms lasting for a few seconds only.

The structure of the intracranial arteries differs from those elsewhere in important respects. Once the carotid and vertebral arteries enter the cranial cavity, they lose some of their adventitia and all of their lymphatics, but they retain their vasa vasorum. The anterior, middle, and posterior cerebral arteries have thinner walls than arteries of comparable diameter elsewhere; there is no external elastic lamina, the media is thin, and *there are no vasa vasorum* in these vessels (Clarke, 1965). The fragility of the

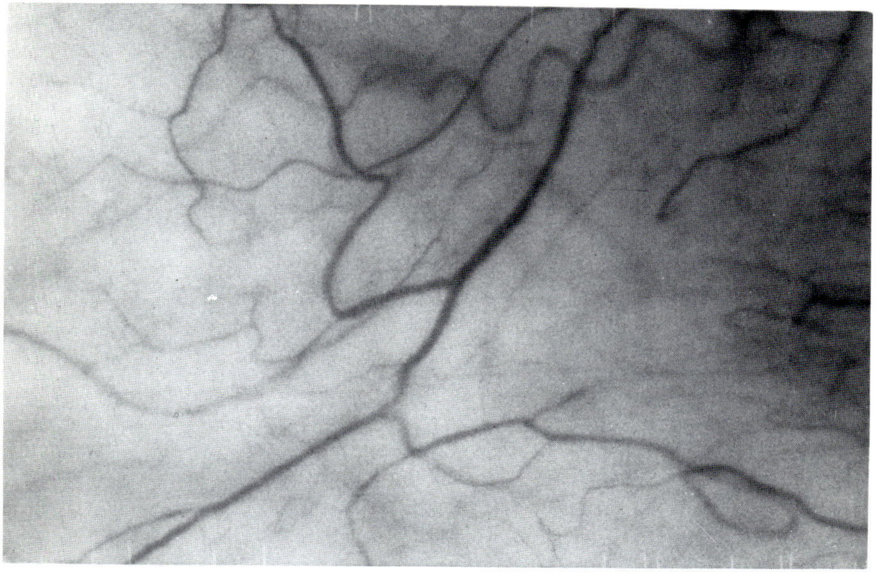

Fig. 1. Normal conjunctival vessels. Age 29.

cerebral arteries may explain the presence of military aneurysms on intracerebral arteries measuring 150 to 300 μm in diameter, and their tendency to rupture, especially but not exclusively, in the presence of arterial hypertension (Ross Russell, 1963).

The capillaries of the central nervous system present unique structural and physiologic features. They are invested in over 85% of their circumference by the footplates of glial cells which lie on the basement membrane. Second, the endothelial cells overlap and are sealed together, without fenestrations, so that in health large molecules cannot pass between the cells to reach the intercellular spaces of the parenchyma. This contributes to the blood–brain barrier. It is probable that the glial footplates also have a barrier function. The effect of the barrier in health is to prevent the passage into the brain of some solutes and to delay the transport of others (Bakay, 1968). The efficiency of the barrier can be reduced by trauma, hypoxia, hypercapnia, inflammation, tumors, uremia, convulsions, etc., allowing the transport of substances which are normally excluded from the parenchyma and increasing the passage of molecules which normally reach the brain in small quantities. The breakdown of the barrier is not wholly harmful in that it allows for an increase in the passage of drugs and antibiotics, (e.g., penicillin) into the brain and cerebrospinal fluid.

It is probable that neurons derive some of their nutrition via the glial footplates. If this were so, it would be expected that alterations of capillary permeability and the rheologic factors that compromise capillary flow would have an effect on the health of the neurons, not only by impairing their nutrition but also by allowing the passage into the parenchyma of substances which are excluded completely under normal conditions or are allowed through in concentrations lower than those in the plasma. These principles apply also to the blood–retinal barrier (Ashton, 1965).

The capillaries of the choroid plexus and their ependymal covering also possess discriminative functions (the blood–CSF barrier). As in the case of the blood–brain barrier, impairment of this barrier allows passage into the spinal fluid of substances which are normally kept out. The cerebrospinal fluid also receives a considerable contribution of fluid and solutes which pass through the capillaries of the brain and spinal cord, traverse the intercellular spaces, and reach the subarachnoid space through the ependyma. Therefore, the breakdown of the blood–brain barrier and the blood–CSF barrier are jointly responsible for the presence of abnormal solutes and cells in the cerebrospinal fluid.

Another feature of the microcirculation of the brain is that the arterioles are extremely sensitive to changes in the concentration of pCO_2; hypercapnia produces intense vasodilatation. In man, inhalation of 5% carbon dioxide increase cerebral blood flow by approximately 50% (Reivich, 1971), but in conditions causing chronic hypercapnia, a process of adaptation seems to occur which limits the effect of pCO_2 on the cerebral circulation.

It is probable that other agents, some humoral and some of local origin, influence flow through the cerebral microvasculature as they do in other vascular beds. According to Altura (1971), blood-borne agents include the catecholamines, amines such as serotonin, histamine, and acetylcholine, a variety of polypeptides, glucocorticoids, and estrogens. Locally produced factors include adenosine and adenine nucleotides, hypoxia, a fall of pH, potassium ions, inorganic phosphate, carbon dioxide, Kreb's Cycle intermediates, prostaglandins, and hyperosmolarity. The situation is further complicated by four circumstances. First, the local response to any of these agents may differ from one vascular bed to another. Second, there are species differences, so it is imprudent to extrapolate from, say, experiments on the rat's tail to the human brain. Third, glucocorticoids, estrogens, and prostaglandins can modify vascular responses to other vasodilator and vasoconstrictor agents. Last, some of these agents have side effects which can modify flow. For instance, epinephrine and norepinephrine, liberated in conditions of stress, cause a steep rise in free fatty acids, especially in obese subjects, which increases sludging and platelet adhesiveness, thereby compromising flow through capillaries. Similarly, serotonin causes clumping of platelets, which can impair flow.

The effect of raised intracranial pressure on the cerebral vessels has important clinical effects. When the intracranial pressure exceeds 450 mm Hg of water, cerebral blood flow is reduced as the result of the pressure on the microcirculation. Venules and capillaries are compressed—an outflow obstruction—and as the pressure rises still higher, arterial input is completely blocked and the cerebral circulation ceases. This sequence of events depends on the fact that the brain is enclosed in a rigid box. Similarly, the spinal cord is enclosed in the tough and inelastic pia, and this circumstance probably explains why compression of the cord by tumors and by spondylitic ridges causes local myelomalacia, although at autopsy the spinal arteries are found to be patent; it is the microvasculature which is compressed.

II. Rheologic Factors Affecting Capillary Flow

Traditional emphasis on the importance of the arterial input in maintaining perfusion of the brain has obscured the fact that obstruction to the outflow from capillaries can be almost as lethal. At the level of the macrocirculation, dural sinus thrombosis and cortical venous thrombosis can cause massive hemorrhagic infarction. Similarly, obstruction of the veins of the microcirculation can cause death of tissue, as in retinal venous thrombosis, while massive obstruction of the capillaries and venules, as in cerebral malaria, sickle cell crises, fat embolism, decompression sickness, and Waldenstrom's macroglobulinemia, can cause damage to the brain and retina. Other factors, less exotic and much more common, play a considerable role in reducing capillary flow, such as the elevated hematocrit in the polycythemias, agglutination of circulating erythrocytes and platelets, and rigidity of the erythrocytes.

The influence of an elevated hematocrit is most dramatically seen in severe polycythemia vera, where cerebral blood flow may be reduced by 50%. Myocardial infarction and strokes are common. This disease, however, is less common than the symptomatic polycythemias, resulting from unilateral renal artery stenosis, stress, etc. In these conditions the hematocrit commonly lies between 50 and 56%—a figure which is apt to be disregarded because it is usually accepted that the upper limit of the hematocrit in a normal male is 54%. However, it is doubtful whether this figure can be regarded as physiologically acceptable because study of the conjunctival vessels shows that when the hematocrit reaches approximately 50%, capillary flow slows, and areas of complete stasis may be seen. I have often observed a dramatic improvement of capillary flow a day or two or after phelebotomy in such cases.

There is clinical and epidemiological evidence that a modest elevation of the red cell count can be harmful. The Framingham study has disclosed that individuals with a hemoglobin above 15 gm in a man and 14 gm in a woman are twice as liable to stroke as those with lower hemoglobin values. Heyman *et al.* (1971) confirm an increased liability to stroke and myocardial infarction in subjects with modest elevation of the hematocrit. Moreover, the effort threshold for intermittent claudication is lowered by minor elevation of the hematocrit (47 to 54%) and is increased by phlebotomy (Cranley *et al.,* 1963). Liability to transient ischemic attacks in patients with polycythemia and vertebral-basilar insufficiency is decreased by lowering the red cell count.

While it is obvious that a high hematocrit will increase viscosity at low rates of shear, thereby slowing the flow in capillaries and venules, it has little or no effect at high rates of shear, as in the large arteries. Therefore, the question remains why there is an increased incidence of thrombosis of *large* arteries in the polycythemias (high altitude erythrocytosis excepted). Is it because of reduced perfusion in the microcirculation of the arterial wall, i.e., in the vasa vasorum, with consequent ischemic damage to the artery? The increased incidence of arterial thrombosis in polycythemia vera has been attributed to the increased number of platelets which occurs in this condition, but this does not apply to the symptomatic polycythemias in which there is also an increased liability to thrombosis.

The second common cause of elevated viscosity at low rates of shear is intravascular agglutination of circulating red cells, sometimes referred to as sludging (Fig. 2). Since most of the conditions which increase the adhesiveness of red cells have the same effect on platelets, it is likely that platelet aggregation accompanies agglutination of the erythrocytes.

Sludging is a nonspecific response to trauma, infection, diabetes, the lipidemias (including alimentary lipemia), tissue necrosis, extensive skin disease, etc. It also occurs during stress, probably as a result of the mobilization of free fatty acids by catecholamines. The aggregates are rarely firm enough to plug arterioles, but they often block capillaries and postcapillary venules. When sludging is severe and generalized, it causes outflow obstruction, with perivascular edema and occasional microhemorrhages. These

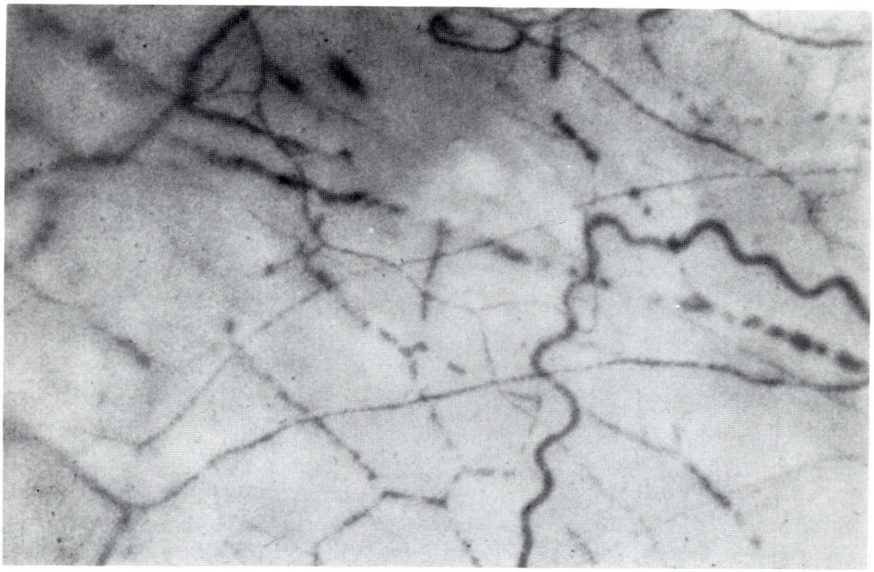

Fig. 2. Sludge and stasis in the conjunctiva of a man of 55 with cerebral and coronary atherosclerosis.

phenomena can be seen in the bulbar conjunctiva with the aid of a microscope or a conventional slit-lamp, preferably equipped with a red-free filter to aid contrast and to protect the eye from the heat of the examining lamp, which causes artifacts (Fink *et al.*, 1961). Similar events have been seen in the pial vessels following a large fatty meal in experimental animals.

Whereas mild degrees of red cell and platelet aggregation probably do no harm, there is ample experimental evidence that *severe* sludging is damaging (Swank and Bartsch, 1971). In the hamster, alimentary lipemia causes aggregation of red cells, reduced oxygen uptake by the brain, and changes in the electrocardiogram. In patients with coronary disease, a fatty meal increases liability to angina (Kuo and Joyner, 1955), and Plotz (1949) has recorded an increased incidence of myocardial infarction in patients on a high fat (Sippy) diet. Sludging induced by the repeated intravenous administration of high molecular weight dextran can give rise to visceral microinfarcts (Stalker, 1962; Bergentz *et al.*, 1965). It can also give rise to intramural arterial hemorrhages from vasa vasorum; mural thrombi are found attached to the intima overlying some of these hemorrhages (Elliott and Leonberg, 1971). Obstruction of the vasa vasorum of the aorta by platelet aggregates gives rise to edema of the intima, followed by thickening of the intima and degeneration of the media (Nakata, 1967). Myocardial infarction has been produced in the pig by obstruction of myocardial capillaries by platelet aggregates (Glynn *et al.*, 1966). It is important to note that the obstruction of the microcirculation in these experiments lasted only a few minutes. Thereafter, the emboli broke up, leaving a patent microcirculation. Bicher (1969) has reported that sludging produced in animals by high molecular weight dextran causes electrocardiographic and histologic evidence of myocardial damage and that these effects can be avoided by the administration of a ketolactone derivative (substance "86") which inhibits red cell and platelet aggregation.

Clearly, agglutination of red cells and of platelets, which occurs intermittently throughout life as a result of trauma, disease, stress, lipemia, etc., can compromise blood flow through the microcirculation, including the vasa vasorum of arteries.

A third rheologic factor which can reduce flow in capillaries is loss of the normal deformability of red cells. Rigidity of erythrocytes results from acidosis, hyperosmolarity, and hypoxia (Wells, 1971), and is, therefore, likely to occur in conditions of stasis, such as are produced by sludging and polycythemia.

Another condition which influences the flow properties of blood in the microvasculature is the condition of the blood vessels themselves. Both dilatation of venules and constriction of arterioles reduces the rate of shear, thereby favoring aggregation. Second, experimental studies on animals have shown that when normal blood passes into capillaries and venules which have been injured by chemical or thermal agents, or by bacterial endotoxins, leukocytes and platelets stick to the endothelium and both red cells and platelets form into clumps (Lutz, 1951; Kreyberg, 1963). It is, therefore, pertinent to ask to what extent naturally occurring disease of the microvasculature is responsible for the sludging which is seen within such vessels. Clearly, there are complex reciprocal relationships between the state of the vessel and the physical characteristics of the blood within it. All observers agree, however, that when sludging is seen in small arteries and arterioles, it is the result of systemic disease or hyperlipidemia. In this connection it should be noted that severe sludging is the rule in advanced generalized atherosclerosis. This fact raises the interesting possibility of a vicious cycle whereby atherosclerosis of the aorta and large vessels, as in other systemic diseases, produces sludging which in its turn impairs blood flow through the microcirculation, including the vasa vasorum, thus increasing arterial damage.

III. Pathology and Pathogenesis of Microangiopathy

It is generally agreed that arteries narrower than 200 μm in diameter do not devlop atherosclerosis, which is a disease of larger vessels. Nevertheless, occlusion or narrowing of arteries can give rise to secondary changes, resulting from hypoxia, in the microcirculation distal to the obstruction. This is seen in the eye, where atheromatous stenosis of the central retinal artery causes tortuosity and congestion of capillaries and venules, microaneurysms, edema, and hemorrhages. The same thing is sometimes seen in the retina as the result of stenosis of the internal carotid artery, in which case it can be accompanied by an ischemic uveitis.

A different type of sclerosis affects arteries ranging in diameter from 150 to 600 μm. They exhibit fibrosis of the adventitia and media, with little or no intimal change (Baker and Ianone, 1959; Ellington, 1970). This process, like atheroma, starts in the third decade, advances throughout life, and is aggravated by hypertension and diabetes. A similar sclerotic process occurs in the small arteries of the retina, and Heisig and Lindner (1965) have found it in the bulbar conjunctival vessels.

The microvasculature is also involved in the arteriolosclerosis of severe hypertension. In cats and monkeys, a steep rise in blood pressure is accompanied by focal waistlike contractions of small pial arteries, which disappear when the blood pressure is reduced. In man, severe hypertension is associated with degenerative changes in the microvasculature; the first histologic changes appear in the capillaries, which display increased cellularity around the basement membrane and hyperplasia of the endothelium (Scheinker, 1948). It is likely that the changes in the capillaries are due to hypoxia, the result of reduced blood flow from arteriolar constriction. However, even in the absence of hypertension, degenerative changes appear in veins, venules, capillaries, arterioles, and small arteries. They can be seen during life in the retinal and bulbar conjunctival vessels. (Section 5.)

Microaneurysms are a feature of degenerative vascular disease in the brain, retina, and bulbar conjunctiva. In the brain, they arise from small penetrating arteries 150 μm or more in diameter. In the retina and conjunctiva, they are much smaller. In the retina, capillary microaneurysms and aneurysmal dilatation of small veins occur in both diabetics and nondiabetics, and in both hypertensives and normotensives, but they are most numerous in diabetics and hypertensives. In nondiabetics they tend to be situated in the periphery of the retina and are often too small to be seen with the ophthalmoscope, but they can be demonstrated *in vivo* by fluorscein angiography (Hodge and Dollery, 1964) and postmortem by perfusing the vessels with India Ink.

Using the latter method, Ashton (1951) found them in 34% of 174 eyes from nondiabetic patients ranging in age from 27 to 81. In the bulbar conjunctiva, capillary microaneurysms appear in some apparently healthy persons in the third decade (Luedde, 1913; Labram and Lestradet, 1961) and become more common as life advances; Davis and Landau (1969) found them to be almost three times more common in patients under 65 with ischemic heart disease than in healthy controls. They can also occur in the conjunctiva in diabetes (Ditzell, 1962) in sickle cell crises (Fink *et al.*, 1961), in the course of general infections, including syphilis (Luedde, 1913), and in hypercholesterolemia. I have seen them in three healthy young women when taking oral contraceptive agents; they disappeared within 2 weeks of stopping the medication.

The causes of degenerative microangiopathy are not understood. The microvasculature appears to react in a somewhat stereotyped way to insults as dissimilar as hypertension, hypoxia, bacterial endotoxins, and other vasotoxic agents; one aspect of this stereotypy is the fact that under experimental conditions the endothelium of venules and capillaries reacts more intensely to both local and systemic insults than the epithelium of arterioles (Zweifach, 1959), a situation which is reproduced in the conjunctival vessels of man. It is also clear that the vascular response to any given insult depends on the size and structure of the vessel in question (and perhaps on its metabolic endowment as well). Thus, hyperlipidemia accelerates atherosclerosis in large arteries, but gives rise to microaneurysms in capillaries and venules. Syphilis produces aneurysms of capillaries (Luedde, 1913), endarteritis of small arteries, and aneurysm of the aorta. Diabetes produces aneurysms and thickening of the basement membrane of the capillaries, sclerosis and endothelial proliferation of arterioles, and increased liability to thrombosis in large arteries.

It has been questioned whether conjunctival microangiopathy could be the result of exposure to local irritation—sunlight, dust, conjunctivitis, etc.—and this has led some ophthalmologists to discount the possible systemic implications of these changes. However, we have looked for and failed to find a consistent correlation between conjunctival microangiopathy and pingueculae and pterygia, both of which are supposedly related to environmental irritation. Second, recurrent attacks of conjunctivitis have left no permanent abnormalities in several cases we have examined. Third, the theory of local irritation does not explain why microangiopathy is more common in young men than in young women (Labram and Lestradet, 1961) or why its incidence is affected by heredity and its severity by

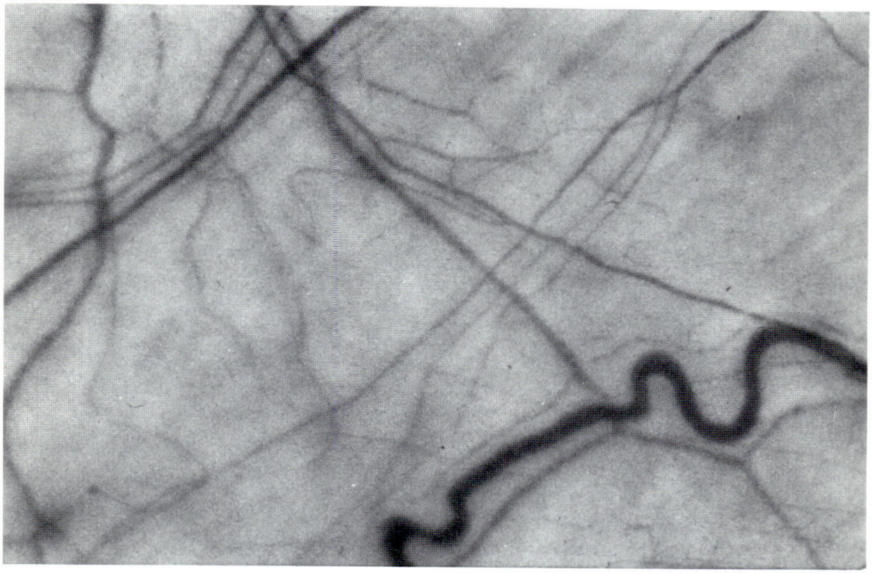

Fig. 3. Normal conjunctival vessels. Age 70.

hypertension (Lack *et al.*, 1949), or why it is sometimes absent in elderly individuals who have led outdoor lives (as in a weatherbeaten woman aged 70 whose vessels are depicted in Fig. 3).

IV. Vasa Vasorum

If it be accepted that compromise of blood flow through the microcirculation can damage tissues, it is logical to consider whether obstruction of the vasa vasorum by disease or by decrease in the flow properties of blood, contributes to degenerative arterial disease, as suggested by Köster and other nineteenth century pathologists (Ramsey, 1936). This possibility is supported by a considerable body of experimental evidence, a miniscule fragment of which is mentioned in Section II. It has been found that although the vasa vasorum supply only the adventitia and the outer part of the media of healthy arteries, obstruction of the vasa can cause edema and subsequent thickening of the intima, medial sclerosis, and arterial thrombosis. Since atherosclerosis occurs in the anterior, middle, and posterior cerebral arteries, which lack an intrinsic microcirculation, disease of the vasa vasorum is by no means a *sine qua non* for atherogenesis. At best, it can only be a contributory factor. Nevertheless, the hypothesis raises interesting questions. Is the enhanced tendency to arterial thrombosis in diabetics due, in some measure at least, to diabetic microangiopathy of the vasa vasorum? Does the vasoconstrictor effect of cigaret smoking on some vascular beds, in some individuals, apply to the microvasculature of the arterial wall? Does the vasodilator effect of certain estrogens apply to the vasa vasorum, and if so could this explain the relative rarity of vascular catastrophes in premenopausal women? Does atherosclerosis appear later in the cerebral vessels than in the coronary and peripheral arteries because, lacking vasa vasorum, they are vulnerable to atherogenic factors only at the blood–intima interface?

Living atheromatous plaques derive some of their nutrition from the blood within the lumen of the artery and some from new capillaries which originate in the vasa vasorum, penetrate the media, and supply areas of thickened intima (Geiringer, 1951). Winternitz and his associates (1938) concluded from their studies of human material that failure to maintain this blood supply could be responsible for necrosis and ulceraton of plaques, events which promote thrombosis. Clearly, information is needed as to whether obstruction of the tenuous blood supply of atheromatous plaques by factors such as sludging, an elevated hematocrit, or the mechanical effects of hypertension lead to ulceration of plaques.

V. Microangiopathy of the Bulbar Conjunctival Vessels

The conjunctival microvasculature, an outgrowth of the intracranial vascular system, deserves notice because it is the only place in the human body where arterioles, capillaries, and veins, and the circulation within them, can be observed in the natural state.

For almost 100 years it has been recognized that degenerative disease of the aorta and large arteries is usually accompanied by retinal "arteriosclerosis"—a misleading term for a condition which involves veins and capillaries as well as arteries. It is less well known that the vessels of the bulbar conjunctiva exhibit similar changes in patients with degenerative vascular disease (Fig. 4). This association, first described by Bajardi at the turn of the century, has been confirmed by Zeller (1921), Ruedemann, (1933), Kittel (1960), Davis and Landau (1969), and many others.

The earliest changes in the conjunctival vessels are seen in the veins, venules, and capillaries. The veins become wide and tortuous and may form loops, and the venules sometimes exhibit aneurysmal dilatations. The capillaries become kinked, tortuous, and uneven in caliber. Capillary microaneurysms often appear, and sometimes the capillary itself becomes

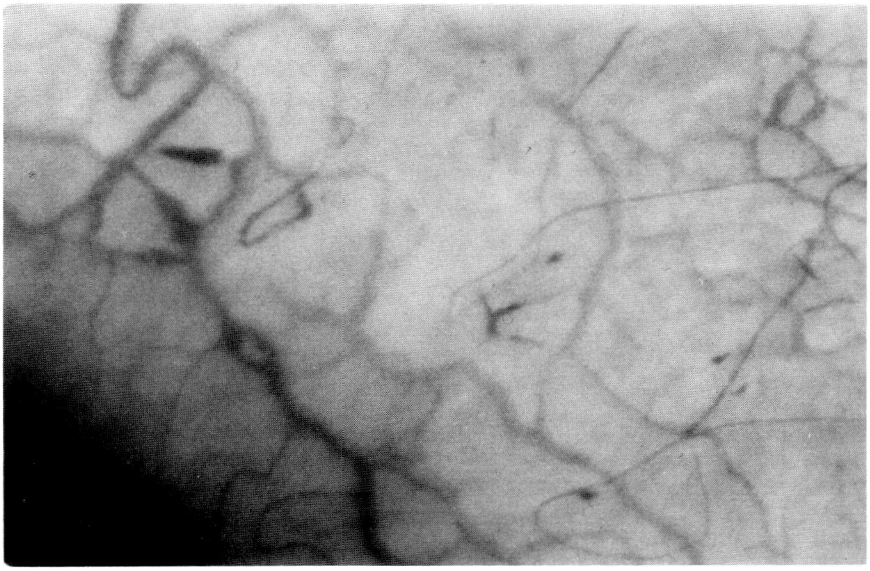

Fig. 4. Venous dilatations, microaneurysms, and a carrot-shaped hemorrhage in the conjunctiva—a case of cerebral thrombosis, age 68.

virtually invisible so that the aneurysm appears to be detached from the vascular network. Arteries and arterioles become straighter, with narrowing of the lumen, and they lose their translucency so that it is sometimes difficult to discern blood flow within them. Sludging is usually present in venules and capillaries (Fig. 2) and is often seen in arterioles as well, but it may be slight or absent if the patient is taking aspirin or aspirin-containing drugs, which reduce aggregation of both erythrocyte and platelets (F. A. Elliott, unpublished). When sludging is severe, areas of stasis and perivascular edema appear. Microhemorrhages are occasionally present in both hypertensives and normotensives.

These morphologic changes are not peculiar to the conjunctival vessels. Corkscrew tortuosity of small veins, capillary aneurysms, and sclerosis of small arteries occur in the retina and brain, as well as in the conjunctiva (Baker and Ianone, 1959; Hassler, 1965; Fang, 1967; Ellington, 1970).

Morphologic changes and abnormal flow may appear years before visible changes are expected in the retinal vessels (Luedde, 1913; Dennis, 1918; Ruedemann, 1933), but this discrepancy may be more apparent than real because the earliest changes to appear are in capillaries and venules, which are too small to be seen with the ophthalmoscope. The same is true of some microaneurysms (Ashton, 1951). Moreover, except for exudates and perivascular infiltrates, the white sclera provides a more favorable background for observation than the red retina; the importance of the background is illustrated by the difficulty in identifying early microangiopathy in negroes, in whom the sclera commonly contains patches of pigment.

Conjunctival microangiopthy is virtually always present in patients with overt cerebrovascular disease, irrespective of age. It was severe, for instance, in a man of 28 with stenosis of the right carotid and left vertebral arteries and type IV hyperlipoproteinemia and in a woman of 35 with carotid stenosis who developed sudden hemiplegia. Conversely, experience over the years has shown that it is unwise to ascribe neurologic symptoms to cerebrovascular disease in the presence of a normal conjunctival microcirculation. Further evidence linking conjunctival microangiopathy to atherosclerosis of larger vessels is supplied by Heisig and Lindner (1965) who found that the degree of conjunctival microangiopathy correlated well with the severity of cerebral atherosclerosis as determined by autopsy in eight cases, while Wells and his associates (1971) found morphologic changes and abnormal flow in the conjunctival vessels of all members of a group of patients with angiographically proved coronary sclerosis.

Some elderly individuals exhibit a normal or nearly normal conjunctival microvasculature (Fig. 3). They are usually exceptionally vigorous in mind and body and look younger than their chronological age. Knisely and his associates (1957) found normal vessels and normal flow in 5% of a group of 150 "functioning" individuals over the age of 60. It would be useful to know whether these elderly individuals are also free from atherosclerosis. Moses (1963) found no atherosclerosis of the cerebral vessels in 30% of subjects over 70 years who had died of causes other than a vascular catastrophe. Both Corsellis (1962) and Howell (1966) reported absence of atherosclerosis throughout the body in 4% of subjects in the ninth and tenth decade, while Baker and Resch (1965) found that the vessels of the Circle of Willis were healthy in 4% of subjects over the age of 80.

Vascular changes are to be found in the conjunctiva of apparently healthy individuals in the third decade, or even earlier. Luedde (1913) found microaneurysms and aneurysmal dilatations of small veins in 22% of a large group of healthy army recruits whose average age was 23.5 years (Fig. 5). Labram and Lestradet (1961) found that in the 20- to 40-age group men are more often affected than women, an observation we have confirmed. In a study of healthy adults aged 21 to 39 years, Elliott and Leonberg (1972) found conjunctival microangiopathy in 56% of the men

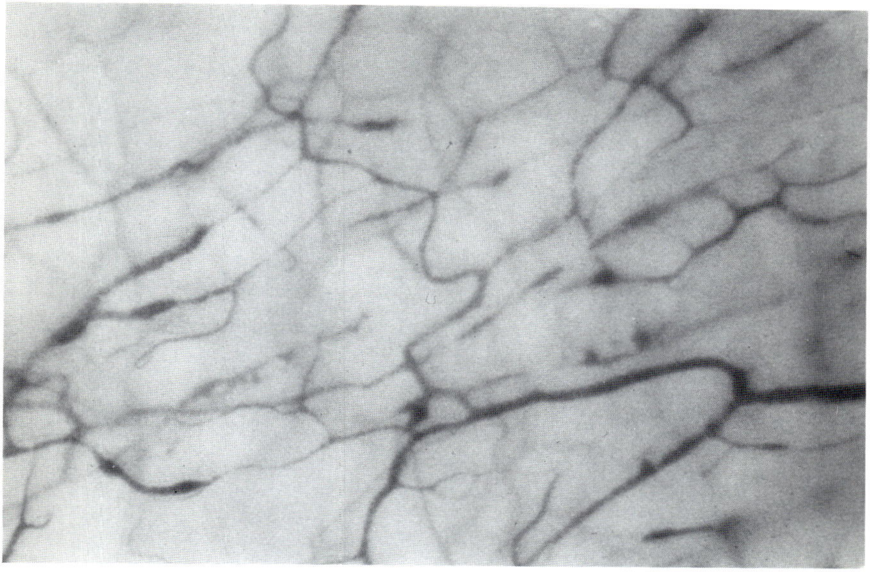

Fig. 5. Venous dilatations, sludge, and stasis in the conjunctiva of a "healthy" man age 27.

and 26% of the women, and no less than 88% of men and 45% of women with a family history of early parental death from vascular disease of the heart or brain.

The parallel between conjunctival microangiopathy and atherosclerosis of large arteries is obvious. Both start in or before the third decade, and both become worse as life advances, but both are absent or minimal in a few elderly subjects. Both are more severe in young men than in young women, and both are influenced by heredity. Like atherosclerosis, microangiopathy is aggravated by hypertension (Lack *et al.*, 1949).

It is unlikely that these are chance associations. A more acceptable explanation is that microangiopathy, like atherosclerosis, represents a nonspecific vascular response to diverse insults in susceptible persons. In view of the clinical and experimental evidence, it appears probable that the presence of persistent changes in the bulbar conjunctival microvessels of healthy young adults is an index to the vulnerability of the arterial system, and that conjunctival biomicroscopy may provide a simple screening test for the identification of the individuals who are a special risk.

References

Altura, B. M. (1971). Chemical and humoral regulation of blood flow through the precapillary sphincter. *Microvasc. Res.* **3,** 361–384.

Ashton, N. (1951). Retinal micro-aneurysms in the non-diabetic subject. *Brit. J. Ophthalmol.* **35,** 189–212.

Ashton, N. (1965). The blood–retinal barrier and vasoglial relationships in retinal disease. *Trans. Ophthalmol. Soc. U. K.* **85,** 199–230.

Bakay, L. (1968). Changes in barrier effect in pathological states. *Prog. Brain Res.* **29,** 315–341.

Baker, A. B., and Ianorie, A. (1959). Cerebrovascular disease. II. The smaller intracerebral arteries. *Neurology* **9,** 391–396.

Baker, A. B., and Resch, J. A. (1965). An approach to the etiologic mechanism of atherosclerosis. *In* "Cerebral Vascular Diseases" (R. G. Siekert and J. P. Whisnant, eds.), pp. 168–171. Grune & Stratton, New York.

Bergentz, S. E., Fajers, C. M., Gelin, L. E., and Rudenstam, C. M. (1965). Intravascular aggregation of long duration and its consequences. *Bibl. Anat.* **7,** 207–217.

Bicher, H. I. (1969). The prevention of sludge-induced myocardial damage by an antiadhesive drug. *Eur. Conf. Microcirc.,* 1968, pp. 202–207.

Clarke, J. A. (1965). An x-ray microscopic study of the vasa-vasorum of the intracranial arteries. *Z. Anat. Enkwicklungsgesch.* **124,** 396–400.

Corsellis, J. A. M. (1962). "Mental Illness and the Aging Brain." Oxford Univ. Press, London and New York.

Cranley, J. J., Fogarty, T. J., and Krause, R. J. (1963). Phlebotomy for moderate erythrocythemia. Improvement in peripheral circulation and myocardial function in patients with obliterative arterial disease of the lower extremities. *J. Amer. Med. Ass.* **186,** 206–210.

Davis, E., and Landau, J. (1969). Conjunctival micropools ("microaneurysms") in clinical arteriosclerosis. *Eur. Conf. Microcir., 5th.* 1968, pp. 385–388.

Dennis, D. N. (1918). Study of the conjunctival circulation to determine early signs of arteriosclerosis. *Trans. Amer. Ophthalmol. Soc.* **16,** 313–321.

Ditzell, J. (1962). "Konjunctivalkarrene Ved Diabetes Mellitus." Munksgaard, Copenhagen.

Ellington, A. L. (1970). The smaller intracerebral vessels. *Stroke* **1,** 128–134.

Elliott, F. A., and Leonberg, S. C. (1971). The affect of sludge on the arterial wall. *Eur. Conf. Microcirc., 6th.,* 1970, pp. 371–375.

Elliott, F. A., and Leonberg, S. C. To be published.

Fang, H. C. H. (1967). Microangiopathies of the brain in diabetic patients: A contribution to the study of pathogenetic factors underlying increased vulnerability to vascular complications. *Circulation* **36,** Suppl. 2, 106.

Fink, A. I., Funahashi, T., Robinson, M., and Watson, R. J. (1961). Conjunctival blood flow in sickle cell disease. *Arch. Ophthalmol.* **66,** 824–829.

Geiringer, E. (1951). Intimal vascularization and atherosclerosis. *J. Pathol. Bacteriol.* **63,** 201–211.

Glynn, M. F., Murphy, E. A., and Mustard, J. F. (1966). Platelets and thrombosis. *Ann. Intern. Med.* **64,** 715–719.

Harper, A. M. (1966). Autoregulation of cerebral blood flow: Influence of the arterial blood pressure on blood flow through the cerebral cortex. *J. Neurol., Neurosurg. Psychiat.* **29,** 398–403.

Hassler, O. (1965). Vascular changes in senile brains. A micro-angiographic study. *Acta Neuropathol.* **5,** 40–53.

Heisig, N., and Lindner, J. (1965). Vergleich vitalmikroskopischer und histopathologischer Befunde an der terminalen Strombahn bei degenerativen Gefässerkrankungen. *Bibl. Anat.* **7,** 530–536.

Heyman, A., Karp, H. R., Heyden, S., Bartel, A., Cassel, J. C., Tyroler, H. A., Cornoni, S., Hames, C. G., and Stuart, W. (1971). Cerebrovascular disease in the bi-racial population of Evans County Georgia. *Stroke* **2,** 509–518.

Hodge, J. V., and Dollery, C. T. (1964). Retinal soft exudates. A clinical study by colour fluorescence photography. *Quart. J. Med.* **33,** 113–117.

Howell, T. H. (1966). Neurological problems of the elderly. *Gerontol. Clin.* **8,** 77–94.

Kittel, V. (1960). "Die Biomikroskopie der Bulbusbindehautgefäbe des Menschen und Ihre Klinische Verwertbarkeit." Thieme, Leipzig.

Knisely, M., Barnes, R. H., and Satterwhite, W. (1957). *In vivo* observations on the bulbar conjunctival blood vessels and blood of functioning people 60 years of age and over. *J. Gerontol.* **12,** 429.

Kreyberg, L. (1963). Stasis and necrosis; a brief review. *Scand. J. Clin. Lab. Invest.* **15,** Suppl. 71, 1–26.

Kuo, P. T., and Joyner, C. R. (1955). Angina pectoris induced by fat ingestion in patients with coronary artery disease. *J. Amer. Med. Ass.* **158,** 1008–1013.

Labram, C., and Lestradet, H. (1961). Studies on vascular aging as observed by bimicroscopic examination of the conjunctival vessels. *Rev. Atheroscler. Arteriopathies Peripheriques* **3,** 8–26.

Lack, A., Adolph, W., Ralston, W., Leiby, G., Winsor, T., and Griffith, G. (1949). Biomicroscopy of conjunctival vessels in hypertension. *Amer. Heart J.* **38,** 654–664.

Luedde, W. H. (1913). A microscopic study of the conjunctival vessels. *Amer. J. Ophthalmol.* **30,** 129–192.

Lutz, B. R. (1951). Intravascular agglutination of the formed elements of blood. *Physiol. Rev.* **31,** 107–130.

Moses, C. (1963). "Atherosclerosis: Mechanisms and Prevention." Lea & Febiger, Philadelphia, Pennsylvania.

Nakata, Y. (1967). An experimental study on the vascular lesions caused by obstruction of the vasa vasorum. *Jap. Circ. J.* **31,** 275–287.

Plotz, M. (1949). Possible hazards of high fat diets in coronary disease. *J. Amer. Med. Ass.* **139,** 623–626.

Ramsey, E. M. (1936). Nutrition of the blood vessel wall: Review of the literature. *Yale J. Biol. Med.* **9,** 14–36.

Reivich, M. (1971). Cerebral circulation. *In* "Cardiac and Vascular Diseases" (H. L. Conn and O. Horwitz, eds.), pp. 139–165. Lea & Febiger, Philadelphia, Pennsylvania.

Ross Russell, R. W. (1963). Observations on intracerebral aneurysms. *Brain* **86,** 425–442.

Ruedemann, A. D. (1933). Conjunctival vessels. *J. Amer. Med. Ass.* **101,** 1477–1481.

Scheinker, I. M. (1948). Alterations of cerebral capillaries in the early stage of arterial hypertension. *Amer. J. Pathol.* **24,** 211–217.

Stalker, A. L. (1962). Intravascular erythrocyte aggregation. *Bibl. Anat.* **4,** 108–111.

Swank, R. L., and Bartsch, W. (1971). Influence of aggregated blood cells on cerebrovascular disease. *In* "Cerebral Circulation and Stroke" (K. J. Zulch, ed.), pp. 169–174. Springer-Verlag, Berlin and New York.

Wells, R. (1971). The microcirculation. *In* "Cardiac and Vascular Diseases" (H. L. Conn, Jr. and O. Horwitz, eds.), pp. 108–121. Lea & Febiger, Philadelphia, Pennsylvania.

Winternitz, R. E., Thomas, R. M., and LeCompte, P. M. (1938). "The Biology of Atherosclerosis." Thomas, Springfield, Illinois.

Zeller, K. (1921). Studien an Bindehautgefässen. *Klin. Monatsbl. Augenheilk.* **66,** 609–621.

Zweifach, B. W. (1959). *In* "The Arterial Wall" (A. I. Lansing, ed.), pp. 33–34. Williams & Wilkins, Baltimore, Maryland.

AUTHOR INDEX

Numbers in italic refer to the pages on which the complete references are listed.

SUBJECT INDEX